Rheumatology and Orthopaedics

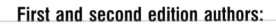

First and second edition authors:

Annabel Coote
Paul Haslam
Daniel Marsland
Sabrina Kapoor

3rd Edition
CRASH COURSE

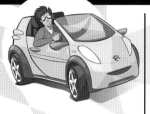

SERIES EDITOR
Dan Horton-Szar
BSc(Hons) MBBS(Hons) MRCGP
Northgate Medical Practice Canterbury
Kent, UK

FACULTY ADVISORS
Max Field
BSc MD FRCP
Reader and Honorary Consultant Rheumatologist,
Centre for Rheumatic Diseases, Institute of Infection,
Immunity and Inflammation,
Glasgow Royal Infirmary, Glasgow, UK

Alistair Gray
FRCS Ed Orth
Consultant Orthopaedic Surgeon,
Glasgow Western Infirmary, Glasgow;
Honorary Clinical Associate Professor,
University of Glasgow, Glasgow, UK

Rheumatology and Orthopaedics

Cameron Elias-Jones
MBChB MRCS(Ed) Specialty Registrar,
Trauma and Orthopaedics, Western Infirmary,
Glasgow, UK

Martin Perry
MBChB BSc(Hons) MRCP(UK) FHEA Consultant Rheumatologist
and Physician, Royal Alexandra Hospital, Paisley, UK

MOSBY

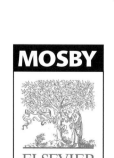

ELSEVIER

Edinburgh London New York Oxford Philadelphia St Louis Sydney Toronto 2015

MT

ELSEVIER
MOSBY

Senior Content Strategist: Jeremy Bowes
Senior Content Development Specialist: Ailsa Laing
Project Manager: Andrew Riley
Designer: Christian Bilbow

First edition 2004

Second edition 2008

Third edition 2013

Updated Third edition 2015

ISBN: 978-0-7234-3867-0

British Library Cataloguing in Publication Data
A catalogue record for this book is available from the British Library

Library of Congress Cataloging in Publication Data
A catalog record for this book is available from the Library of Congress

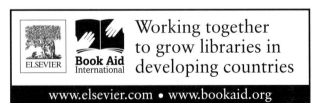
Printed in China

Last digit is the print line: 10 9 8 7 6 5 4 3 2 1

8/1/16

Series editor foreword

The *Crash Course* series was first published in 1997 and now, 16 years on, we are still going strong. Medicine never stands still, and the work of keeping this series relevant for today's students is an ongoing process. These new editions build on the success of the previous titles and incorporate new and revised material to keep the series up to date with current guidelines for best practice and recent developments in medical research and pharmacology.

We always listen to feedback from our readers, through focus groups and student reviews of the *Crash Course* titles. For the new editions we have completely rewritten our self-assessment material to keep up with today's 'single-best answer' and 'extended matching question' formats. The artwork and layout of the titles have also been largely reworked to make the text easier on the eye during long sessions of revision.

Despite fully revising the books with each edition, we hold fast to the principles on which we first developed the series. *Crash Course* will always bring you all the information you need to revise in compact, manageable volumes that integrate basic medical science and clinical practice. The books still maintain the balance between clarity and conciseness, and provide sufficient depth for those aiming at distinction. The authors are medical students and junior doctors who have recent experience of the exams you are now facing, and the accuracy of the material is checked by a team of faculty advisors from across the UK.

I wish you all the best for your future careers!

Dr Dan Horton-Szar

Preface

Musculoskeletal problems represent an increasing problem in primary and secondary care as a result of an ageing population, the anticipated obesity epidemic and active sporting young adults. It is inevitable that all doctors will encounter patients with orthopaedic and rheumatological problems. Musculoskeletal medicine is a rapidly changing field, subject to much clinical and basic science research.

This *Crash Course* has been redesigned, rewritten and reformatted to help medical students develop a basic knowledge of diseases that affect the musculoskeletal system and the new understanding that underlies their pathologies and treatments.

We hope you enjoy reading and learning from this book and that it will help you pass your exams, and perhaps stimulate you toward a career in orthopaedics or rheumatology.

Cameron Elias-Jones, Martin Perry, Max Field and Alistair Gray

Acknowledgements

Our sincere thanks to:

Ms Hannah Corinthians Tan, Medical Student, The University of Glasgow, Glasgow, UK for help with the development of self-assessment questions.

The Glasgow Orthopaedics and Rheumatology Society for reviewing self-assessment questions.

Dr Anna Ciechomska, Associate Specialist, Rheumatology, Inverclyde Royal Hospital, Greenock, UK for supplying ultrasound images.

Dr Nigel Raby, Consultant Radiologist, Western Infirmary Glasgow, UK for supply of radiology images.

Dr David Colville, Specialty Trainee, Nuclear Medicine, Glasgow Royal Infirmary, Glasgow, UK for provision of isotope bone scan images.

Dedications

To Audrey, my family and all those who supported me while I was writing this book.

Cameron Elias-Jones

To my wife Jennifer and our family – Charis, David and Rhianna – for the joy and inspiration they are to me. Also to my father and mother, for their steadfast support and guidance throughout my life. Soli Deo gloria.

Martin Perry

To Vicky, my wife, for her constant support, and to the University of Glasgow medical students who show boundless enthusiasm.

Max Field

To my wife and family, for their patience and support.

Alistair Gray

Contents

Contents

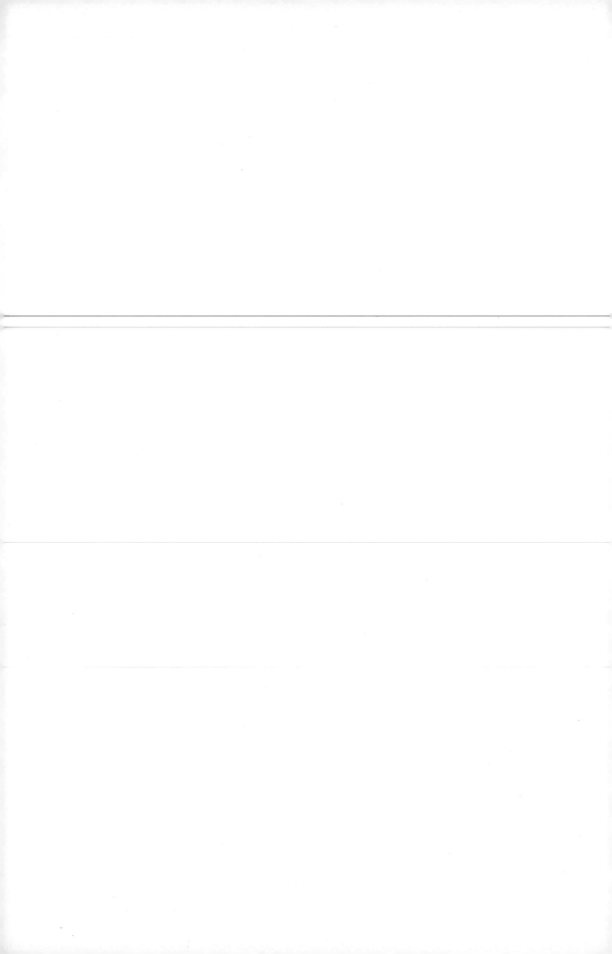

Taking a history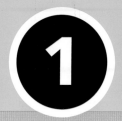

Objectives

After reading this chapter you should be able to:
- Understand why history taking is so important in making a diagnosis.
- Take a detailed history of a presenting complaint using open and closed questions and determine the functional impact of a condition.

Good history taking is a valuable skill and crucial to making a correct diagnosis. It is important to establish a good rapport with patients. A relaxed, trusting patient will find it easier to share information with you and answer your questions.

The first things to document in your history are:
- The patient's name, age, date of birth, sex and hospital number.
- The date, time and place of the consultation (e.g. accident and emergency department).
- The source of referral, e.g. GP referral.

PRESENTING COMPLAINT

This should be a short statement, summarizing the patient's presenting symptoms. The following are some examples:
- Painful right knee.
- Pain and stiffness of both arms.

HISTORY OF THE PRESENTING COMPLAINT

COMMUNICATION

Begin your history with open questions, e.g. 'Tell me about your pain', then ask closed questions if necessary, e.g. 'Does your knee ever give way?'

This should contain details of the patient's presenting symptoms from their onset to the current time. The following areas should be discussed when taking a history.

Symptom onset
- Date and time of symptom onset.
- Speed of onset – was it acute or gradual?
- Presence of any precipitating factors, such as trauma, commencement of a new drug, etc.

Pain, swelling and stiffness

Establish the following points:
- Site and radiation.
- Nature – e.g. whether sharp or dull.
- Periodicity – is it continuous or intermittent?
- Exacerbating and relieving factors.
- Timing – is it worse at any particular time of day?

As a rule, pain and stiffness due to inflammatory conditions such as rheumatoid arthritis are worse first thing in the morning and improve as the day progresses. The duration of the early-morning stiffness is quite a good guide to the severity of the inflammation. In contrast, pain due to a mechanical or degenerative problem tends to be worse later in the day and associated with a milder degree of stiffness and is worse with activity.

Warmth/erythema

Inflamed joints may appear red and feel warm.

Deformity

Some patients consult their doctor because they have developed a deformity and are concerned. This may or may not be associated with pain.

Weakness

It is important to ascertain whether this is localized or generalized. Localized weakness suggests a focal problem, such as a peripheral nerve lesion, whereas generalized weakness is more likely to have a systemic cause.

Numbness

The distribution of numbness or paraesthesia should be documented, as well as any precipitating factors. For example, if numbness affects the radial 3½ fingers, it is probably due to carpal tunnel syndrome. If it affects all the digits, is associated with pallor and is provoked by cold weather, Raynaud phenomenon is more likely.

Functional loss and disability

Loss of function refers to a person's inability to perform an action, such as gripping an object or walking. This is usually the reason why someone presents to a doctor. Disability is the result of functional loss on the individual's ability to lead a full and active life.

HINTS AND TIPS

Always record a patient's level of function in the notes. It is a good marker of progress.

Any restriction that a patient's disease has on activities of daily living should be documented.

PAST MEDICAL HISTORY

Ask about all current and previous medical and surgical disorders, including any musculoskeletal problems. In certain situations, it is worth asking about specific illnesses. For example, a patient with carpal tunnel syndrome may have underlying hypothyroidism or diabetes mellitus.

DRUG HISTORY

The drug history is always important, but it sometimes has great relevance to orthopaedic and rheumatological problems. Acute gout can be precipitated by the initiation of diuretic therapy, and long-term corticosteroid use can cause osteoporosis.

SOCIAL HISTORY

Record relevant information about the patient's occupation, domestic situation, degree of independence, smoking and alcohol intake. Asking which is the patient's dominant hand is also important.

FAMILY HISTORY

Ask particularly about a family history of musculoskeletal disease.

SYSTEMIC ENQUIRY

This should include a brief review of any symptoms affecting other systems of the body. It is particularly relevant if you think the patient might have a connective tissue disease.

After reading this chapter you should be able to:
- Establish a rapport with the patient and show consideration if the patient is in pain.
- Use the Regional Examination of the Musculoskeletal System (REMS).
- Know how to examine the major joints of the upper and lower limbs and spine.
- Describe special examination tests for each joint.

GENERAL PRINCIPLES

It is important to establish a rapport with the patient. Dress smartly, be polite and have some identification.

Introduce yourself and start by asking if any area is painful before you touch the patient. One of the first things to notice is how the patient walks. Pathological gait patterns are shown in Figure 2.1. Note any aids or appliances, such as wheelchair, zimmer frame or stick.

Watch how reliant patients are on relatives during simple tasks such as getting undressed or getting up from a chair.

Start your examination by looking at the patient's hands first and then moving to the face, and so on. A thorough general examination is required for patients presenting with:

- Polyarthritis – these patients may have an inflammatory arthropathy, and a general examination is tailored towards looking for extra-articular manifestations. Examination of the cardiovascular system, respiratory system and abdomen is required.
- Widespread aches and pains – these patients may have an inflammatory arthritis, connective tissue disorder or malignancy. Examination of other systems is required.

HINTS AND TIPS

As a general principle, always examine the joints above and below.

CLINICAL EXAMINING

- Start with adequate exposure.
- Stand and walk the patient.

- Position the patient for the joint(s) to be examined. Make the patient comfortable and make sure you can get to the correct side of the patient.

HINTS AND TIPS

When examining joints, ensure you observe both passive movement (examiner moves the joint) and active movement (patient moves the joint).

- Look:
  - Check for swelling, muscle wasting, scars, erythema or deformity.
- Feel:
  - Palpate the joint systematically, noting any effusion and any tenderness over the joint line or other prominent features of the joint.
- Move:
  - Demonstrate joint movement actively and passively.
- Examine joints above and below.

Practise a routine on your friends.

HINTS AND TIPS

Using these basic principles and applying the same basic rules, you can examine any joint.

Peripheral nervous examination

Abnormalities of the structures of the back such as intervertebral disc prolapse can cause abnormalities of the peripheral nervous system due to compression on nerve roots. The most commonly affected are the L5 and S1 nerve roots.

Fig. 2.1 Pathological patterns of gait

Gait	Features	Cause
Trendelenburg	Waddling gait	Loss of hip abductor function
Antalgic (painful)	The patient tries to offload the painful limb by quickening and shortening the weight-bearing stance phase of the gait cycle	Any painful condition
Short-leg gait	Dipping of shoulder on affected side	Any condition causing significant leg length discrepancy
High stepping	Knee is flexed and foot is lifted high to avoid foot dragging on the floor	Nerve palsy (peroneal or sciatic)
Stiff knee	Knee cleared of floor by swinging out away from the body	Fusion of knee

Fig. 2.2 Testing lower-limb muscle function (myotomes)

Muscle action	Nerve roots tested
Hip flexion (iliopsoas)	L1, L2
Knee flexion (quadriceps)	L3
Ankle dorsiflexion (tibialis anterior)	L4
Great toe extension (extensor hallucis longus)	L5
Ankle plantar flexion (soleus/ gastrocnemius)	S1

Lower limb

Tone

Lower limb tone is usually normal but is reduced in spinal cord compression (flaccid paralysis).

Power is assessed by Medical Research Council grade:

0 Nothing.
1 Flicker.
2 Power to move limb with gravity eliminated.
3 Power to move limb against gravity.
4 Reduced from normal.
5 Normal.

Test muscle function as shown in Figure 2.2.

Reflexes

Always compare the reflexes with the opposite limb and make sure the patient is relaxed. Reflexes can be reduced, brisk or absent.

Three reflexes are commonly tested:

- Knee L3–L4: flex both knees over the couch and tap lightly on the patellar ligament.
- Ankle L5, S1: dorsiflex the ankle with the knees flexed and the leg externally rotated. Tap the Achilles tendon.
- Plantar: this is performed by stroking the plantar skin with the handle of the tendon hammer. If the toes extend this is abnormal and called 'up going', indicating an upper motor neuron lesion.

Sensation

Ask the patient if the sensation is normal and the same as on the other side. Dermatomes are shown in Figure 2.3.

Anal tone and perianal sensation

In cauda equina syndrome anal tone is lost and perianal sensation reduced; therefore an examination per rectum is an important part of any spinal examination.

EXAMINATION OF THE HIP

Hip disease is common and examination follows the pattern of look, feel, move. True hip pain is often felt in the groin, and on movement and may radiate to the knee.

The examination starts by observing the patient walking from the waiting area to the consultation room. A Trendelenburg gait (waddling) is due to failure of the hip abductors to elevate the pelvis on weight bearing, causing a dipping or rolling gait (Fig. 2.4). To compensate for this the trunk is swung over the weight-bearing hip, which maintains balance.

Failure of hip abduction can be due to pain or ineffectual muscle function following hip surgery.

The patient may also have an antalgic gait (see Fig. 2.1).

Look

Scars from previous surgery could be present anteriorly, laterally or medially. Look for erythema, obvious deformity and muscle wasting, especially over the quadriceps muscles. As the hip is a deep joint, swelling can be difficult to see. Look at both sides of the hip by turning the patient to the prone position.

True leg length discrepancy

Ensure the patient is lying comfortably on the examination couch with the knees straight.

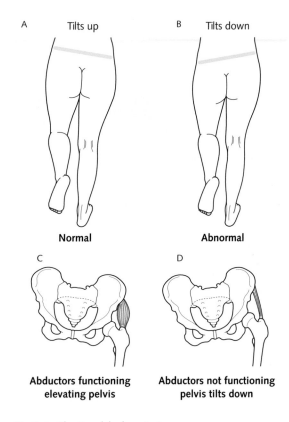

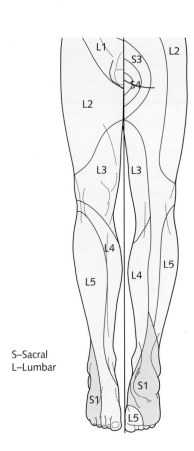

Fig. 2.3   Dermatomes of the lower limb.

S–Sacral
L–Lumbar

Fig. 2.4   The Trendelenburg test.

Measure both limbs from the anterior superior iliac spine to the medial malleolus and compare the values.

An idea of where any leg length discrepancy lies can be obtained by flexing both hips and knees and placing them together. Look from the side and determine the relative positions of the knees.

If one knee is higher than the other then this suggests tibial shortness; however, if one knee lies behind the other it suggests a femoral discrepancy (Fig. 2.5).

Feel

The hip is deeply situated and few features are palpable.

The greater trochanter is easily felt laterally, over which bursitis may be present.

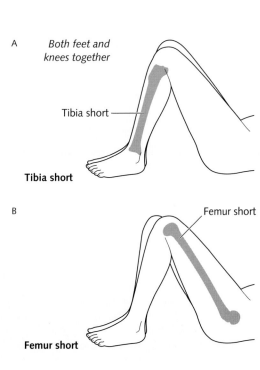

Fig. 2.5   Assessing leg length discrepancy.

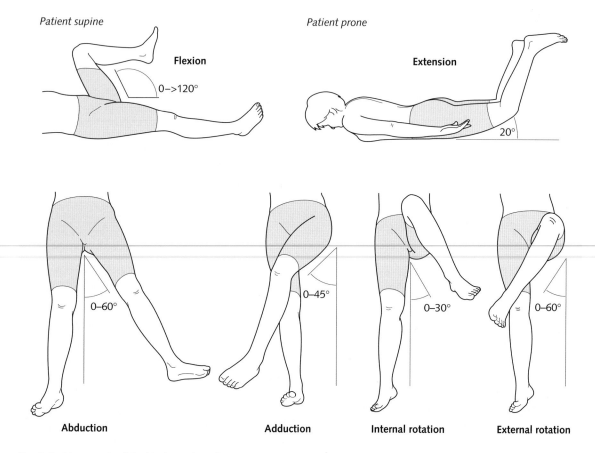

Fig. 2.6 Movements of the hip (note that all ranges are approximate and vary from patient to patient). When assessing hip movement, the pelvis should be stabilized with a hand to prevent pelvic tilting.

Move

Normal movements are shown in Figure 2.6.

> **HINTS AND TIPS**
>
> When assessing hip movements, remember to stabilize the pelvis with a hand to ensure that pelvic tilting does not occur.

Trendelenburg test

This is used to assess the function of the hip abductors.

Stand face on to the patient and put your hands on the patient's pelvis, then ask the patient to place the hands on your forearms to steady him- or herself. Ask the patient then to lift each leg in turn and watch for pelvic tilt. Remember it is the standing leg you are testing and show the patient he or she should lift up the leg behind them by bending at the knee. (If the hip is flexed, this can tilt the pelvis.)

If the abductors are not functioning the pelvis tilts downwards towards the unsupported leg (Fig. 2.4B and D).

Thomas test

This is a test for fixed flexion of the hip.

The idea of the test is to abolish the natural lumbar lordosis of the spine and visualize the true degree of flexion deformity at the hip.

To perform the test, the patient is positioned supine (flat on the back) and the opposite hip is flexed fully. This manoeuvre fully corrects the lordosis that is felt by placing a hand under the spine. Now simply observe the degree (if any) of hip flexion (Fig. 2.7).

EXAMINATION OF THE KNEE

The knee lies superficially and many landmarks are easily palpable.

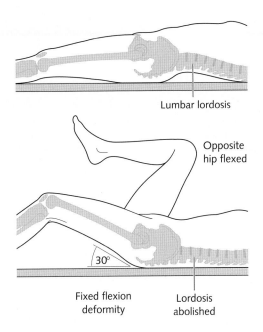

Lumbar lordosis

Opposite hip flexed

30°

Fixed flexion deformity   Lordosis abolished

Fig. 2.7   The Thomas test for fixed flexion of the hip.

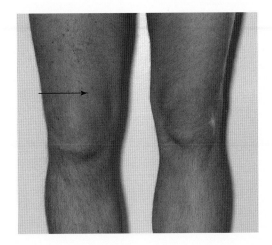

Fig. 2.8   Right knee effusion. Note the loss of dimples in the thigh and under the patella.

Look

- Look for quadriceps wasting, which can be assessed by measuring the thigh circumference and comparing it with the measurement on the other side.
- Localized swelling anteriorly or posteriorly may be visible (remember to inspect the back of the knee – this is easily done with the patient standing).
- Note an effusion (which can be seen by loss of normal skin dimples at the joint line), scars, erythema or evidence of psoriasis.
- Look for surgical scars.
- Ask the patient to stand and walk, and note any gait abnormality.
- Deformities (varus, valgus and fixed flexion) are more obvious on standing.

Feel

A knee effusion is important to recognize (Fig. 2.8), as it always indicates pathology. There are two tests commonly used: the patellar test and the wipe test.

Patellar tap

Fluid is milked down from the suprapatellar pouch, which lifts the patella away from the femur. The patella is then pushed down on to the femur, producing a 'tap' (Fig. 2.9).

Wipe test

Fluid is milked out of the medial dimple. The examining hand then sweeps the fluid from the lateral side of the knee, refilling the medial dimple with a visible bulge.

Flexing the knee to 90° allows structures to be palpated more easily.

Feel for warmth in the knees with the back of the hand.

Be methodical, starting distally over the tibial tubercle and moving proximally, palpating in turn the patellar tendon, proximal tibia, medial and lateral joint lines, femoral condyles, patella and quadriceps tendon (Fig. 2.10). The collateral ligaments are also palpable.

Remember to palpate the posterior aspect of the knee. A Baker cyst or bursa may be present.

Move

Both active and passive movement should be tested. The normal range is 0–150° (Fig. 2.11). Note any fixed flexion or hyperextension of the knee. Feel for patellar crepitus during flexion.

Medial and lateral collateral ligaments

Different patients have different degrees of laxity of the ligaments. It is therefore important to compare your examination with the normal side. Flex the knee to 15° and alternately stress the joint line on each side. Place one hand on the opposite side of the joint line to that which is being tested and apply force to the lower tibia (Fig. 2.12).

Anterior cruciate ligament (ACL)

Anterior drawer test

This is also a test for ACL deficiency but can be misleading (the anterior drawer test can be positive after medial meniscectomy or in posterior cruciate ligament (PCL) deficiency).

Fig. 2.9   Patellar tap sign.

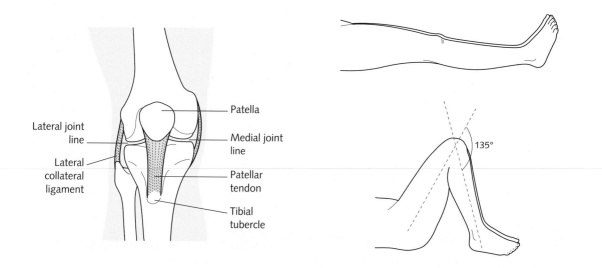

A

B

Patellar tap

Knee with
tense
effusion

Hand placed on
knee and fluid
milked down

Second hand tap
pushes down on
patella

Lateral joint
line

Lateral
collateral
ligament

Patella

Medial joint
line

Patellar
tendon

Tibial
tubercle

135°

Fig. 2.10   Anatomical structures easily palpated around the knee.

Fig. 2.11   Range of movement of the knee.

The knee is flexed to 90° and the hamstrings are relaxed. The examiner sits carefully on the patient's foot and both thumbs are placed on the proximal tibia and over both joint lines. The tibia is pulled forward and, if movement is excessive, the test is positive.

Posterior cruciate ligament

The posterior drawer test is performed exactly as the anterior drawer but the knee is pushed backwards.

The classic sign for a PCL rupture is the posterior sag. This is demonstrated by flexing both knees to 90° and comparing the knee contour (Fig. 2.13). A sag occurs as the tibia falls posteriorly and the tibial tubercle becomes less prominent.

EXAMINATION OF THE ANKLE AND FOOT

Look

Inspect the ankle and foot with the patient in both resting and weight-bearing positions. Observe nails and skin for psoriatic changes. Look at the distribution of any swelling. Synovitis of the ankle usually produces diffuse swelling, obscuring the contours of the medial and lateral malleoli. Swelling in the region of the Achilles tendon is more likely to be due to Achilles tendinopathy or tendon rupture.

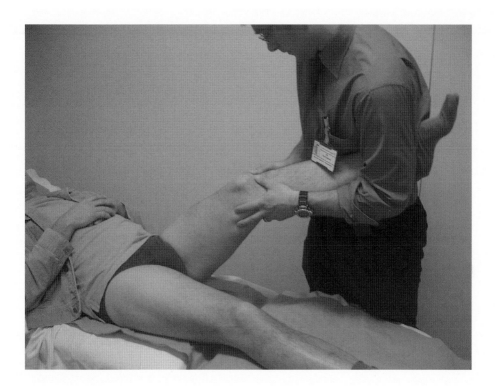

Fig. 2.12 Collateral ligament examination.

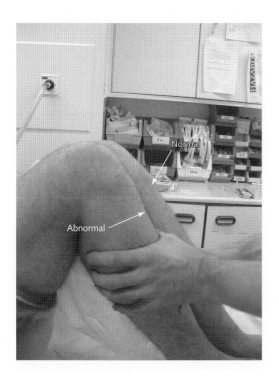

Fig. 2.13 Posterior sag sign. The right knee shows the positive sign. Note that the tibial tuberosity is more prominent on the left.

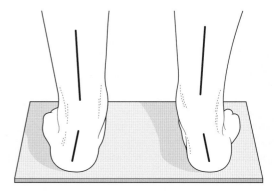

Fig. 2.14 Pes planus with pronation of the feet and hindfoot valgus.

Disease of the subtalar joint or abnormalities of the longitudinal arch of the foot may disrupt the alignment of the heel and Achilles tendon. This should be vertical and is seen easily from behind whilst the patient is standing. Pes planus (flat foot) can cause pronation of the foot and valgus deformity of the heel (Fig. 2.14).

Forefoot problems are common. Hallux valgus is a deformity of the great toe, which becomes abducted at the metatarsophalangeal (MTP) joint. Excessive pressure on the medial side can lead to formation of

Fig. 2.15 Common deformities of the forefoot. MTP, metatarsophalangeal; PIP, proximal interphalangeal; DIP, distal interphalangeal.

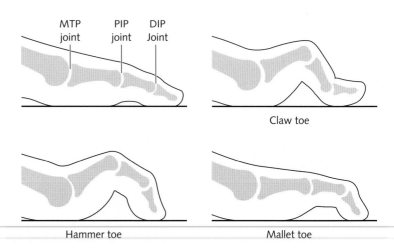

a bursa, often referred to as a 'bunion'. Look at the patient's footwear for signs of excessive wear. Figure 2.15 shows other deformities that commonly affect the forefoot.

The MTP joints are commonly affected by rheumatoid arthritis and may sublux. The metatarsal heads become prominent and callosities often form in the overlying skin. Clawing of the toes may occur.

Feel

Feel for warmth. Palpate the ankle joint, subtalar joint and forefoot, squeezing the MTP joints to elicit any discomfort.

Move

Test plantar flexion and dorsiflexion of the ankle with the knee flexed. The subtalar joint allows inversion and eversion of the hindfoot. This is tested by stabilizing the tibia with one hand and turning the calcaneus inward and outward with the other. Midtarsal movements contribute to plantar flexion, dorsiflexion, inversion and eversion. These are tested by stabilizing the heel with one hand and moving the forefoot with the other. Movements of the MTP, proximal interphalangeal (PIP) and distal interphalangeal (DIP) joints are best examined actively whilst the patient is lying or sitting.

EXAMINATION OF THE SPINE

When examining the spine always remember also to perform a peripheral nervous system examination.

Look

Assess the patient's posture. Check for cervical lordosis, thoracic kyphosis and lumbar lordosis. If the patient has sciatica the affected leg is often flexed and the patient is stooped. Muscle wasting, assymetry and scoliosis may be present.

- Kyphotic deformity is best visualized from the side.

> **HINTS AND TIPS**
>
> In scoliosis the rib hump deformity is more clearly seen when the patient bends forwards (see Fig. 9.14, p. 62).

Feel

Palpation is performed standing and with the patient lying prone.

Feel over the spinous processes, paraspinal muscles and the sacroiliac joints for tenderness.

Move

Cervical spine

Movements of the cervical spine (Fig. 2.16) are usually stated as percentage loss when compared with normal, if possible.

Flexion
Ask the patient to bend the head forward to put the chin on the chest.

Extension
Ask the patient to look up at the ceiling.

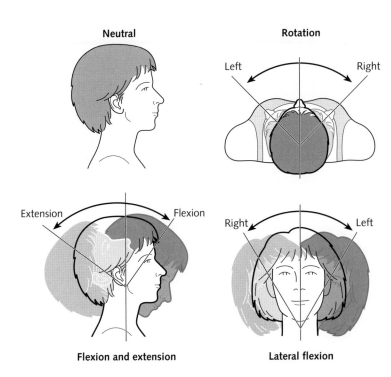

Fig. 2.16 Movements of the cervical spine.

Lateral flexion
Ask the patient to put the ear down to the shoulder.

Rotation
Ask the patient to look to either side.

Thoracolumbar spine (Fig. 2.17)

Flexion
Often patients are reluctant to flex the spine if it is acutely tender. Ask patients to bend over, keeping knees extended, and reach as far as they can.

Look and feel for movement of the lumbar spine. This can be measured by marking two points on the lumbar spine and observing the increase in the distance between them on flexion (see p. 84).

Extension
Get the patient to arch the back backwards. In conditions such as spinal stenosis this can exacerbate the pain.

Rotation
With the patient sitting on a couch to fix the pelvis and arms crossed in front, thoracic rotation is assessed.

Lateral flexion
Ask the patient to slide one hand down the side of the leg.

Special tests

Straight-leg raising
Straight-leg raising is a test for nerve root irritation (radiculopathy).

With the patient supine, elevate the affected leg passively, keeping it straight. If the patient complains of pain down the leg, look at the angle that the leg makes with the couch, e.g. 30°. The next step is to bend the knee as this will abolish the symptoms by relieving tension on the nerve.

For the test to be positive the pain must radiate to the foot (often patients will complain of back pain when elevating the leg).

EXAMINATION OF THE SHOULDER

Movement of the shoulder occurs at four joints (Fig. 2.18). The majority of the total range of movement arises from the glenohumeral and scapulothoracic joints.

Look

Look at the position and contours of the shoulder from front, the side and behind and compare with the opposite side.

• Swelling of the shoulder is uncommon. When it does occur, it is best seen anteriorly.

Fig. 2.17 Thoracolumbar movements.

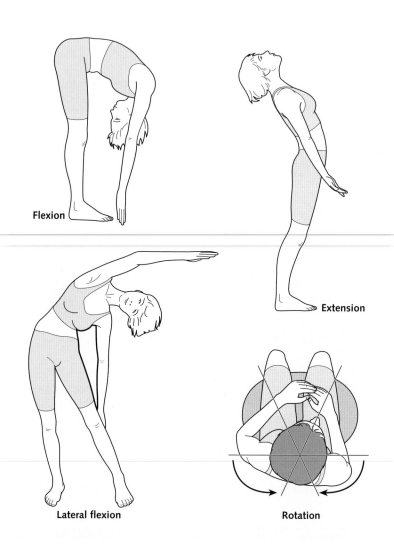

Flexion

Extension

Lateral flexion

Rotation

- Muscle wasting may be due to chronic shoulder pathology, such as chronic rotator cuff tendinopathy.
- Scars from shoulder replacements are also anterior.

Feel

Feel for tenderness and swelling of the acromioclavicular, sternoclavicular and glenohumeral joints. A gap on palpation of the acromioclavicular joint indicates dislocation. Feel for warmth, comparing left and right. Palpate surrounding muscles for tenderness.

Move

Examine active and passive movements, looking at the range of abduction, forward flexion, and internal and external rotation.

A quick way to evaluate active shoulder movements is by asking patients to:

- Put their hands behind their head, with the elbows back. (external rotation/abduction, flexion).
- Reach behind their back, as if to fasten a bra strap (internal rotation, adduction, extension).
- Raise their arms behind them (extension) and to the front (flexion).

A normal range of passive movements suggests that glenohumeral disease is very unlikely.

HINTS AND TIPS

Normal passive movements with painful or restricted active movements indicate a muscle or tendon problem.

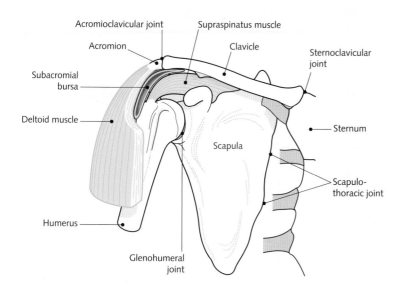

Fig. 2.18 Anatomy of the shoulder.

Acromioclavicular joint — Supraspinatus muscle — Acromion — Clavicle — Sternoclavicular joint — Subacromial bursa — Deltoid muscle — Sternum — Scapula — Scapulo-thoracic joint — Humerus — Glenohumeral joint

- A 'hitch-up' of the shoulder on active abduction of the arm is a sign of reduced glenohumeral range (Fig. 2.19).
- Loss of passive external rotation and abduction are highly indicative of adhesive capsulitis ('frozen shoulder').
- Scapular movements should be assessed from behind during the range of shoulder movements.

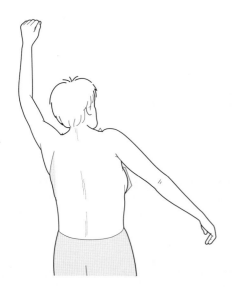

Fig. 2.19 A 'hitched' shoulder. The patient is unable to elevate her arm to the side properly, so is 'cheating' by shrugging her right shoulder.

The rotator cuff

The supraspinatus, infraspinatus, teres minor and subscapularis muscles make up the rotator cuff. They hold the head of the humerus in the glenoid cavity, maintain stability and initiate shoulder abduction. Rotator cuff inflammation, injury and degeneration are common. Disease of the supraspinatus especially causes pain on abduction when the tendon becomes compressed under the acromion. The pain is felt at between 60° and 120° of abduction. This is referred to as a 'painful arc' (Fig. 2.20).

Resisted shoulder movements should be examined. Pain or weakness on resisted movements suggests involvement of the rotator cuff muscles and tendons.

- Supraspinatus is tested with the arm abducted to 30°, flexed to 30° and internally rotated with the thumb pointing downwards. Abduction is then resisted.
- Resisted internal rotation tests the subscapularis.
- Resisted external rotation tests the infraspinatus and teres minor.

EXAMINATION OF THE ELBOW

The elbow joint consists of two articulations. The first is between the humerus, radius and ulna, which allows flexion to a range of 150°. The second is the superior radioulnar joint, which allows rotation of the wrist through 180°.

Look

Examine the elbow in flexion and extension for scars, muscle wasting, fixed flexion, swelling, erythema,

Fig. 2.20 Demonstration of the painful arc.

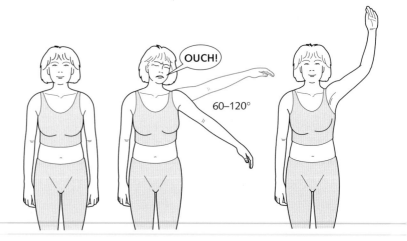

OUCH!

60–120°

rheumatoid nodules and psoriatic plaques. Olecranon bursitis may be seen as a swollen 'golf ball' over the elbow.

Feel

Feel for warmth. Palpate the olecranon process and medial and lateral epicondyles. The former will be tender in golfer's elbow, the latter in tennis elbow. The radial head is usually felt easily in the lateral aspect of the joint and its movement can be assessed during pronation and supination.

Move

Test flexion, extension, pronation and supination. Extension of the elbow is to 180° or beyond in almost all normal people. The inability to straighten the elbow to 180° is therefore considered pathological, even if it is painfree and unnoticed by the patient. On the other hand, many people can extend another 5–10°, so hyperextension (as in hypermobility) is defined as extension beyond 190°.

It is best to assess pronation and supination with the elbow flexed to 90° and held close to the side of the body. If you suspect the patient may have epicondylitis, examine resisted movements of the wrist for pain (see Fig. 24.1).

EXAMINATION OF THE WRIST AND HAND

Rest the patient's hands on a pillow.

Look

Inspection of the hands is an important part of the musculoskeletal examination. Look at skin, nails, joints and muscles.

Skin

Check for psoriasis, rheumatoid nodules and tight skin (scleroderma) or skin thinning (steroids). Nail fold infarcts and digital ulcers can occur as a consequence of vasculitis and scleroderma. Scars from carpal tunnel decompression are seen on the volar aspect of the wrist.

Nails

Look for pitting or onycholysis in psoriasis, and splinter haemorrhage in vasculitis.

Joints

- Look for deformity, swelling and scars of joint replacement.
- The pattern of any deformity aids diagnosis – osteoarthritis tends to affect DIP/PIP joints (see Ch. 11), whereas rheumatoid arthritis affects metacarpophalangeal (MCP)/wrist/PIP (see Ch. 12).

Muscle

- Wasting of thenar and hypothenar eminences suggests median (carpal tunnel) or ulnar pathology respectively or disuse secondary to joint disease.
- Atrophy of the dorsal interossei occurs in rheumatoid arthritis.

Feel

- Palpate each joint systematically for the boggy and spongy feeling of synovitis. Bony overgrowth such as osteophytosis will feel hard. A bimanual approach is best, with the examiner's fingertips placed at either side of the joint, feeling for soft-tissue swelling. Synovitis at the PIP joint bulges out either side of the extensor expansion.

Tenosynovitis of the finger flexors can be associated with tendon nodules, which can be felt moving on finger flexion:

- Feel for warmth.
- Squeeze the metacarpal joints to elicit any tenderness.
- Check sensation for median, ulnar and radial nerve (see Chapter 10).

Move

It is important to assess hand function. Active and passive movement of the wrist and digits should be tested, as well as the patient's ability to perform certain tasks. The muscles responsible for various movements of the hand and wrist are shown in Figure 2.21.

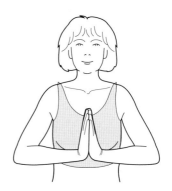

Fig. 2.22 The 'prayer' sign.

- The 'prayer' sign is useful when assessing hand and wrist function. Ask the patient to extend both wrists and place the palms of the hands flat against each other, as if praying (Fig. 2.22). Patients with limited wrist extension, deformities or synovitis of their MCP or PIP joints will find this difficult. Then ask the patient to flex the wrists, and point fingers downwards, apposing fingers.
- Ask the patient to make a fist, tucking fingers into the palm.
- Ask the patient to straighten the fingers against resistance.
- Abduct fingers and check power with the corresponding finger of the examiner's hand pressing against the patient's finger.
- Check interossei by asking the patient to hold a sheet of paper between the fingers.
- Abduction of the thumb against resistance checks median nerve motor function.

Fig. 2.21 Muscles responsible for hand and wrist movement.

Movement	Muscle(s) responsible (nerve supply)
Wrist flexion	Flexor carpi radialis (median) Flexor carpi ulnaris (ulnar) Palmaris longus (median)
Wrist extension	Extensor carpi radialis longus and brevis (both radial) Extensor carpi ulnaris (radial)
DIP joint flexion	Flexor digitorum profundus (median and ulnar)
PIP joint flexion	Flexor digitorum superficialis (median)
MCP joint flexion and IP joint extension	Lumbricals (median and ulnar)
Finger abduction	Dorsal interossei (ulnar)
Finger adduction	Palmar interossei (ulnar)
Extension of MCPs, PIPs and DIPs	Extensor digitorum (radial)
Thumb abduction	Abductor pollicis brevis (median)
Thumb adduction	Adductor pollicis (ulnar)
Thumb opposition	Opponens pollicis (median)
Thumb extension	Extensor pollicis longus (radial)

DIP, distal interphalangeal; PIP, proximal interphalangeal; MCP, metacarpophalangeal; IP, interphalangeal.

HINTS AND TIPS

Ask the patient to pick up a penny from the table or fasten a button. This will give you a good idea of what the patient's hand function is like. It is surprising how well some people can perform fiddly tasks, despite having hand deformities.

Special tests

Tinel and Phalen tests should be performed in patients who have symptoms suggestive of carpal tunnel syndrome. These tests are described in Chapter 10.

Further reading

MacLeod, J., 2009. MacLeod's Clinical Examination, eleventh ed. Elsevier, Edinburgh.

Regional Examination of the Musculoskeletal System (REMS) hand book. Available online at www.arthritisresearchuk.org.

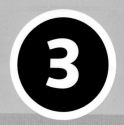

Investigations **3**

● Objectives

After reading this chapter you should be able to:
- Understand which general and specific blood tests are useful for most orthopaedic and rheumatological conditions.
- Describe what tests can be done on a joint fluid aspirate to help make a diagnosis.
- Describe common tests used to diagnose osteoporosis and understand the difference between an isotope and a dual-energy X-ray absorptiometry (DEXA) bone scan.
- Understand the uses and indications for X-ray imaging, ultrasound, computed tomography (CT) and magnetic resonance imaging (MRI).

BLOOD TESTS

The following blood tests are useful in the investigation of rheumatic disease.

Full blood count

- Anaemia may be due to chronic inflammatory disease or iron deficiency from non-steroidal anti-inflammatory drug (NSAID) therapy. Haemolytic anaemia can occur in autoimmune disease where red cells are destroyed in the peripheral circulation (see Ch. 12 for anaemia in rheumatoid arthritis).
- A polymorphonuclear leukocytosis may be a consequence of infection, such as septic arthritis or osteomyelitis. It can also be a sign of inflammation such as gout. Prolonged corticosteroid use can also cause a raised white cell count.
- Leukopenia can be a feature of systemic lupus erythematosus (SLE) or bone marrow suppression from disease-modifying antirheumatic drugs.
- Thrombocytosis often occurs in active inflammatory disease. It is sometimes referred to as a 'reactive thrombocytosis'. Thrombocytopenia occurs in SLE and antiphospholipid syndrome.

HINTS AND TIPS

A low or normal leukocyte count does not exclude sepsis if the clinical situation suggests otherwise.

Erythrocyte sedimentation rate (ESR) and C-reactive protein (CRP)

- These are non-specific markers of inflammation and will rise in infectious and inflammatory disorders.
- The ESR measures aggregation of erythrocytes, which increases with the concentration of plasma proteins such as fibrinogen and immunoglobulins.
- The upper limit of normal for the ESR increases with age.
- CRP is synthesized by the liver and rises within 6–10 hours of an inflammatory event.

HINTS AND TIPS

The CRP responds more rapidly than the ESR to inflammation.

Urea and electrolytes

Renal impairment might occur in gout or connective tissue disease. NSAIDs can cause interstitial nephritis.

Liver function tests

- A raised level of alkaline phosphatase is seen in Paget disease.
- Some drugs used for musculoskeletal problems can be hepatotoxic, such as methotrexate, sulphasalazine and NSAIDs.

Uric acid

- Uric acid is raised in many patients with gout, but can be normal during acute flare.

Calcium

- Hypocalcaemia (and low vitamin D) occurs in osteomalacia.
- Hypercalcaemia can be a feature of malignancy.

Creatine kinase

- This muscle enzyme is raised following muscle trauma or inflammation.

Autoantibodies

Some autoantibodies can occur in healthy people (false positives) and tests for them have little diagnostic value unless they are done in appropriate circumstances.

HINTS AND TIPS

Autoantibody tests should only be requested if there is real clinical suspicion of an autoimmune disease.

Fig. 3.1 Antinuclear antibodies against specific nuclear antigens and their associated diseases

Autoantibodies	Disease
Histone	Drug-induced systemic lupus erythematosus (SLE)
Double-stranded DNA (dsDNA)	SLE
RNP	Mixed connective tissue
Jo-1	Antisynthetase syndrome
Ro, La	Sjögren syndrome, SLE
Scl-70 (topoisomerase)	Diffuse cutaneous scleroderma
Anti-centromere	Localized cutaneous scleroderma

Rheumatoid factor

- Rheumatoid factor is an antibody directed against the Fc fragment of human immunoglobulin G (IgG).
- Rheumatoid factors may be of any immunoglobulin class, although IgM anti-IgG is most commonly measured.
- It is present in 75% of patients with rheumatoid arthritis.

Anticitrullinated peptide antibodies (ACPA)

- ACPAs are highly specific for rheumatoid arthritis and may be detected years before onset of the disease.
- They are associated with joint erosion, and more aggressive disease.
- They can be present in patients who are rheumatoid factor-negative.

Antinuclear antibodies (ANAs)

These are antibodies to nuclear antigens. They are detected by labelling methods, such as indirect immuno-fluorescence. A positive ANA simply indicates that the patient's blood contains antibodies, which will bind to the nuclei of a sample of cells used in the test.

If an ANA test is positive, it is important to examine which nuclear antigens the antibodies are binding to. The pattern of fluorescence gives a clue. The titre of antibody is also important: significance is increased if antibody is detectable after multiple dilutions.

Figure 3.1 lists the ANAs against specific nuclear antigens and the diseases with which they are associated. Antibodies to double-stranded DNA (dsDNA) are very specific for SLE. They are also useful measures of disease activity.

Antineutrophil cytoplasmic antibodies (ANCA)

These antibodies are directed against enzymes present in neutrophil granules. They are associated with vasculitic and inflammatory conditions. Two main patterns of immunofluorescence are seen: cytoplasmic (c-ANCA) and perinuclear (p-ANCA).

c-ANCA and p-ANCA bind to several proteins, the most common being proteinase 3 (PR3) and myeloperoxidase (MPO) respectively. Antibodies to PR3 are found in about 80% of patients with Wegener granulomatosis. Those against MPO are found in polyarteritis nodosa. A positive MPO can also be found with malignancy and certain infections.

Antiphospholipid antibodies

Lupus anticoagulant and anticardiolipin antibodies are found in the antiphospholipid syndrome. They are associated with venous and arterial thrombosis and recurrent miscarriage.

Complement

Activation of the complement system leads to reduced serum levels of complement proteins as they fix to vessel walls and tissue. Reduced C3 and C4 occurs in active lupus and in some types of vasculitis.

Urine tests

Urine dip test gives a quick guide to protein and blood in the urine, but more formal quantification requires a sample to be sent for protein/creatinine ratio.

Proteinuria can suggest glomerulonephritis found in connective tissue diseases, vasculitis and amyloidosis.

Free light chains can be found in myeloma.

SYNOVIAL FLUID ANALYSIS

This is the most important investigation for suspected septic or crystal arthritis. Synovial fluid can be aspirated from most peripheral joints and only a small amount is needed for analysis.

Macroscopic appearance

Normal synovial fluid is pale yellow and clear. Changes in the macroscopic appearance can give clues to the underlying joint pathology (Fig. 3.2).

Gram stain and culture

This should be performed if there is any suspicion of septic arthritis. The absence of organisms on microscopy does not exclude infection.

Polarized light microscopy

For accurate identification of crystals, synovial fluid should be examined under a polarizing light microscope. Urate crystals are needle-shaped and show strong negative birefringence. This means that crystals parallel to the plane of light appear yellow, whereas those at right angles are blue. Calcium pyrophosphate dihydrate crystals are either rhomboid or rod-shaped and show weak positive birefringence (see Fig. 16.4).

NERVE CONDUCTION STUDIES (NCS) AND ELECTROMYOGRAPHY (EMG)

These electrophysiological tests are used to diagnose and assess neuromuscular problems. They help to differentiate between primary muscle disease and neuropathic disorders, for example, carpal tunnel syndrome, myositis and steroid myopathy. NCS measure the conduction velocity of motor and sensory nerves and can localize and assess the severity of peripheral nerve lesions. EMG records the spontaneous and voluntary electrical activity of muscle.

BIOPSY

Biopsies are occasionally performed in the investigation of musculoskeletal disease. Muscle is biopsied in cases of suspected myositis. Evidence of vasculitis can be obtained from biopsy of blood vessels, nerves and skin. Renal biopsies can assess the extent of renal involvement in connective tissue diseases and guide prognosis. Bone biopsy is necessary in the diagnosis of primary bone tumours. Synovial biopsy may be indicated in unexplained monoarthritis.

IMAGING

X-rays

A plain X-ray (radiograph) is usually the first-line investigation of any musculoskeletal disease. X-rays are good at visualizing bone. For detail of ligamentous or cartilage structures other investigations are necessary.

A radiograph involves the use of electromagnetic radiation produced by electrons striking a rotating metal target in an X-ray tube. A narrow beam of X-rays is produced, which then passes through the patient, and the image is formed on an X-ray-sensitive film placed behind the patient (Fig. 3.3).

The amount of the X-ray beam absorbed by the tissues determines the overall appearance of the image. Bone absorbs the most and appears white on the image; muscle absorbs some and appears dark grey; fat is darker grey and air appears black (see Fig. 4.6).

The X-ray machine is controlled by a radiographer who will determine the amount of exposure and the correct position of the patient.

HINTS AND TIPS

Any X-ray causes a small radiation exposure. Pelvic X-rays lead to far higher radiation exposure than peripheral joints. Avoid unnecessary X-rays to minimize cumulative risk of malignancy. Avoid X-rays in pregnancy unless absolutely necessary.

Fig. 3.2 Significance of changes in appearance of synovial fluid

Synovial fluid appearance	Pathology
Yellow and clear	Normal
Blood-stained	Haemarthrosis or puncture of a blood vessel on aspiration
Cloudy	Increased cell count due to inflammation or septic arthritis
Frank pus	Septic arthritis or occasionally crystal arthritis
Chalky	Gout crystals

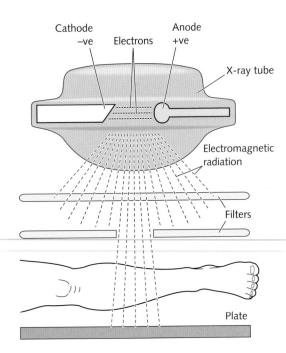

Fig. 3.3 Production of a radiographic image.

Two views are required for fracture identification, taken at 90° to each other, of the joint or bone to be examined (usually anteroposterior and lateral). Sometimes special views are taken (scaphoid).

Fluoroscopy (also known as screening) uses the same principles as radiography but the image is obtained on a screen and is in real time (i.e. moving). Screening is commonly used intraoperatively in orthopaedic surgery when fixing fractures and as guidance for joint injections.

Ultrasound

Ultrasound is used widely and has the advantage of being cheap, portable and safe, and it allows dynamic images.

The image is produced using a transducer that emits a beam of high-frequency sound (ultrasound) and detects the sound waves reflected from the soft tissues of the patient. Different tissues absorb or reflect different amounts of the sound beam, and the reflections are analysed to produce a black and white image.

Over recent years detection of synovitis and early erosions by ultrasound has helped tailor medical therapy in rheumatoid arthritis. Other areas commonly imaged in this way include the shoulder for rotator cuff tears, the hip for joint effusion and extra-articular structures around the knee, such as the patellar tendon.

Ultrasound can also be used for guidance, for example for joint aspiration and injection.

Computed tomography

CT uses the basic principles of an X-ray machine but the image is obtained when the X-ray tube is circled around the patient in the scanner. Instead of an X-ray plate the CT scanner has detectors within the machine to collect images. A large number of images are acquired and processed by the computer and the resulting images are in the form of cross-sectional slices taken in different planes.

The main role for CT is the study of bones, particularly complex fractures, and intervertebral discs to help diagnose discitis.

Remember that CT scans also produce a significant radiation exposure.

It is also possible to reconstruct images in three dimensions. Three-dimensional reconstructions are useful in orthopaedics when planning complex pelvic or hip surgery.

Magnetic resonance imaging

MRI gives excellent images of soft tissues and bone marrow.

The images are generated by the use of a powerful magnet, which aligns protons in the body with the electromagnetic field. A pulse of radiofrequency energy then causes the protons to 'flip' (change alignment) and images are acquired when energy is released as the protons realign themselves within the magnetic field. A coil collects data, which are then reconstructed with complex computer software to produce the image.

As a large magnet is used, any metal components or foreign bodies may become dislodged. Patients with cardiac pacemakers and intraocular metallic foreign bodies must not have an MRI scan.

MRI is commonly used around the knee to look for meniscal or ligamentous injuries (Fig. 3.4), the shoulder for capsule or rotator cuff lesions, and the spine for inflammatory back disease, disc prolapse and nerve root compression. In rheumatology it can be used to assess synovitis and erosive damage (see Fig. 12.12).

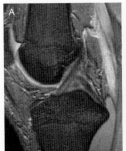
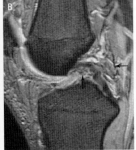

Fig. 3.4 Magnetic resonance imaging scans of the knee. (A) Normal. (B) Rupture of both cruciate ligaments (arrows).

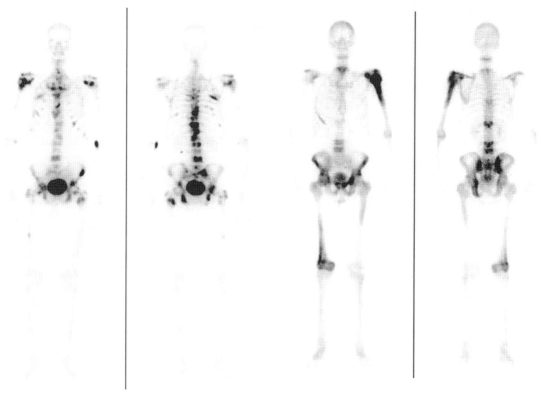

Fig. 3.5 Bone scan showing metastatic deposits (left: anterior, right: posterior view).

Fig. 3.6 Bone scan showing Paget disease (left: anterior, right: posterior view).

MRI is also good at assessing bone changes such as in infection, tumour and osteonecrosis.

Isotope bone scan

An isotope bone scan involves the use of a radioactive tracer injected intravenously and taken up by physiologically active bone. The most commonly used is technetium-99m and its decay is measured with a gamma camera. The procedure is divided into three phases depending on the time after injection: blood flow (initial); blood pool (30 minutes); and delayed (4 hours).

The images obtained show an outline of the body with areas highlighted where the isotope has accumulated.

Bone scans are useful as a tool for identifying the presence of a disease process (sensitive) but not very good at giving a diagnosis (non-specific). Increased uptake occurs typically in growth plates, arthritis, fractures, metastases (Fig. 3.5) (commonly used in malignancy), infection and Paget disease (Fig. 3.6). Decreased uptake occurs in some tumours (haemopoietic) and also in avascular bone.

Measurement of bone mineral density

Bone densitometry (DEXA scanning) uses two X-ray beams to determine the density of bone relative to age- and sex-matched controls and is used in detecting osteoporosis. It is further explained in Chapter 15.

Arthrography

Arthrograms are investigations in which the patient also has contrast or air injected into the joint. Plain X-ray arthrograms have largely been superseded by other investigations but are still used for hip conditions in the child. MRI arthrograms are useful tools for the diagnosis of intra-articular pathology, particularly in the hip and shoulder.

Regional pain 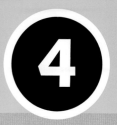 4

Objectives

After reading this chapter you should be able to:
- Give a differential diagnosis for back pain, including sinister causes, and appreciate appropriate investigations.
- Recognize important features in the history and examination for back pain.
- Understand the relevant anatomy of the knee and ankle and be able to list a differential diagnosis for pain.
- Know how to investigate regional pain in the spine and upper and lower limbs appropriately.
- Recognize patterns of upper-limb and neck pain in order to be able to make an accurate diagnosis.

BACK, HIP AND LEG PAIN

One of the most common presentations to a GP is that of back, hip and/or leg pain. Eighty per cent of the population will have an episode of back pain at some time in their lives.

An important point to note is that many patients do not appreciate the location of the hip joint and may even point to the iliac crest or further posteriorly towards the sacroiliac joint and tell you that this is their hip! Other misconceptions abound: one patient may tell you his sciatica is playing up or another that her slipped disc has 'popped out again'.

So when faced with such a patient the physician must decide on the basis of history and examination whether the pain is from the back or the hip joint.

Differential diagnosis

- Simple low back pain (see Ch. 9).
- Osteoarthritis (see Ch. 11).
- Prolapsed intervertebral disc/degenerative disc disease (see Ch. 9).
- Inflammatory spondyloarthropathy (see Ch. 13).
- Vertebral crush fracture (see Ch. 18).
- Spinal stenosis/spondylolisthesis (see Ch. 9).
- Malignancy (see Ch. 22).
- Discitis (see Ch. 9).
- Avascular necrosis of hip.
- Trochanteric bursitis.
- Paget disease (see Ch. 15).
- Abdominal causes (referred, e.g. pancreatitis/dissecting aortic aneurysm).

History focusing on back, hip and leg pain

There are essentially four different presentations (Fig. 4.1):
1. Back pain.
2. Back and leg pain.
3. Hip pain with or without leg pain.
4. Leg pain.

Back pain

Mechanical low back pain
Acute low back pain without radiation into the leg suggests mechanical low back pain – particularly if the patient gives a history of lifting or straining, and the pain is worse on movement and activity. The pain is usually described as a band across the back and may be extremely severe.

Signs of sinister back pain
Figure 4.2 shows 'red flag' signs that should alert the clinician to the possibility of serious spinal pathology. Malignancy such as spinal metastases is not uncommon. A history of fever might suggest discitis. Night sweats and weight loss are associated with malignancy and also tuberculosis.

Pain may radiate to the back from intra-abdominal pathology.

Fig. 4.1 Patterns of pain around the back, leg and hip.

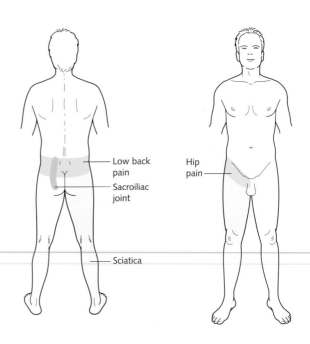

Low back pain	Hip pain
Sacroiliac joint	
Sciatica	

Fig. 4.2 Red flag signs of sinister back pain
Age of onset <20 or >55 years
History of malignancy
Persistent, non-mechanical pain
Night pain
Fever/unexplained weight loss
Bladder/bowel dysfunction
Progressive neurology, abnormal gait, saddle anaesthesia

Back and leg pain

Back and leg pain suggests that there is nerve root entrapment.

Sciatica
True sciatica radiates from the low back down the back of the leg and into the foot. It may be of acute onset from a specific incident, and is typically constant with acute exacerbations lasting seconds. The nature of the pain is like an electric shock and can be very severe. It is aggravated in certain positions such as standing straight and by sneezing or coughing. Over time the pain usually settles.

Spinal stenosis
In spinal stenosis the patient typically has back pain, and the leg pain comes on after walking and is relieved by rest and leaning forward – so-called spinal claudication.

Facet joint osteoarthritis
Facet joint osteoarthritis of the spine can also radiate into the leg but the pain does not extend below the knee and is aching in character.

Hip pain with or without leg pain

True hip joint pain is felt in the groin and can radiate down the front of the thigh to the knee. The pain of an arthritic hip is of gradual onset, deep and gnawing. It can be unrelenting and persistent. Night pain may be present.

Leg pain

Occasionally a prolapsed intervertebral disc presents with leg pain only (sciatica) without the back pain.

Muscular conditions such as muscular dystropy or myositis may present with leg pain or weakness, often gradual in onset and felt as a constant ache.

Peripheral vascular disease gives crampy leg pain on walking – claudication, usually relieved by rest.

Osteoarthritis of the hip may produce leg pain distally.

Loss of function/degree of disability

Patients will complain of limitation of certain activities, which may be recreational, work-related or more basic activities of daily living.

It is important to know how much impact the disorder has on normal day-to-day living.

Back pain is the leading cause of sickness from work.

Associated symptoms

It is essential to ask about urinary or bowel disturbance in any patient with back pain. Incontinence of urine or faeces suggests a cauda equina syndrome needing urgent investigation and surgical decompression.

Numbness, pins and needles and weakness of the foot should be elicited in the history and suggest true sciatica.

Weight loss, sweats and a history of previous malignancy indicate possible tumour.

Examination of the back and hip and investigations are described in Chapter 9. However a few specific investigations are worth noting.

Plain X-ray

These should not be done for mechanical back pain as there is minimal diagnostic yield and they expose the patient to radiation. Usually, normal appearances occur in simple low back pain, prolapsed disc and even in malignancy or infection if early in the disease process. When back or sacroiliac pathology is suspected in a young patient, magnetic resonance imaging (MRI) is the investigation of choice.

Where red flags are found the following are significant and warrant further investigation:

- Osteoarthritic changes in the hip and spine.
- 'Squaring' of vertebral bodies and bridging syndesmophytes (see Fig.13.6) in ankylosing spondylitis.
- Spondylolisthesis.
- Lytic lesions, destruction of the vertebral body, classically the pedicle (winking-owl sign) (Fig. 4.3), indicating malignancy.

Fig. 4.3 Malignancy of the spine. The winking-owl sign occurs when the pedicle is destroyed due to metastasis. The missing 'eye' represents bony destruction of the pedicle by tumour, so always look closely at the pedicles.

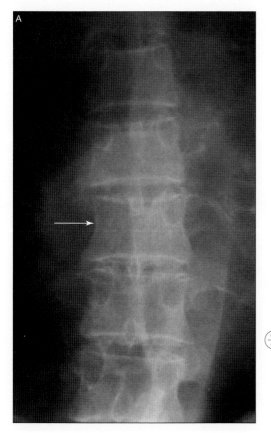

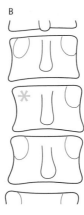

missing 'eye' represents bony destruction of the pedicle by tumour, therefore always look closely at the pedicles

- Fracture.
- Erosion of vertebral body around the disc due to infection.

Isotope bone scanning, computed tomography (CT) and MRI can be used where doubt remains, especially infection, malignancy and spinal cord compression.

KNEE PAIN

Knee pain is a very common presenting complaint, accounting for over a third of all referrals to orthopaedic surgeons.

Differential diagnosis

- Meniscal injuries.
- Ligament injury.
- Osteochondritis.
- Bursitis.
- Osteoarthritis.
- Septic arthritis.
- Rheumatoid or other inflammatory arthritis
- Anterior knee pain/patellofemoral disorders.
- Referred from hip or spine.

History focusing on knee pain

The first thing to consider is the patient's age and occupation. A young athletic patient with a recent injury is unlikely to have rheumatoid arthritis (think of meniscal/ligamentous injuries). Similarly, an elderly patient with gradual onset of pain over many years will most likely have osteoarthritis.

Characteristics of pain

The mode of onset is usually gradual, over a few weeks or months. If there is a sudden onset the most likely cause is an injury to the knee such as a meniscal tear or fracture. A history of spontaneous pain over days is most likely due to septic or crystal arthritis but could signal a flare-up of inflammatory arthritis.

Pain and stiffness in the morning improving through the day suggest an inflammatory arthritis.

Pain originating from knee pathology rarely radiates but hip pain is commonly felt in the knee, particularly in children.

Nature of pain

Meniscal tear often gives a sharp stabbing pain.

Arthritic pain is usually a deep gnawing pain.

Constant pain that is not affected by activity is often a feature of anterior knee pain.

Aggravating/relieving factors

Osteoarthritic pain is generally worse on activity and relieved by rest; inflammatory pain eases with use of the joint.

Classically patellofemoral pain is worse on walking up or down stairs.

Meniscal tears may give more trouble on full flexion or when twisting.

In an acute crystal or septic arthritis the pain is intense and any movement exacerbates this considerably.

Pain from prepatellar bursitis is worse on kneeling.

Site of pain

Pain can be generalized or localized.

Generalized pain ('all over') suggests an arthritic process affecting the whole joint. Large effusions such as after an injury or in sepsis also give a tense painful joint.

Localized pain depends on the site. Commonly painful areas around the knee are shown in Figure 4.4:

- Anterior: patellofemoral pain is felt here. Pain is felt at the front of the knee in prepatellar and infrapatellar bursitis.
- Medial or lateral: localized pain to either joint line could be osteoarthritis (particularly so in varus knees on the medial joint line) or from meniscal tears and collateral ligament sprains.
- Posterior pain is less common but could be related to a large Baker cyst or bursitis.
- Pain down the back of the knee could be referred from the spine.
- Pain down the front of the thigh and into the knee suggests hip pathology.

Loss of function

Patients may have significant disability due to their knee pain. They may notice decreased movement or loss of full extension.

Athletic patients with a meniscal tear or cruciate ligament injury will tell you they don't trust the knee during certain sporting activities and may be unable to do them at all.

Associated symptoms

It is important to ask some closed questions when taking a history in a patient with knee pain.

Ask about any generalized symptoms of ill health such as a fever.

Any history of injury is important.

- Ask if the patient heard a 'snap'.
- Ask how long the swelling took to appear.
- A history of locking suggests meniscal injury or loose body.

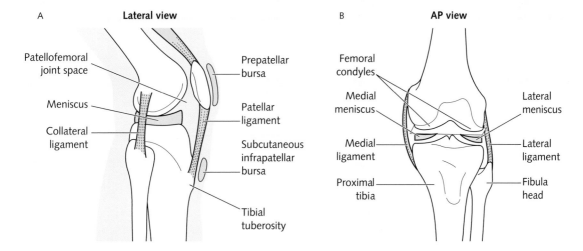

A   Lateral view

Patellofemoral joint space

Meniscus

Collateral ligament

Prepatellar bursa

Patellar ligament

Subcutaneous infrapatellar bursa

Tibial tuberosity

B   AP view

Femoral condyles

Medial meniscus

Medial ligament

Proximal tibia

Lateral meniscus

Lateral ligament

Fibula head

Fig. 4.4 Anatomical structures in the knee that cause pain. AP, anteroposterior.

- Giving way may be due to a ligamentous problem such as anterior cruciate ligament rupture.

Examination is described in Chapter 2.

Investigations

Figure 4.5 provides an algorithm for the investigation of knee pain.

Further imaging

This is only warranted under certain conditions:

- MRI: useful to confirm meniscal or ligamentous pathology.
- CT: gives detailed information on bony structures; also useful to visualize patellar tracking.
- Isotope bone scanning: occasionally used if unsure about diagnosis. It will show 'hot spots' due to increased activity in many conditions such as inflammatory arthritis but also rarer causes such as osteomyelitis and bone tumours. It is a sensitive test but not specific. A normal bone scan is reassuring if one suspects sinister pathology.
- Ultrasound: for confirmation of synovitis, effusion or for guided injections

Aspiration

Aspiration of joint fluid is a very simple method of investigation and can give clues to the diagnosis.

Using aseptic technique, feel the upper and lower border of the patella. From the midpoint, feel laterally until you can identify the patellofemoral joint space. This is the easiest landmark to use, and the needle should be inserted at 90° to the lateral aspect of the

knee, angled slightly proximally. Inject local anaesthetic and aspirate fluid.

Look at the fluid obtained:

- Straw/yellow fluid: likely to be a simple effusion or possibly a crystal arthropathy (send for polarized light microscopy to identify crystals).
- Green or dirty fluid: likely to be pus, and septic arthritis is likely.
- Blood: a haemarthrosis occurs after injury or occasionally in bleeding disorders or patients on warfarin. Blood and fat globules (a lipohaemarthrosis; Fig. 4.6) are present in fracture or anterior cruciate ligament rupture.

Arthroscopy

Knee arthroscopy involves 'keyhole' surgery to look into the joint to see if there is any pathology.

> **HINTS AND TIPS**
>
> Always send fluid obtained to microbiology for microscopy, culture and sensitivities and ask the laboratory to look for crystals.

ANKLE AND FOOT PAIN

The complexity of structures in the foot and ankle combined with the relative difficulty in examining individual joints make diagnosis in the foot and ankle more challenging. Biomechanical aspects play a particularly important part in ankle and foot problems.

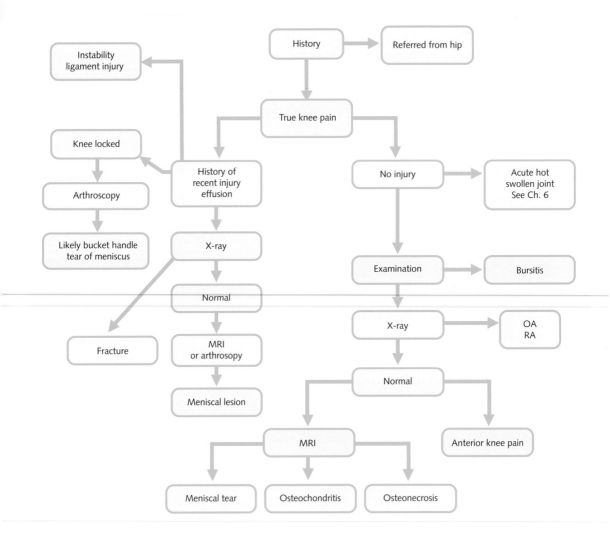

Fig. 4.5 Algorithm for the investigation of knee pain. MRI, magnetic resonance imaging; OA, osteoarthritis; RA, rheumatoid arthritis.

Fig. 4.6 A lipohaemarthrosis in the suprapatellar pouch secondary to a tibial plateau fracture. A fluid level is seen as the fat 'floats' on the blood.

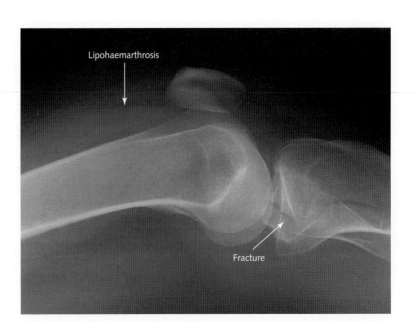

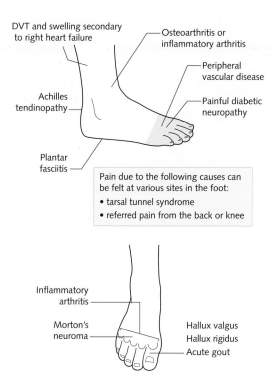

DVT and swelling secondary to right heart failure

Osteoarthritis or inflammatory arthritis

Peripheral vascular disease

Achilles tendinopathy

Painful diabetic neuropathy

Plantar fasciitis

Pain due to the following causes can be felt at various sites in the foot:
- tarsal tunnel syndrome
- referred pain from the back or knee

Inflammatory arthritis

Morton's neuroma

Hallux valgus
Hallux rigidus
Acute gout

Fig. 4.7   Differential diagnosis of ankle and/or foot pain. DVT, deep vein thrombosis.

Differential diagnosis

The differential diagnosis of pain in the ankle and/or foot is shown in Figure 4.7.

History focusing on ankle pain

The following points should be covered when taking a history from patients with ankle or foot pain.

Characteristics (see Fig. 4.7)

- Recurrent self-limiting pain suggests crystal arthropathy (e.g. gout).
- Chronic pain with soft-tissue swelling suggests inflammation or infection.
- Posterior pain on walking may be due to Achilles tendinopathy, while discomfort on the sole of the foot may be due to plantar fasciitis.

COMMUNICATION

It is important to enquire what impact pain in the ankle or foot has on a patient's function and lifestyle. Achilles tendinopathy can ruin the career of an athlete, but may interfere little with the activities of a patient who leads a more sedentary lifestyle.

Presence of associated symptoms

- Back or knee pain suggest that the pain may be referred.
- Coldness and pallor of the foot may be due to peripheral vascular disease.
- Paraesthesiae or 'burning' pain can occur with Morton neuroma, painful diabetic neuropathy or tarsal tunnel syndrome (compression of the tibial nerve passing through the tarsal tunnel).
- Plantar fasciitis is associated with spondyloarthropathies, so ask about a history of psoriasis or inflammatory bowel disease.
- Repetitive trauma due to running, jumping or other athletic activities can predispose to Achilles tendinopathy, plantar fasciitis ('policeman's heel') and ligamentous laxity.
- A recent illness or initiation of diuretic therapy may trigger an acute attack of gout.

Examination

Regional Examination of the Musculoskeletal System (REMS) relating to the foot and ankle is described in Chapter 2.

HINTS AND TIPS

The ankle and foot should be inspected during weight bearing as well as in the neutral position. Some clinical signs are more obvious when the patient is standing.

Investigations

For blood investigations, see p. 32.

Radiological investigations

- Plain X-rays may show erosions of inflammatory arthritis or characteristic degenerative change.
- Ultrasonography can identify synovitis (with power signal), effusion, gout crystals, arthritis, tendinopathy and Morton neuromas.
- MRI can also be used to assess the above; it is less operator-dependent but more expensive.

Synovial fluid examination

See knee section, above.

Nerve conduction studies

These are useful in confirming the diagnosis of tarsal tunnel syndrome or peripheral neuropathy.

NECK AND/OR UPPER-LIMB PAIN

A careful history is especially required when the patient presents with problems in this region due to the wide differential which includes cardiac and neurological causes of pain.

Differential diagnosis

Figures 4.8–4.11 give the differential diagnoses that should be considered when patients present with neck, shoulder, elbow, or wrist and hand pain.

Neck pain

History

Trauma or impact injuries to the neck require careful assessment for fracture or neurological signs. Carotid artery dissection produces sudden anterior pain secondary to trauma. Chronic stiffness may suggest an inflammatory cause. Shooting pain radiating down the arms implies nerve root entrapment. Weakness or clumsiness of the lower limbs or urinary symptoms may result from cervical cord compression. Dizziness may occur as a result of vertebral artery compression in severe degenerative disease. Fever, weight loss and general malaise

---

Fig. 4.8 Differential diagnosis of neck pain

- Mechanical neck pain
- Cervical spondylosis
- Ankylosing spondylitis
- Cervical disc prolapse
- Cervical discitis
- Metastatic vertebral deposits
- Referred pain from:
  - Local structures (e.g. thyroiditis, cervical lymphadenopathy)
  - Distant structures (e.g. ischaemic heart disease, subphrenic abscess)

Fig. 4.9 Differential diagnosis of shoulder pain

- Rotator cuff pathology (impingement, tendinopathy or tear)
- Capsulitis
- Arthritis of the acromioclavicular joint
- Arthritis of the glenohumeral joint
- Bicipital tendinopathy
- Polymyalgia rheumatica
- Referred pain from:
  - Neck pathology
  - Cardiac ischaemia
  - Pancoast tumour
  - Intra-abdominal pathology (e.g. subphrenic abscess)

Fig. 4.10 Differential diagnosis of elbow pain

- Lateral epicondylitis (tennis elbow)
- Olecranon bursitis
- Crystal arthropathy
- Osteoarthritis
- Inflammatory arthritis
- Medial epicondylitis (golfer's elbow)
- Referred pain from the neck or shoulder

Fig. 4.11 Differential diagnosis of pain in the hand and wrist

- Osteoarthritis
- Carpal tunnel syndrome
- Tenosynovitis
- Inflammatory arthritis
- Crystal arthropathy
- Ulnar nerve entrapment
- Raynaud phenomenon
- Complex regional pain syndrome
- Referred pain from the cervical spine, shoulder or elbow

---

raise the possibility of sepsis, malignancy or inflammatory conditions such as polymyalgia rheumatica.

- Some symptoms will give a clue to the presence of disease that may be causing referred pain (e.g. haemoptysis in a patient with a Pancoast tumour).

Examination

REMS in Chapter 2 outlines the examination technique. Remember to examine for bony tenderness following trauma, and lymphadenopathy when there are concerns over infection or malignancy. Loss of the normal cervical lordosis may be seen due to cervical spondylosis or muscle spasm.

Shoulder pain

History

This is a common site of pain but referred pain is also common, such as from the diaphragm in cholecystitis and the neck in nerve root irritation. Reduction in the range of movement with associated pain may occur in frozen shoulder and painful arc syndrome, the latter having exacerbation of pain on abduction. The site of pain may give a clue to its origin. Figure 4.12 shows how the site of shoulder pain varies with the cause.

Examination

REMS in Chapter 2 outlines technique. Anterior dislocation will produce an obvious bulge, while frozen shoulder tends to produce a globally restricted joint.

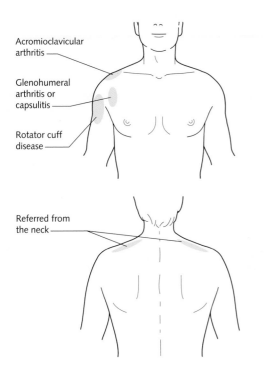

Acromioclavicular arthritis

Glenohumeral arthritis or capsulitis

Rotator cuff disease

Referred from the neck

Fig. 4.12 Many structures can give rise to shoulder pain. These diagrams show how the site of pain varies with the origin.

Wasting of the shoulder muscles may occur in chronic rotator cuff injuries. A reduction in passive and active movement suggests arthritis or capsulitis of the joint. A reduction in active movement, with normal passive movement, suggests a rotator cuff problem.

Elbow

History

Repetitive movement (pronation) can trigger lateral epicondylitis (tennis elbow).

Examination

Movement of the elbow in lateral epicondylitis will probably be normal, but resisted dorsiflexion of the wrist will exacerbate the pain.

Wrist and hand

History

Precipitants may be important: Raynaud phenomenon is provoked by cold weather.

Acute gout may be precipitated by drugs such as diuretics or initiation of allopurinol.

Examination

Look for:

- Heberden or Bouchard nodes, seen in osteoarthritis (see Ch. 11).
- Synovial swelling of the small hand joints or tendon sheaths in rheumatoid arthritis.
- Rheumatoid nodules.
- Plaques of psoriasis.
- Gouty tophi
- Wasting of the thenar or hypothenar muscles resulting from median or ulnar nerve compression respectively.
- Ischaemic changes in the digits due to Raynaud phenomenon.
- Changes in skin colour, with atrophy and reduced hair growth as features of complex regional pain syndrome.

As well as accurately identifying tender structures, palpation helps in the assessment of swelling. Hard, bony swelling as seen in osteoarthritis should be distinguished from the softer boggy, synovial swelling of inflammatory arthritis. Inflamed tendon sheaths in the hand or wrist may feel thickened or nodular and palpation may produce crepitus. A suggested algorithm for the examination and investigation of patients with neck and/or upper-limb pain is shown in Figure 4.13.

Examination of other body systems

Neurological examination of the cranial nerves and all four limbs is essential in a patient with neck pain and any neurological symptoms. Cervical radiculopathy and cord compression should be excluded. Motor and sensory function of the median and ulnar nerves should be assessed in cases of hand and wrist pain (Fig. 4.14). Tinel and Phalen tests may be abnormal in carpal tunnel syndrome (see Fig. 10.3).

Examination of the cardiovascular, respiratory and abdominal systems may reveal a source of referred pain.

Investigations

The choice of investigations depends on the clinical examination findings. In some cases, the diagnosis is obvious from examination and further investigation is not required. For example, a 75-year-old man who complains of pain in his digits and has squaring of his first carpometacarpal joint and Heberden nodes has osteoarthritis. Plain X-rays will confirm the diagnosis, but will not alter his management in any way.

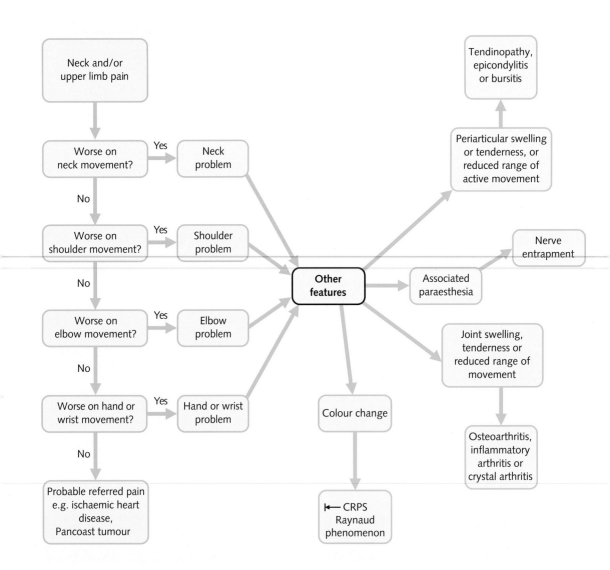

Fig. 4.13 Algorithm for the diagnosis of neck and/or upper-limb pain. CRPS, complex regional pain syndrome.

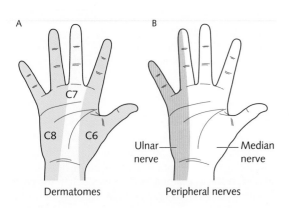

Fig. 4.14 Nerve entrapment in the upper limb can cause pain, paraesthesiae or sensory loss in the hand. The digits affected give a clue as to which nerve is involved.

Blood tests

- Erythrocyte sedimentation rate and C-reactive protein may be raised in inflammatory, infectious or malignant conditions.
- The finding of a positive rheumatoid factor (or citric citrullinated peptide antibody) in a patient with synovitis is suggestive of rheumatoid arthritis.

Radiological investigations

X-rays

Plain X-rays may show signs of:

- Degenerative or inflammatory arthritis.
- Calcification due to tendinopathy.
- Periosteal reaction due to enthesitis.
- Bony metastasis.

HINTS AND TIPS

X-rays are of little value in cervical spondylosis. There is poor correlation between the severity of radiographic signs and symptoms. Many people develop radiographic signs of spondylosis with increasing age, yet never suffer from neck pain.

Ultrasound scans

Ultrasound scanning can demonstrate thickening and oedema of tendon sheaths in tenosynovitis, and can identify synovitis, effusion and tears in the rotator cuff apparatus.

MRI

MRI is useful in the following circumstances:

- Imaging the cervical cord and nerve roots.
- Detecting rotator cuff inflammation or degeneration.

Isotope bone scans

Isotope bone scans show increased tracer uptake in areas of accelerated bone turnover, such as inflammation, infection, malignancy or fracture. The finding of a 'hot spot' should be followed by MRI or CT scanning.

Nerve conduction studies

These can help to exclude cervical radiculopathy in patients with neck pain and upper-limb paraesthesiae. Reduced nerve conduction velocities are seen in median and ulnar nerve entrapment.

Complex regional pain syndrome

This is also referred to as reflex sympathetic dystrophy, algodystrophy or Sudeck atrophy. It is not common, but can affect any part of the musculoskeletal system. The distal forearm and hand are most often involved. The key features are of pain, hypersensitivity and autonomic disturbances, which can affect the integrity of the skin. Allodynia may be present (pain felt from a stimulus that would not normally produce pain, e.g. light touch). A preceding injury has invariably occurred. Treatment is with bisphosphonates.

Further reading

Da Silva, J.A.P., Woolf, A.D., 2010. Rheumatology in Practice. Springer, London.
NICE low backpain guideline, 2009. Available online at: http://www.nice.org.uk/nicemedia/pdf/CG88NICEGuideline.pdf.
www.jointzone.com.

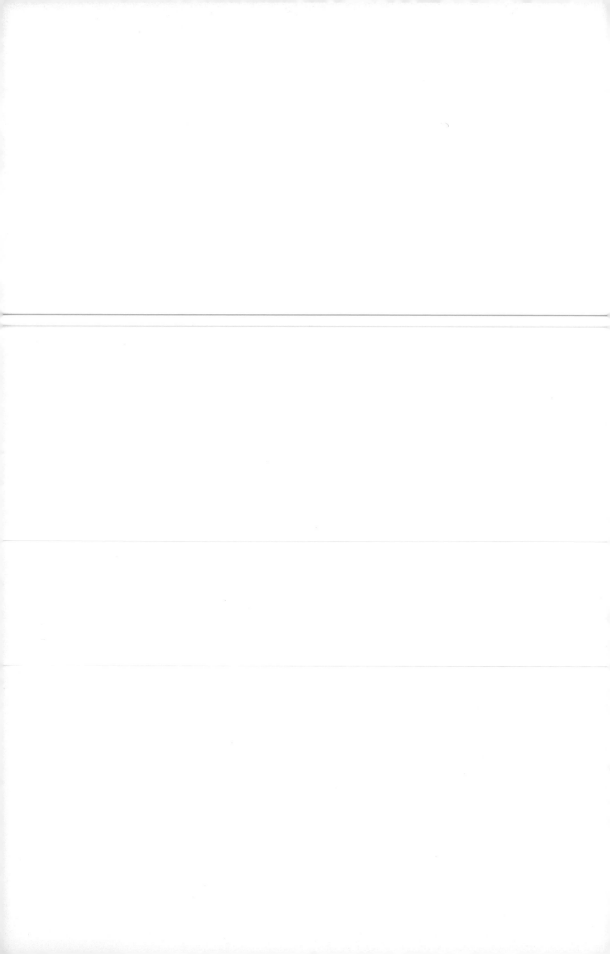

Widespread musculoskeletal pain

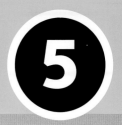

Objectives

After reading this chapter you should be able to:
- List the causes of widespread musculoskeletal pain.
- Recognize how pain and stiffness due to inflammatory disease vary in severity throughout the day.
- Select appropriate investigations for the assessment of patients with widespread musculoskeletal pain.
- Recognize the common symptoms of fibromyalgia.
- Understand the strategies employed in the management of patients with fibromyalgia.

DIFFERENTIAL DIAGNOSIS

Patients sometimes present with widespread musculo-skeletal pain. The differential diagnosis is shown in Figure 5.1.

The age, sex and race of the patient will give some guide to the likely diagnosis. For example, polymyalgia rheumatica (PMR) rarely affects people under the age of 60 years, fibromyalgia and systemic lupus erythematosus (SLE) are more common in women than in men and osteomalacia is more prevalent in Asian than in Caucasian populations.

PARANEOPLASTIC RHEUMATIC SYNDROME

This is a rare, but important, cause of musculoskeletal pain. Patients with lymphoma, leukaemia or other malignancies sometimes present with rheumatic symptoms. These can mimic inflammatory polyarthritis or PMR. Equally widespread bony metastases can present as bone or joint pain. Primary tumours that spread to bone include breast, lung, kidney, thyroid and prostate.

History

A thorough history should be taken, covering the following points.

Onset of pain

This will nearly always be insidious, but rarely SLE and PMR can give pain developing over a few days.

Timing of pain

As a rule, pain that is worse in the mornings and improves throughout the day is more likely to be inflammatory in origin.

Site of pain

Patients may find it hard to distinguish whether the pain is arising from their muscles or joints. Remember that pain can be referred from a proximal joint.

Presence of stiffness

Patients with musculoskeletal pain due to any cause may complain of stiffness. Significant stiffness that is maximal in the mornings and lasts for more than 30 minutes suggests inflammatory arthritis, SLE or PMR.

Associated symptoms

- Temporal headaches or jaw claudication are suggestive of giant cell arteritis associated with PMR.
- A history of skin rashes, mouth ulcers or Raynaud phenomenon raises the possibility of SLE.
- Psychiatric problems, such as anxiety and depression, can be features of fibromyalgia.
- Abdominal pain and confusion can occur in hypercalcaemia.

Examination and investigation

A suggested algorithm for the examination and investigation of patients with widespread musculoskeletal pain is shown in Figure 5.2.

Fig. 5.1 The differential diagnosis of widespread musculoskeletal pain
Inflammatory polyarthritis
Fibromyalgia
Systemic lupus erythematosus
Myositis
Polymyalgia rheumatica
Metabolic bone disease (osteomalacia, hypercalcaemia)
Paraneoplastic rheumatic syndrome
Widespread skeletal metastasis
Thyroid disease
Vitamin deficiency – B_{12}/folate
Drugs – e.g. statins

Examination

Examination can help make the decision as to whether the pain is arising from the joints, muscles or soft tissues. The joints should be examined for signs of inflammation. Power in all four limbs should be measured and the soft tissues palpated for areas of tenderness. Examination of other systems is also important.

Investigation

Investigations should be guided by the examination findings. It is important to remember that they may be normal in the early stages of disease.

Blood tests

- The ESR is likely to be raised in cases of PMR, inflammatory arthritis, SLE or malignancy.
- Serum calcium levels may be low in osteomalacia, and high in malignancy.
- Parathyroid hormone levels should be checked in the presence of hypercalcaemia to exclude hyperparathyroidism.
- Serum alkaline phosphatase may be elevated in Pagets' disease. It can also rise in response to inflammation.
- An immunology screen, including measurement of antinuclear and anti-double-stranded DNA antibodies, may be abnormal in active SLE.

Radiological investigations

X-rays of the small joints may show the erosive changes of inflammatory arthritis. Radiographs of the long bones and pelvis should be taken if the patient has risk factors for osteomalacia, such as reduced sunlight exposure or intestinal malabsorption. Looser's zones may be seen.

Other radiological tests (e.g. chest X-ray, isotope bone scan, abdominal ultrasound scan) may be necessary if there is any suspicion of malignancy.

FIBROMYALGIA

Definition

Rheumatologists meet many patients suffering from chronic widespread pain which cannot be explained. There are often associated symptoms such as depression, fatigue, poor concentration and sleep disturbance. Fibromyalgia is a condition of chronic pain accompanied by the finding of soft-tissue tenderness on examination, located over a number of trigger points. However, the existence of fibromyalgia as an organic 'disease' remains controversial. Many physicians recognize the above clinical features, but feel that giving patients a 'label' may reinforce their illness behaviour. However, there is evidence that referral rates and investigations lessen once patients have been diagnosed.

Prevalence

Fibromyalgia is common. The prevalence is estimated to be between 2 and 5%.

Aetiology

The aetiology of fibromyalgia is unknown, but several risk factors for the condition are recognized. These include:

- Female sex.
- Middle age.
- Stress.

There is some overlap between the features of fibromyalgia and other syndromes that have a functional component (Fig. 5.3).

Pathogenesis

The roles of various neurotransmitters, hormones and peptides have been examined in fibromyalgia; in spite of much research, the pathogenesis has not been explained.

Clinical features

Fibromyalgia predominantly affects women between the ages of 30 and 60 years. Patients usually report a long history of widespread pain which responds poorly to analgesia. Other common symptoms are shown in Figure 5.4.

Fatigue is often severe and follows minimal exertion. Sleep disruption is common and patients frequently complain that they wake feeling unrefreshed. Psychiatric problems, such as anxiety and depression, are thought to affect as many as 20% of fibromyalgia sufferers.

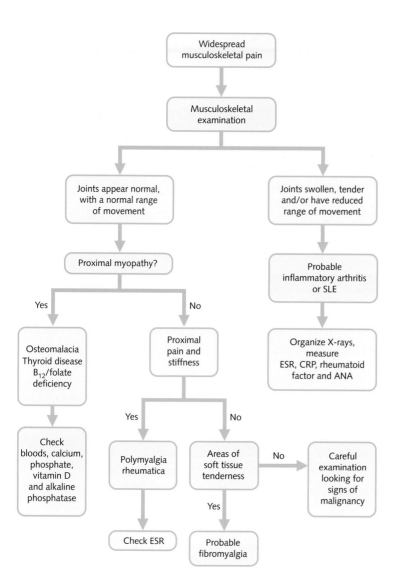

Fig. 5.2 Algorithm for the investigation of widespread musculoskeletal pain. ANA, antinuclear antibody; CRP, C-reactive protein; ESR, erythrocyte sedimentation rate; SLE, systemic lupus erythematosus.

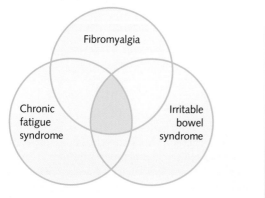

Fig. 5.3 Overlap between fibromyalgia and other syndromes.

Fig. 5.4 Common symptoms of fibromyalgia
Fatigue
Sleep disturbance
Poor concentration
Headache
Paraesthesia
Anxiety
Depression
Altered bowel habit
Widespread pain

Fig. 5.5 The 'tender points' of fibromyalgia.

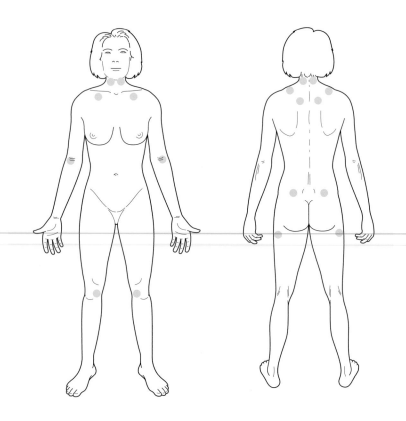

The only significant finding on musculoskeletal examination is the presence of soft-tissue tenderness, usually at multiple sites. Common sites of tenderness are shown in Figure 5.5.

Investigations

Fibromyalgia is a clinical diagnosis based on recognition of symptoms and tender points. The only role of investigations is in the exclusion of other conditions.

Management

There is no specific treatment. Quality of life for most patients remains poor. Addressing social stressors and depression is essential if better outcomes are to be obtained. The following treatment strategies may help.

Education

- Inform patients about the condition.
- Reassure them that they do not have a destructive arthritis.

- Emphasize that they will not harm their joints by exercising.

Physiotherapy/exercise

A graded aerobic exercise regime can improve fitness and reduce pain and fatigue.

Cognitive behavioural therapy

This encourages patients to develop mechanisms to cope with their symptoms.

Drug therapy

A series of drug therapies have been used, with modest success. These include tricyclic antidepressants such as amitriptyline, dual reuptake inhibitors (duloxetine), anticonvulsants (pregabalin, gabapentin) and analgesics such as tramadol. There is no role for anti-inflammatory drugs.

Further reading

Clauw, D.J., 2009. Fibromyalgia: an overview. Am. J. Med. 122 (Suppl.), S3–S13.

Fibromyalgia Association UK, www.fmauk.org.

Firestein, G.S., Budd, R.C., Gabriel, S.E., et al., 2013. Kelley's Textbook of Rheumatology, nineth ed. Elsevier, Philadelphia.

An acute hot swollen joint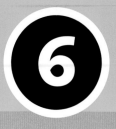

Objectives

After reading this chapter you should be able to:
- Give a list of differential diagnoses for a hot swollen joint.
- Take a history from a patient, picking out relevant details.
- Understand how to investigate a hot swollen knee.

DIFFERENTIAL DIAGNOSIS

The phrase 'acute hot swollen joint' implies that the patient has presented as an emergency with rapid onset of symptoms and a large painful effusion. While there are many causes of a swollen and hot joint, the most important cause to exclude in the acute setting is septic arthritis:

- Septic arthritis.
- Crystal arthropathy:
  - Gout.
  - Pseudogout.
- Inflammatory arthritis (rheumatoid arthritis or seronegative spondyloarthropathy).
- Transient synovitis.
- Haemarthrosis.

HISTORY FOCUSING ON THE ACUTE HOT SWOLLEN JOINT

Pain

Patients with acute gout or septic arthritis classically have very severe pain. However, it is difficult to differentiate these conditions from other causes of hot swollen joints as the majority of patients will present with intense pain that is worse on movement.

Patient age and sex

All of the above conditions could present in the adult patient, whereas only septic arthritis, reactive arthritis and possibly inflammatory arthritis are likely causes in children.

Gout is more common in men, and rheumatoid arthritis is more common in women.

Which joint?

Certain joints are more commonly affected by specific disorders (Fig. 6.1):

- Gout commonly affects the first metatarsophalangeal joint of the foot.
- Pseudogout is common in the knee and wrist.
- Multiple joint involvement points to an inflammatory disorder such as rheumatoid arthritis or juvenile idiopathic arthritis.

Is the patient ill?

Fever, night sweats, rigors and general flu-like symptoms suggest likely infection but it is possible to have the same symptoms in an acute flare-up of an inflammatory arthropathy.

Previous history

This is likely in gout as 90% of patients with an acute attack will have recurrent episodes.

It is unlikely in septic arthritis unless the patient has a predisposing factor such as diabetes mellitus, immunosuppression or sickle cell disease.

HINTS AND TIPS

Be careful. Patients with known inflammatory or crystal arthritis can present with joint infection. Patients on immunosuppressant drugs may not mount the usual inflammatory responses so the joint may not have the typical features associated with infection.

Associated symptoms

Patients with an inflammatory disorder may have systemic features of the disease process, such as sacroiliac

Fig. 6.1 Likely diagnosis for each joint in a patient presenting with an acute hot swollen joint.

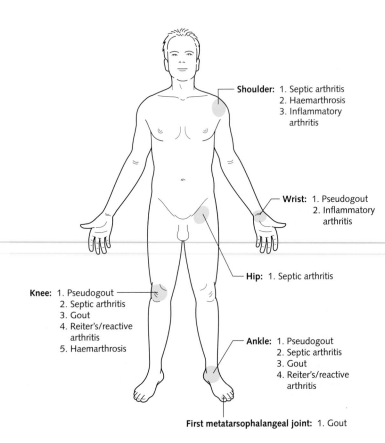

Shoulder: 1. Septic arthritis
2. Haemarthrosis
3. Inflammatory arthritis

Wrist: 1. Pseudogout
2. Inflammatory arthritis

Hip: 1. Septic arthritis

Knee: 1. Pseudogout
2. Septic arthritis
3. Gout
4. Reiter's/reactive arthritis
5. Haemarthrosis

Ankle: 1. Pseudogout
2. Septic arthritis
3. Gout
4. Reiter's/reactive arthritis

First metatarsophalangeal joint: 1. Gout

joint pain in ankylosing spondylitis or painful metacarpophalangeal joints in rheumatoid arthritis.

Eye symptoms can occur in:

- Reiter syndrome (conjunctivitis).
- Rheumatoid arthritis (keratoconjunctivitis).
- Juvenile idiopathic arthritis (uveitis).

Patients with a history of recent sexually transmitted disease or diarrhoea may have Reiter syndrome.

Also consider gonococcal arthritis in patients with a history of sexually transmitted diseases.

A recent viral illness can result in a reactive arthritis.

Past medical history

Patients with diabetes mellitus are at an increased risk of septic arthritis, as they are of any other infection.

Gout is linked with increased cell turnover and therefore any illness can predispose to it due to catabolism; however it is particularly common in myeloproliferative disease.

Patients with malignancy having chemotherapy are particularly prone to gout due to vast numbers of cells being 'killed' (see Ch. 22).

Certain conditions also predispose to joint infection, e.g. intravenous drug use.

Patients with a bleeding disorder (such as haemophilia) or on warfarin are at risk of developing an acute haemarthrosis (bleeding into a joint). These patients can present with an acutely swollen tender joint after only a trivial injury.

Drug history

Diuretics, particularly thaizides, and low-dose aspirin can increase uric acid levels, predisposing to gout.

Patients on steroids or other immunosuppressants are at increased risk of infection.

Social history

Alcohol excess and high-purine diets predispose to gout.

EXAMINATION OF A PATIENT WITH AN ACUTE HOT SWOLLEN JOINT

General

- Most patients presenting in such a way will look unwell, be uncomfortable and may be agitated.
- Pyrexia suggests infection but mildly elevated temperatures can be present in gout and inflammatory arthritis.
- In severe cases of sepsis, the patient may show signs of cardiovascular compromise, such as tachycardia and hypotension – septicaemic shock.
- The patient should be examined for general signs of inflammatory arthritis.
- Patients with gout may have gouty tophi; these are commonly found on extensor surfaces of the elbow and fingers.

The joint

- The knee is the most commonly affected joint overall.
- Any affected joint will have a tense effusion and be tender to palpation, and passive and active movement. Typically a septic joint will be exquisitely tender, with the patient holding the joint rigidly still to minimize discomfort. The other causes of arthropathy, whilst tender, tend not to be as severe.

- A full examination of the joint is unnecessary and impossible.
- A thorough examination of other joints should be performed to make sure the patient has a mono-arthritis (i.e. no other joints are involved).

INVESTIGATION OF A PATIENT WITH AN ACUTE SWOLLEN JOINT

An algorithm for the investigation of a patient with an acute swollen joint is shown in Figure 6.2.

Blood tests

The aim of initial investigation is to confirmor exclude septic arthritis. Do *not* rely on blood tests alone, which may be normal:

- A raised white cell count (WCC) suggests infection but can be raised due to inflammatory causes. WCCs tend not to be raised, or only very slightly raised, in cases of crystal arthropathy.
- Inflammatory markers C-reactive protein and erythrocyte sedimentation rate can be raised in all the conditions listed above, particularly septic arthritis and inflammatory arthritis.
- In cases of immunosuppression, blood results may not demonstrate a significant inflammatory response. Consequently their result should be treated with caution.

Fig. 6.2 Algorithm for the investigation of an acute hot swollen joint. CRP, C-reactive protein; ESR, erythrocyte sedimentation rate; FBC, full blood count.

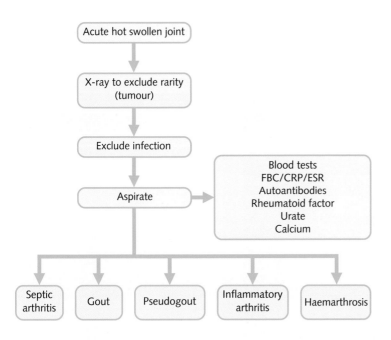

Normal inflammatory markers cannot completely exclude infection:

- Serum urate may be elevated, normal or low in patients with acute gout.
- Serum calcium should be checked as pseudogout can be caused by hyperparathyroidism.
- If haemarthrosis is suspected a clotting screen should be performed and patients on warfarin should have their international normalized ratio checked.

X-rays

Plain X-rays of the affected joint may show:

- Normal appearances.
- Chondrocalcinosis (found in pseudogout due to calcium deposition in menisci).
- Bony erosions associated with gout or inflammatory arthritis.

HINTS AND TIPS

Of all the investigations, the most important is aspiration of the joint.

Aspiration/synovial fluid analysis

- A superficial joint such as the knee is simple to aspirate, particularly when there is a tense effusion.
- Deeply situated joints such as the hip require ultrasound or X-ray guidance.
- Aspiration should be done before antibiotics are given. In every case fluid aspirated must be sent to microbiology for an urgent Gram stain, though a negative Gram stain does not definitively exclude infection. The aspirate should also be sent for culture and sensitivity, though the results may take some days to be available. It is important to ask for microscopy for crystals, which may be performed by microbiology, or a separate sample may need to be sent to histology.
- The general appearance of the aspirate should be described (see Ch.3).

Ultrasound

Ultrasound scanning is useful to detect an effusion, particularly in the hip.

Objectives

After reading this chapter you should be able to:
- Give a list of the most likely differential diagnoses according to the age of the child.
- Understand what to look for on examination of the neonate, infant and child.
- Investigate a child with a limp to rule out serious conditions.
- Differentiate between an ill and a well child.

There are many causes of a limping child. However, it is most important in the acute phase to exclude septic arthtitis as this can cause major morbidity and even mortality if missed.

DIFFERENTIAL DIAGNOSIS

- Septic arthritis.
- Irritable hip.
- Developmental dysplasia of the hip (DDH).
- Perthes disease.
- Slipped upper femoral epiphysis (SUFE).
- Osteomyelitis.
- Occult trauma.
- Neuromuscular causes.
- Juvenile idiopathic arthritis (JIA: see Ch. 17).
- Malignancy (very rare).

HISTORY FOCUSING ON THE CHILD WITH A LIMP

There is a big difference between an infant aged 15 months and an adolescent aged 15 years. Infants will not give an accurate history and if very unwell may be distressed and uncooperative. The majority of children do, however, give a good history.

Age

The most important factor in assessing a child with a limp is the age of the child. Figure 7.1 shows the likely differential diagnosis depending on the age of the child.

Sex

The sex of the child can also give clues to the diagnosis; for example, Perthes disease is much more common in boys than in girls.

Is the child ill?

To answer this question the general state of the child must be noted. Systemically unwell children will show little interest in play or food and simply will not be themselves. Fever, rigors and night sweats should be noted as well as duration of symptoms. An unwell child suggests infection or JIA (see Ch. 17).

Pain

Most children limp because of pain:
- More sudden onset of pain is more likely due to trauma or infection.
- The history in Perthes disease is often of a vague gradual onset of pain and limp.
- The classic history for a SUFE is often a background of hip pain for weeks followed by sudden increase in pain.
- Transient synovitis of the hip gives pain in the groin and mimics septic arthritis.
- Any child complaining of knee pain must be suspected of having hip pathology.

Occasionally sinister causes of pain (such as bone tumours) present with gradually increasing pain (including night pain) not relieved by simple analgesia.

Painless limp

- Late-presenting DDH presents with a limp and leg length discrepancy.
- Neuromuscular disorders such as cerebral palsy result in poor gait due to muscle imbalance rather than pain.
- Cerebral palsy can present as developmental delay but milder forms can present later in childhood as the weakness becomes more apparent.
- Muscular dystrophy can also present with gradual onset of weakness and limp.

Fig. 7.1	Diagnosis by age in a child with a limp
All ages	Infection (septic arthritis or osteomyelitis) Juvenile idiopathic arthritis
Infant (1–3 years)	Late-presenting developmental dysplasia of the hip (DDH) Irritable hip Neuromuscular Occult trauma (including non-accidental injury)
Childhood (3–11 years)	Perthes disease Irritable hip Neuromuscular Slipped upper femoral epiphysis (SUFE) Non-accidental injury
Adolescence (12–16 years)	SUFE infection

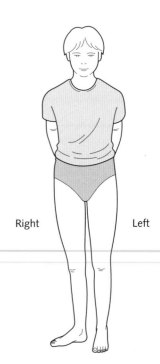

Fig. 7.2 External rotation deformity: a child with externally rotated right leg in slipped upper femoral epiphysis.

Associated symptoms

History of injury may be elicited in occult trauma but in non-accidental injury this will not be forthcoming.

A recent history of upper respiratory tract infection or otitis media is often found in patients with transient synovitis.

Multiple joint aches and pains suggest juvenile arthritis. In JIA the eyes can be involved as part of the systemic effects of the disease. If left untreated blindness can result (see Ch. 17).

Past medical history

Any previous history of Perthes disease or SUFE is very important as these patients are at increased risk of developing disease in the opposite hip.

Family history

A family history of Perthes disease, DDH and SUFE also leads to an increased risk.

EXAMINING A CHILD WITH A LIMP

Systemic features of illhealth such as pyrexia, drowsiness and irritability should be noted and will point towards infection as the cause.

Multiple joint problems may be obvious initially, suggesting JIA.

Neuromuscular disorders may be obvious or detected on neurological examination.

Inspection

Gait

- An antalgic gait is present in painful conditions.
- A Trendelenburg gait (see Ch. 2) is present in a toddler with late DDH or some neuromuscular conditions.
- Neuromuscular disorders give a variety of patterns of gait abnormality.
- A worrying sign is a child too ill or in too much pain to weight-bear.

Standing

- An abnormal single large posterior skin crease is present in DDH.
- In SUFE or infection, the hip is often held in an abnormal position of external rotation and flexion (Fig. 7.2).

Further inspection could reveal scars, swelling or erythema.

Fixed flexion

If the Thomas test is positive (a fixed flexion deformity), suspect significant pathology such as advanced Perthes, DDH or SUFE.

Limb length discrepancy

- A short leg is typical of DDH.
- Apparent shortening will be present if there is any fixed flexion deformity.

Palpation

Palpate any tender areas for effusion, warmth and localized pain.

The hip joint cannot be palpated directly because it is a deep joint; it is important to palpate the groin and greater trochanter for tenderness.

Palpation around the knee will reveal joint line tenderness in conditions such as osteochondritis or, in older children, meniscal tears.

Tenderness over the tibial tubercle is likely to be due to Osgood–Schlatter disease.

Movement

- Loss of hip movements indicates pathology.
- DDH results in loss of abduction compared with the other side.
- Perthes disease results in loss of abduction and flexion. Complete loss of abduction is a worrying sign in Perthes as this may indicate subluxation of the joint.
- In septic arthritis any movement gives extreme pain. A child will hold a joint rigid to avoid pain.

INVESTIGATING A CHILD WITH A LIMP

Blood tests

Markedly raised white cell count, erythrocyte sedimentation rate and C-reactive protein are present in infection but these inflammatory markers can also be mildly increased in transient synovitis or JIA.

Very rare causes of abnormal blood tests include leukaemia. Creatinine kinase is raised in muscular dystrophy.

X-rays

A plain X-ray is often unnecessary in the younger child, particularly in cases of transient synovitis.

A hip radiograph may show:

- Subluxation in the case of DDH.
- Perthes disease.
- SUFE.
- Evidence of infection (remember, X-rays are initially normal).
- A fracture.

HINTS AND TIPS

If a SUFE is suspected, request a frog lateral X-ray.

If you are sure the problem is from the knee then anteroposterior and lateral knee X-rays should be performed and may show:

- Osgood–Schlatter disease.
- Osteochondritis dissecans.
- A fracture.

Ultrasound

Ultrasound is a very useful investigation for suspected joint problems, particularly of the hip, which is deeply situated.

The scan will show an effusion in:

- Septic arthritis.
- Transient synovitis.
- Perthes disease (early).

Isotope bone scanning

If hot, this is likely to be significant and possible causes are:

- Osteomyelitis – the scan will also show any seeding of infection.
- Malignancy.

Magnetic resonance imaging (MRI)

MRI is not a first-line investigation in children. It is difficult for a young child to stay still for the scan. MRI is useful in:

- Diagnosis of knee disorders (see Ch. 17).
- Bone and soft-tissue tumours.
- Osteomyelitis.

Objectives

After reading this chapter you should be able to:
- Give a list of differential diagnoses for a limb swelling.
- Take a focused history from a patient with a limb swelling.
- Examine and describe a limb swelling.
- Know how to investigate a limb swelling.
- Recognize sinister features of a limb swelling.

DIFFERENTIAL DIAGNOSIS

It is helpful to consider differential diagnoses in relation to the anatomical location:

- Skin or subcutaneous:
  - Rheumatoid nodule.
  - Lipoma.
  - Bursitis.
  - Neurofibroma.
  - Cyst.
  - Ganglion.
- Joint:
  - Joint effusion.
  - Ganglion.
  - Baker cyst.
- Bone:
  - Osteophytes.
  - Bone tumour.
- Muscle/deep soft tissues:
  - Sarcoma.

Patients commonly present with lumps, bumps and swellings. The majority of these are benign, but it is important not to overlook very rare tumours presenting in this way.

HISTORY FOCUSING ON A SWELLING

The following points are important.

Duration of symptoms

How long has the patient had the lump or swelling, and when did the patient first notice the lump?

Increase in size

Has it grown rapidly, or recently incresed in size? Tumours may present in this way.

Solitary or multiple

Does the patient have more than one lump or swelling and if so, where? Neurofibromata or rheumatoid nodules are often multiple. Multiple lipomas may represent a hereditary lipomatosis.

Variability

Does the swelling come and go and if so, over what period? Classically a ganglion will disappear and then recur. A joint effusion will be larger during an exacerbation of the underyling joint disease.

Is it painful?

The majority of lesions are not painful. A tense effusion will be painful, as may bursitis. Deep pain related to a bony or soft-tissue mass may be sinister. Also pain worse at night is a symptom suspicious of malignancy.

Loss of function

Does the swelling or lump inhibit the patient in any way? Swellings around the hand can be a nuisance to patients and those on the foot can rub when shoes are worn.

Associated symptoms

Usually there will be none.

The general health of the patient should be ascertained, with weight loss, fatigue, night sweats and poor health being sinister symptoms.

Very occasionally large swellings or masses can compress vessels or nerves, e.g. in the case of malignant lesions.

Patients presenting with joint swelling may have other symptoms related to the underlying disease process, such as pain in the joint if arthritic.

A patient may have painless joint swelling as a presenting feature of a more generalized inflammatory condition. It is important therefore to ask about other joints such as those in the hand.

A patient with a Baker cyst may have pain in the knee.

Occupational history

Patients who kneel frequently, such as carpet fitters, are very prone to developing prepatellar bursitis.

COMMUNICATION

Patients will often think that their swelling is a cancer. Ask them if they are worried about it and once you are sure it is nothing to worry about (as the vast majority are) then tell them! Often patients don't mind having a small lump such as a lipoma or ganglion and just need reassurance.

EXAMINATION FOCUSING ON A SWELLING

The affected area or joint should be examined and also the local lymph nodes.

The following points relate to a swelling or mass rather than a joint effusion, which should be obvious on clinical examination.

When examining a lump or swelling the following points should be elicited.

Site

Which limb is affected and where is the lesion?

Size

Sinister pathology should be suspected in any lump larger than 5 cm.

Depth of lesion

- Is the lesion within the skin, in the subcutaneous tissue or deep to the fascia? Painful deep lesions are suspicious and need investigation.
- Is the skin normal over the lesion, inflamed or abnormal?

Consistency

Is the lesion soft, firm or hard? A lipoma is often described as firm.

Diffuse or discrete

Some swellings are large without clear margins and appear to merge with the surrounding structures, whereas others are more easily palpable.

Surface

Is the surface of the lesion smooth or irregular?

Mobile or fixed

A discrete mass may be fixed to the underlying structures, like a ganglion, or more mobile, e.g. a lipoma.

Fluctuance

Fluctuant lesions contain fluid, such as a Baker cyst.

Pulsatile

Pulsatile and expansile lesions are vascular aneurysms.

Transillumination

Fluid-filled or soft lesions (e.g. lipoma) will transilluminate when tested with a pen torch if the fluid is clear.

The patient presenting with joint swelling only

Occasionally a patient will present with swelling of a single large joint and this can be the onset of a generalized condition such as rheumatoid arthritis.

Therefore it is important to examine other joints, such as the hand (if rheumatoid arthritis is suspected) or the spine (if ankylosing spondylitis is suspected).

INVESTIGATION OF A PATIENT WITH A SWELLING

We will consider joint swelling as a separate condition from a discrete swelling or mass.

Joint swelling (effusion)

Exclude infection (see Ch. 20).

Blood tests should be carried out; including inflammatory markers and urate, as well as rheumatoid factor and autoantibodies to look for inflammatory arthritis.

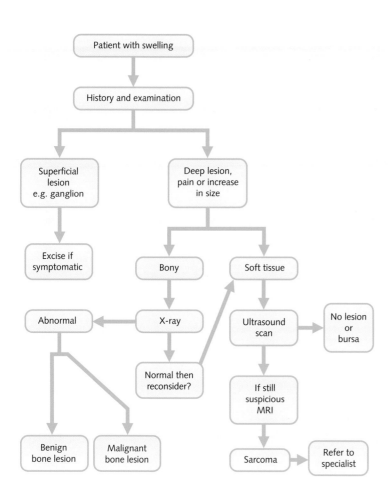

Fig. 8.1 Algorithm for the investigation of a limb swelling. MRI, magnetic resonance imaging.

X-rays may show osteoarthritis or rheumatoid arthritis or be normal.

Synovial fluid microscopy is performed looking for crystals indicating gout and pseudogout.

A limb swelling or lump

Further investigation may be unnecessary.

For example, a patient has a cystic lesion on the volar aspect of the wrist, which comes and goes and is fixed to deep structures. The lesion is firm and smooth and transilluminates. This patient probably has a ganglion and this can be confirmed by aspirating jelly-like fluid, or proceeding directly to surgical excision:

Further investigation is necessary if there is doubt about a diagnosis.

- If bony pathology is suspected an X-ray of the affected limb should be performed. A benign or malignant bony lesion may be found.
- A deeply situated soft-tissue lesion may be a sarcoma and if so, needs urgent further investigation.
- An initial ultrasound scan may be useful to confirm the presence of a mass and whether it is fluid-filled or solid.
- However, a magnetic resonance imaging scan with contrast gives detail regarding the exact nature of the lesion.
- If doubt still exists, the patient should be referred to a specialist musculoskeletal oncology service and the next step would be a biopsy.
- An algorithm for the investigation of a limb swelling is given in Figure 8.1.

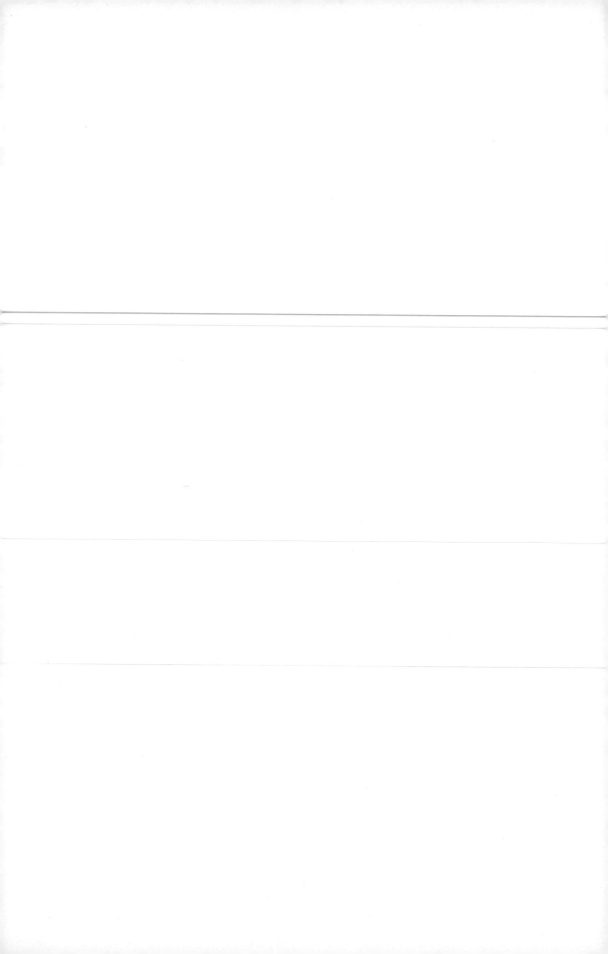

Back pain 9

Objectives

After reading this chapter you should be able to:
- Discuss the likely causes of back pain.
- Give a differential diagnosis for back pain.
- Know 'red flag' signs associated with sinister causes of back pain and how to investigate them.
- Outline the presentation and treatment of musculoskeletal back pain.
- Know how and when to investigate back pain.
- Recognize the difference between spinal stenosis and a prolapsed intervertebral disc.
- Know the difference between spinal claudication and vascular claudication.
- Define spondylolysis and spondylolisthesis.
- Outline the diagnosis and treatment of discitis and vertebral osteomyelitis.

Back pain, or leg pain secondary to pathology in the spine, is extremely common. In fact, as many as 80% of the population will have an episode of back pain in their life. The patient may present with back pain, leg pain or both, and it is important to take a detailed history and perform a detailed examination to try and elicit the casue of the patient's symptoms. There are many pitfalls when assessing a patient with back pain. This may be due to the terms patients use to describe their symptoms: one patient may tell you his sciatica is playing up or another that her slipped disc has 'popped out again'. Another problem is that pain patients attribute to their back may be coming from somewhere else – the hip or sacro-iliac joints, for example.

DIFFERENTIAL DIAGNOSIS

- Mechanical low back pain.
- Osteoarthritis of the spine.
- Prolapsed intervertebral disc.
- Vertebral crush fracture.
- Spinal stenosis/spondylolisthesis.
- Malignancy.
- Infection.
- Discitis.
- Vertebral osteomyelitis.
- Hip causes:
  - Osteoarthritis.
  - Avascular necrosis:
- Abdominal causes.
  - Pancreatitis.
  - Dissecting aortic aneurysm.
  - Renal disease.

Back pain in isolation

Acute low back pain without radiation into the leg suggests simple low back pain, particularly if the patient gives a history of lifting or straining and the pain is worse on movement and activity (so-called 'mechanical pain'). The pain is usually described as a band across the back and may be extremely severe.

Figure 4.2 shows 'red flag' signs that should alert the clinician to the possibility of serious spinal pathology.

EXAMINATION FOCUSING ON BACK AND LEG PAIN

General examination

Look at the patient: weight loss, anaemia and general ill health may suggest malignancy. Look at the posture and gait:

- A stooped posture with flexion of the knee suggests sciatica.
- A frail old woman with a stooped posture may have osteoporotic fractures.
- A very stiff spine may be simple low back pain or ankylosing spondylitis.
- Fixed flexion of the hip with an antalgic or Trendelenburg gait is likely to be hip pathology. There may be a limb-length discrepancy.
- Look for deformity of the spine, previous scars, wasting and any lower-limb deformity.

Perform the Trendelenburg and Thomas tests as described in Chapter 2. These are tests aimed at examining the hip and, if positive, suggest hip pathology.

Palpation

- With the patient standing, palpate the spine centrally and surrounding muscles for tenderness. In simple low back pain, often the area around the posterior superior iliac spine and sacroiliac joint is tender.

Movement

- Assess movements of the spine. Diminished movement is likely if pathology is present. It may be impossible for the patient to comply because of pain.

Special tests

Straight-leg raising will be diminished with a positive sciatic stretch test (Lasegue test) if the nerve root is irritated by a prolapsed disc or spinal stenosis.

A peripheral nervous system examination may show weakness and sensory loss in a single nerve root pattern.

A digital rectal examination is mandatory in all patients with suspected cauda equina syndrome.

INVESTIGATION OF A PATIENT WITH BACK PAIN

Blood tests

These are not always necessary but should be performed to exclude sinister causes in patients over 55 years of age or as guided by clinical suspicion. Full blood count may reveal:

- Raised white cell count if infection is present, such as in discitis.
- Anaemia in malignancy.

Biochemistry is required only to exclude abdominal causes and help confirm cases of malignancy:

- Erythrocyte sedimentation rate (ESR) and C-reactive protein (CRP) are elevated in infection and malignancy. Immunoglobulins and Bence Jones protein should be checked to exclude myeloma.
- Patients presenting with metastatic disease and an unknown primary need thorough investigation. Biopsy specimens may be taken at surgery.

Plain X-ray

Plain X-rays of spine should not be taken routinely except after trauma. This may show:

- Normal appearances in simple low back pain, prolapsed disc and even in malignancy or infection if early in the disease process (it is therefore not a useful test).
- Osteoarthritic changes in the spine.
- A spondylolisthesis.

- Destruction of the vertebral body, classically the pedicle (winking-owl sign) (see Fig. 4.3), indicating malignancy.
- Fracture.
- Erosion of vertebral body around the disc due to infection.

Further special tests may be needed if there is doubt about the diagnosis or to plan surgery:

- Isotope bone scanning: hot spot in infection and malignancy.
- Computed tomography (CT) scanning: for looking at bony structures in detail, e.g. spondylolisthesis.
- Magnetic resonance imaging (MRI): useful for looking at soft-tissue structures, including identification of disc prolapse and nerve root prior to surgery; and early detection of malignancy and infection.

Algorithms for the diagnosis and investigation of back and leg pain and for the investigation of sinister back pain are provided in Figures 9.1 and 9.2.

MECHANICAL LOW BACK PAIN

Back pain is extremely common and causes a significant burden on the resources of westernized societies in terms of lost working days.

Definition

Musculoskeletal back pain is not a single specific disease entity but rather a collection of ill-defined conditions presenting with low back pain. This diagnosis should only be made after other pathological conditions have been excluded.

Incidence

Eighty per cent of the population will have back pain at some stage in their lives.

Aetiology and pathology

As back pain is so common it is difficult to define clear aetiological factors for its occurrence.

It is known, however, that patients with chronic back pain are more likely to smoke, have a medicolegal claim pending and be over 30 at presentation.

There is much controversy about the exact pathology. One problem is that a lot of the pathological changes seen will also be present in the healthy 'normal' population with no symptoms.

Implicated structures are listed in Figure 9.3:

- Facet joint arthritis shows the typical features of osteoarthritis with joint space destruction and osteophyte formation.

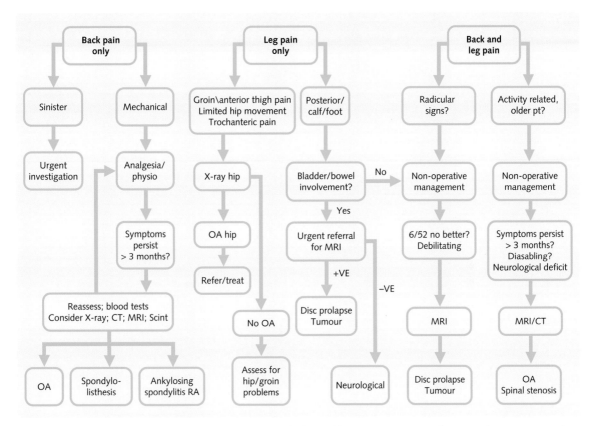

Fig. 9.1 Algorithm for the diagnosis and investigation of back, hip and leg pain. CT, computed tomography; MRI, magnetic resonance imaging; OA, osteoarthritis; RA, rheumatoid arthritis.

- Degenerative disc disease occurs with ageing and is related to decreased water content in the nucleus pulposus. The disc space narrows and the segment is said to become more mobile. It is this abnormal movement, together with an inability to distribute load, that causes pain.

An interesting point is that patients rarely present after the age of 60 and as the patient enters old age usually the symptoms subside. This is said to be due to stiffening of a mobile spine.

Clinical features

There are two typical clinical scenarios: acute back pain over days or weeks, and chronic unrelenting back pain for many years.

Acute back pain over days or weeks

Pain is usually solely located to the back, possibly following a precipitating incident. Pain is severe and the patient may have difficulty getting into a comfortable position. Sometimes the patient has pain referred down the back of the leg but this differs from true radicular pain in that back pain is still the predominant feature and the pain does not typically radiate beyond the knee. The pain is mechanical (i.e. worse on movement).

Clinical examination will show muscle spasm with loss of lumbar lordosis. The patient may find it difficult to walk and spinal movements will be minimal.

Sciatic stretch testing and peripheral nerve examination will be negative.

Chronic unrelenting back pain for many years

The patient will be unable to work, and may be overweight and depressed. Often the patient has seen numerous doctors, physiotherapists and other allied health workers, including alternative medical practitioners.

The back pain is usually unrelenting and does not have any relieving factors. Leg pain may or may not be present.

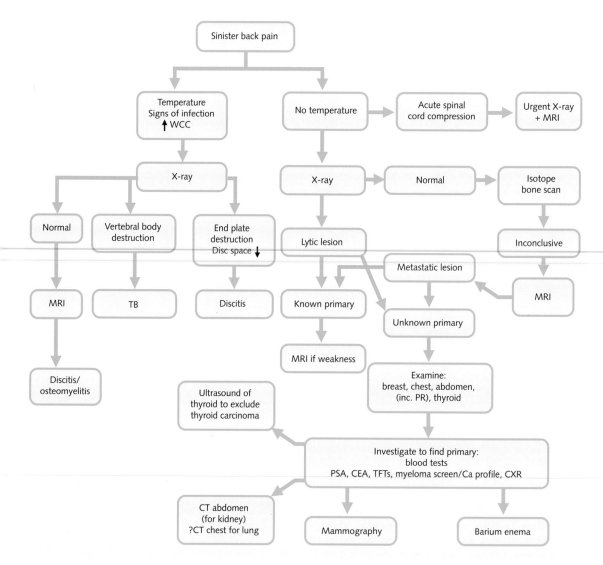

Fig. 9.2 Algorithm for the investigation of sinister back pain. Ca, calcium; CEA, carcinoembryonic antigen; CT, computed tomography; CXR, chest X-ray; MRI, magnetic resonance imaging; PR, per rectum; PSA, prostate-specific antigen; TB, tuberculosis; TFTs, thyroid function tests; WCC, white cell count.

Fig. 9.3 Possible causes of musculoskeletal back pain
Bone/periosteum
Paraspinous muscles spasm/sprain
Facet joint arthritis
Disc/degenerative disc disease
Posterior longitudinal ligament

Clinical examination rarely shows any significant features other than reduced movements. Inappropriate signs (Waddell signs) may be present:

- Superfical tenderness and tenderness not in keeping with the anatomy in question.
- Regional pain not conforming to known neuroanatomy.
- Pain on movements not affecting the lower back, e.g. axial loading and simulated rotation.
- Lack of pain after distraction, e.g. patients being unable to straight-leg raise, but able to sit on the examination couch with legs straight and hips flexed to 90°.
- Overreaction to pain. This is very subjective and should be used with caution.

Diagnosis and investigation

The majority of patients with a short history (less than 6 weeks) and mechanical symptoms need no further investigation.

Prolonged symptoms need investigation to exclude sinister causes of back pain.

Blood tests including full blood count, ESR, liver function tests, calcium/phosphate/alkaline phosphatase, myeloma screen, and CRP should all be normal in mechanical back pain.

X-rays may show:

- Normal appearances.
- Minor disc narrowing.
- Osteoarthritis (Fig. 9.4).

MRI and CT scanning are rarely helpful and may be misleading if they highlight an abnormality that may not be significant.

Treatment

Conservative

Analgesia, non-steroidal anti-inflammatory drugs (NSAIDs) and physiotherapy are used for acute low back pain. Bed rest should be avoided.

Patients with chronic pain are very difficult to treat and need a multidisciplinary approach to try to break

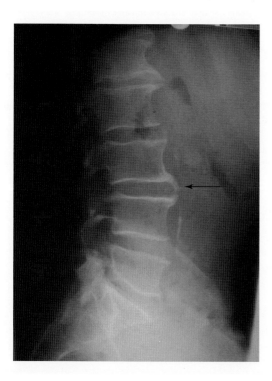

Fig. 9.4 Osteoarthritis of the spine (arrow).

the pain cycle. Psychological input may be required, as may the pain management team. Occasionally facet joint injections for localized disease can relieve symptoms.

Surgical

In the vast majority of patients surgery has no role in the management of mechanical back pain, and the patient must be informed of this. In very few selected patients, some surgeons will advocate surgery in degenerative disc disease, but this is the exception rather than the rule.

Prognosis

Most acute back pain episodes settle spontaneously and the patient returns to normal. Once chronic, the condition becomes extremely difficult to treat.

PROLAPSED INTERVERTEBRAL DISC

Definition

A disc prolapse occurs when part of the nucleus pulposus herniates through the annulus fibrosus and presses on a spinal nerve root.

Incidence

Disc prolapse is common – up to 3% of men and 1% of women will suffer with sciatica related to a prolapsed intervertebral disc. Usual presentation is between 35 and 55 years of age.

Aetiology and pathology

There is good evidence that manual workers involved in heavy lifting have increased incidence of disc prolapse. Regular automobile use is also said to be a risk factor.

The herniation of disc material tends to occur posterolaterally where the annulus is thinner. Central disc prolapse can occur and press on the combined nerve roots, including those supplying the bladder and bowel (cauda equina syndrome). Prolapse can occur without spinal root involvement, in which case the patient will have symptoms of back pain but not true sciatica.

Disc prolapse most commonly occurs at L4–L5 or L5–S1 level but can occur at any level (including cervical and rarely thoracic). The nerve root crosses its space before exiting the spine beneath the pedicle (L4–L5 disc presses on L5 nerve root). See Figure 9.5.

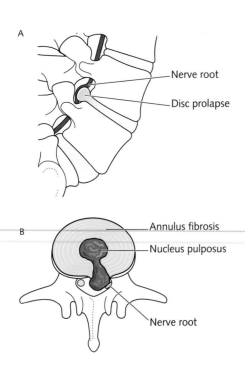

Nerve root

Disc prolapse

Annulus fibrosis

Nucleus pulposus

Nerve root

Fig. 9.5 (A and B) Prolapsed intervertebral disc.

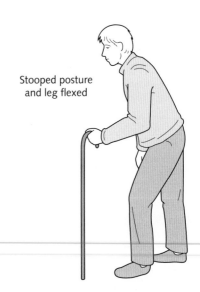

Stooped posture
and leg flexed

Fig. 9.6 Posture in prolapsed intervertebral disc.

Clinical features

Sciatica is a symptom of lower lumbar or sacral nerve root irritation. The patient complains of severe pain radiating down the leg as far as the toes. There may be numbness and tingling or weakness of the foot. Patients find it very uncomfortable to sit, and either stand or lie down. Coughing and sneezing worsen the pain.

In cauda equina syndrome there is bladder and bowel dysfunction with possibly urinary retention and saddle anaesthesia. This is due to compression of the nerves within the cauda equina which supply motor function to the bowel and bladder sphincters, and sensation to the perineum.

HINTS AND TIPS

Bilateral leg symptoms are suggestive of impending cauda equina.

Clinically a patient will have an abnormal posture, stooping to the affected side and standing with the knee flexed to relieve pressure on the dura (Fig. 9.6).

Nerve root tension signs such as straight-leg raising will be positive.

The crossover sign may be positive (elevation of the opposite or normal leg gives pain shooting down the affected leg).

Numbness in a dermatomal distribution and weakness with loss of reflexes may be present.

In cauda equina there is loss of anal tone and reduced perianal sensation on digital rectalexamination.

Check for any sinister features (see Fig. 4.2).

Diagnosis and investigation

In older patients blood tests, described above, should be performed to exclude any sinister causes.

X-rays are usually normal and are performed to exclude bony pathology such as spondylolisthesis.

MRI scanning is now the investigion of choice in patients with persistent symptoms (Fig. 9.7).

Treatment

Conservative

A short period of bed rest followed by gentle physiotherapy with adequate analgesia (including NSAIDs) is the initial treatment for most discs.

Surgical

The only indications for urgent surgical discectomy are cauda equina syndrome and progressively worsening neurological deficit.

If patients have prolonged irretractable back pain (>9 months) then surgery is considered.

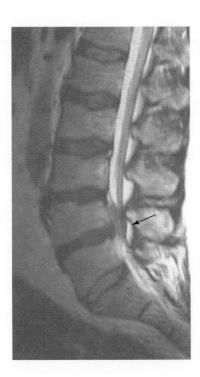

Fig. 9.7 Magnetic resonance imaging scan of prolapsed intervertebral disc at L4–L5 level (arrow).

Prognosis

Seventy per cent of acute disc prolapses settle spontaneously with conservative treatment. It is important to let your patient know acute disc prolapses are usually a self-limiting condition.

SPONDYLOLISTHESIS

Definition

This means slipping of one vertebral body on another.

COMMUNICATION

It is easy to get confused with the terminology. A *spondylolysis* is a defect in the pars interarticularis which may allow the vertebra to slip forward, causing a *spondylolisthesis* (forward slippage of one vertebra on another).

Incidence

The condition is common (approximately 5% of the population) but most are asymptomatic. It is more common in Caucasian males.

Aetiology and pathology

Certain sports predispose to spondylolysis (gymnasts and fast bowlers in cricket). Spondylolisthesis can be caused by spondylolysis and numerous other pathologies.

The slip usually occurs at the L5–S1 level. The degree of slip is normally assessed as a percentage (0–25%, 25–50%, 50–75% or >75%) and graded 1–4. There can be an associated kyphosis or scoliosis.

Clinical features

This condition is the most common cause of persistent back pain in children.

Initially back pain is the sole presentation but if the slip becomes severe then nerve root irritation will occur, causing sciatica. Radicular symptoms are more common in the adult patient.

There is tenderness over the spine but sometimes well-preserved movements (except in the arthritic type of spondylolisthesis); classically hyperextension is painful.

Diagnosis and investigation

Oblique X-rays may show the classic 'collar on Scottie dog' appearance of spondyloysis (Fig. 9.8), and the lateral X-ray will show the degree and angle of slippage (Fig. 9.9).

CT scans clearly demonstrate the lesion.

MRI should be performed if nerve root irritation is suspected.

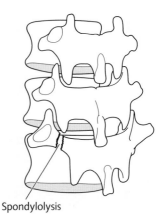

Spondylolysis

Fig. 9.8 Classic 'Scottie dog' appearance of spondylolisthesis.

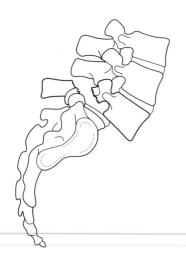

Fig. 9.9 An L5–S1 spondylolisthesis with a pars defect.

Treatment

Conservative

Initial rest and restriction of activities may allow a spondylolysis to heal before a slip occurs.

In adult patients a trial of conservative treatment is advised with physiotherapy, analgesia and activity modification.

Surgical

Persistent pain, radiculopathy and significant deformity are indications for surgery.

Fusion with or without metalwork and bone graft is commonly performed.

Prognosis

The outcome is variable, depending on the type and degree of slip.

SPINAL STENOSIS

Definition

Spinal stenosis is caused by degenerative changes narrowing the spinal canal and causing compression of the nerve roots.

Incidence

This is a common disorder, mainly affecting men over 50 years of age.

Aetiology and pathology

Spinal stenosis is more common in heavy manual labourers.

It is usually secondary to degenerative changes. Thickening of ligaments, osteophytes and posterior disc bulge encroach into the spinal canal (Fig. 9.10).

It is thought that ischaemia of the spinal nerves during exercise produces the classic symptoms.

Clinical features

Typically patients present with discomfort when walking, with pain referred to the buttock, calves and feet. Back pain is usually present. Pain is worse on extension and relieved by rest and flexion of the spine.

Examination will reveal stiffening of the spine but sciatic stretch testing may be normal.

It is important to examine the peripheral vascular system in such patients as vascular claudication presents in a similar way.

Diagnosis and investigation

X-rays will usually show degenerative changes.

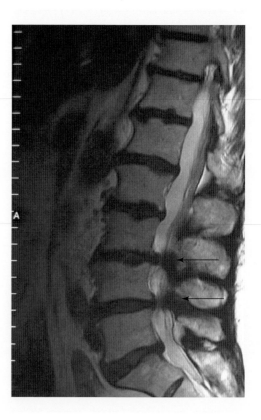

Fig. 9.10 Magnetic resonance imaging scan of spinal stenosis (arrows).

MRI shows the degree of stenosis and nerve root involvement.

If suspected, exclude peripheral vascular insufficiency with Doppler scans.

Treatment

Conservative

Weight loss, physiotherapy, activity modification and NSAIDs may relieve symptoms enough to avoid surgery.

Surgical

Severe symptoms not responding to conservative measures require surgical decompression.

Prognosis

The condition tends to be progressive.

DISCITIS/VERTEBRAL OSTEOMYELITIS

Definition

Discitis is infection of the disc space, and vertebral osteomyelitis is infection of a vertebral body.

Incidence

They are becoming more common, although still rare. Presentation can be at any age.

Aetiology and pathology

Conditions associated with other bone and joint infection (see Ch. 20), particularly intravenous drug use and immunocompromised patients, predispose to spinal infection. Patients with recent sepsis from pneumonia or urinary tract infection can subsequently develop discitis by seeding of infection. It can occur following surgery to the disc.

Common infecting organisms are staphylococci and streptococci in adults, and staphylococci and *Haemophilus* in children. Tuberculosis should also be considered.

Clinical features

Patients are unwell with a pyrexia and complain of severe, unrelenting back pain.

Clinical examination may reveal a swelling and, in severe cases, an angular scoliosis or kyphosis (gibbus). There is pain on palpation, reduced movement and possible abnormal neurology.

Discitis commonly presents late: patients often have 6–12 weeks of symptoms before the correct diagnosis is made.

Diagnosis and investigation

The white cell count, ESR and CRP are elevated.

X-rays show narrowed disc space (discitis) and bony destruction (osteomyelitis) (Fig. 9.11).

An isotope bone scan will be hot in the affected area.

MRI scanning should be performed to detect any epidural abscess.

CT-guided biopsy should be obtained for culture and sensitivity.

Treatment

Conservative

Intravenous antibiotics are given for 6 weeks, with a prolonged course of oral antibiotics if required.

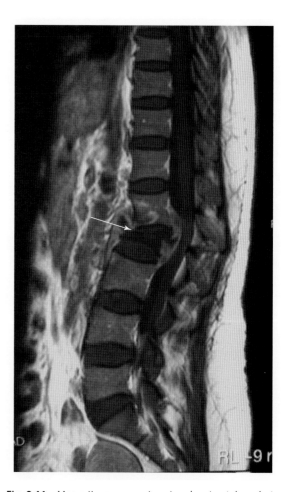

Fig. 9.11 Magnetic resonance imaging showing tuberculosis of the spine. There is complete collapse of the vertebra (arrowed) with resultant kyphosis.

Surgical

Any abscess should be drained and an unstable spine with significant deformity needs stabilization.

Prognosis

Prognosis is variable: childhood cases respond well and should return to normality; severe adult infections can be life-threatening and surgery carries significant risk.

SCOLIOSIS

Definition

This is a lateral deviation and rotational abnormality of the spine.

Incidence

Up to 2.5% of the population are affected by idiopathic scoliosis.

Aetiology and pathology

Causes of scoliosis are listed in Figure 9.12. Curves are thoracolumbar (Fig. 9.13).

Clinical features

Pain is not usually a feature; rather the patient or relatives complain of deformity, in the form of an asymmetrical rib hump, spinal curve and limb length inequality. For clinical examination, the rib hump is more prominent on forward flexion (Fig. 9.14).

Very severe deformity reduces chest expansion, which can be life-threatening.

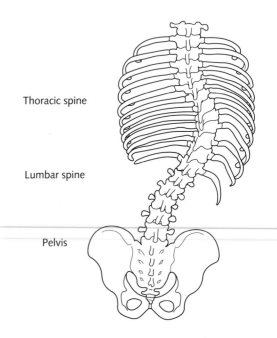

Fig. 9.13 Thoracolumbar curve in scoliosis.

Fig. 9.12	Causes of scoliosis	
Type	**Pathology**	**Example**
Congenital	Abnormal development of spine	Hemivertebra
Idiopathic	Unknown	Adolescent idiopathic scoliosis
Neuromuscular	Abnormal muscle forces acting on the spine	Cerebral palsy
Secondary	Curve develops secondary to another process	Leg length discrepancy

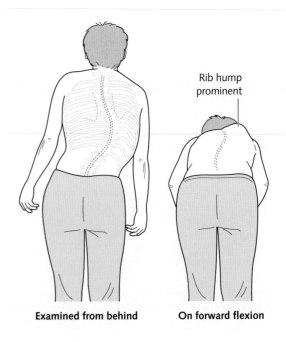

Fig. 9.14 Examination of a patient with scoliosis.

Diagnosis and investigation

Standing X-rays show the curve, and serial films are important to monitor the progress of the curve.

A significant increase in the severity of the curve is often an indication for surgical stabilization.

MRI scans are performed to exclude any associated spinal cord abnormality.

Treatment

Conservative

The treatment depends on the angle of the curve measured on the X-rays. In idiopathic scoliosis the initial treatment is bracing for mild to moderate curves.

Surgical

All congenital, most neuromuscular and severe or progressive idiopathic curves will require surgical stabilization, fusion and correction.

Prognosis

The majority of curves are minor and require little treatment.

Very severe neuromuscular curves can lead to death due to cardiorespiratory compromise.

Further reading

Orthoteers website: http://www.orthoteers.co.uk.

Solomon, L., Warwick, D., Nayagan, D. (Eds.), 2001. Apley's System of Orthopaedics and Fractures, eighth ed. Hodder Arnold, London.

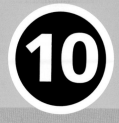
After reading this chapter you should be able to:
* Recognize patterns of neurological pain from the history and examination.
* Give a differential diagnosis for neurological symptoms affecting the upper and lower limbs.
* Know common investigations used to investigate neurological conditions.
* Be aware of the conditions that predispose to carpal tunnel syndrome (CTS).
* Recognize the symptoms and signs of CTS.
* Understand the clinical consequences of damage to the ulnar, radial and common peroneal nerves.

Neurological symptoms occur when there is injury to a nerve. This may be due to chronic compression or an acute injury. Patients may complain of numbness, pins and needles, electric shock-type pain, burning, hypersensitivity, dysaesthesia and weakness. The pattern of these symptoms will help diagnose which nerve is causing the problem.

DIFFERENTIAL DIAGNOSIS

* Peripheral nerve lesions:
    * CTS.
    * Ulnar nerve entrapment.
    * Tarsal tunnel syndrome.
* Spinal pathology:
    * Disc prolapse.
    * Spinal stenosis.
    * Osteoarthritis.
    * Cervical rib.
    * Malignancy.
* Morton neuroma.
* Nerve tumours, e.g. neurofibroma, schwannoma.
* Medical causes, e.g. multiple sclerosis.
* Postsurgery, e.g. superficial radial nerve neuroma.
* Peripheral neuropathy, e.g. alcoholism, diabetes mellitus, drugs, vitamin B_{12} deficiency.
* Complex regional pain syndrome (see Ch. 4).

HISTORY

The following points should be covered.

Site

Global or specific?
Very important in determining which nerve is affected (see examination section, below).

Onset of symptoms

* Acute onset usually occurs with disc prolapse, where pain may be the main feature.
* With gradual onset there is a gradual increase in nerve compression, e.g. spinal stenosis, CTS.
* Onset of symptoms may occur after trauma, e.g. CTS after distal radius fracture.
* Accidental laceration to a nerve during surgery can result in paraesthesia in the distribution of the affected nerve, or a painful neuroma.

Nature of symptoms

Exacerbating features

Sneezing and coughing often exacerbate symptoms of leg pain with disc prolapse.

Relieving features

* Patients with CTS often get night pain which is relieved by hanging their hand down off the bed.
* Patients with lumbar spinal stenosis suffer pain, and numbness in their legs after walking short distances (spinal claudication), which is relieved by bending forward.

Associated features

* Loss of bowel or bladder function in patients with back pain should be treated as cauda equina syndrome until proven otherwise (see Ch. 9).
* Check for constitutional features such as weight loss, malaise or haemoptysis (lung cancer) if malignancy is suspected. Pancoast tumour (an apical lung carcinoma) can present with upper-limb neurological symptoms.

- Patients with undiagnosed diabetes mellitus may have weight loss, polyuria and polydipsia associated with peripheral neuropathy.

Past medical history

The following can predispose to nerve lesions:

- Malignancy.
- Previous surgery.
- Trauma.
- Osteoarthritis and rheumatoid arthritis.
- Systemic lupus erythematosus.

A list of causes specific to CTS can be seen below.

Drug history

Some chemotherapy agents can cause peripheral neuropathy.

Social history

Manual jobs may trigger ulnar or carpal tunnel symptoms. A history of alcohol use may be relevant.

Family history

For example, a family history of neurofibromatosis (von Recklinghausen's disease).

Examination

Knowledge of myotomes and dermatomes will help determine the level of a spinal cord lesion. For peripheral nerve lesions, know the sensory distribution and motor function. Some special tests may reproduce nerve symptoms such as tapping a nerve (Tinel test). Café-au-lait spots are characteristic of neurofibromatosis.

COMMUNICATION

Patients with severe CTS will often be having sleepless nights. They look tired, unhappy and even depressed. It is important not to underestimate the effect this has and take this into consideration when planning treatment. Simple splints may allow them a good night's sleep.

Investigation

Plain radiographs of the spine will show osteophytes causing nerve root compression, or the presence of a cervical rib. Magnetic resonance imaging (MRI) provides very detailed soft-tissue images and is commonly used to investigate spinal pathology such as a disc prolapse. Ultrasound or MRI can diagnose a Morton neuroma.

Nerve conduction studies are used routinely to confirm CTS and can be used to diagnose other peripheral nerve lesions. Blood tests may demonstrate the cause of a peripheral neuropathy – e.g. fasting glucose, thyroid function tests, haematinics.

CARPAL TUNNEL SYNDROME

Definition

CTS results from compression of the median nerve as it passes through the carpal tunnel at the wrist. The carpal tunnel is formed by the space between the transverse carpal ligament and the carpal bones.

Incidence

CTS is common, especially in middle-aged and elderly women.

Aetiology

CTS is usually idiopathic, but can be associated with several underlying conditions (Fig. 10.1).

Clinical features

CTS presents with pain and/or paraesthesia in the median nerve distribution (Fig. 10.2). These symptoms can radiate proximally towards the elbow. They are often worse at night and classically wake the patient from sleep.

Examination may reveal sensory loss in the median nerve distribution, but can be unremarkable. The strength of the thenar muscles should be tested. These may be weak and wasted in advanced disease. The opponens pollicis muscle is tested by asking the patient to touch the thumb to the little finger and resist attempts to separate the two. Phalen and Tinel tests may reproduce the symptoms (Fig. 10.3).

Fig. 10.1 Conditions predisposing to carpal tunnel syndrome
Diabetes mellitus
Hypothyroidism
Rheumatoid arthritis
Pregnancy
Acromegaly
Trauma, e.g. wrist fractures

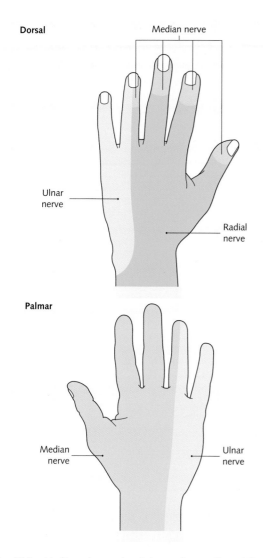

Dorsal

Median nerve

Ulnar nerve

Radial nerve

Palmar

Median nerve

Ulnar nerve

Fig. 10.2 Median, ulnar and radial nerve innervation of the hand.

Investigations

Nerve conduction studies show reduced nerve conduction velocities across the wrist. Investigations such as serum glucose and thyroid function tests should be performed to exclude underlying medical conditions.

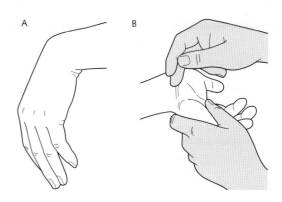

A   B

Fig. 10.3 Provocation tests for carpal tunnel syndrome may reproduce the patient's symptoms. (A) Phalen test: the wrist is held in maximal palmar flexion. (B) Tinel test: tap over the median nerve proximal to the transverse carpal ligament in the wrist.

Management

The most successful treatment is surgical decompression of the carpal tunnel by division of the transverse carpal ligament. This is a very effective procedure and can be performed under local anaesthetic. In less severe cases wrist splints may help nocturnal symptoms, and corticosteroid injection of the carpal tunnel may bring some relief.

ULNAR NERVE ENTRAPMENT

Definition

The ulnar nerve can become compressed as it passes behind the medial epicondyle or through Guyon's canal in the wrist.

Incidence

Ulnar nerve damage at the elbow is fairly common due to its superficial position.

Aetiology

Ulnar nerve entrapment may be idiopathic or due to a precipitating cause (Fig. 10.4).

Fig. 10.4 Precipitating factors for ulnar nerve entrapment
Local trauma, e.g. fractures of the elbow
Prolonged leaning on the elbow
Elbow synovitis

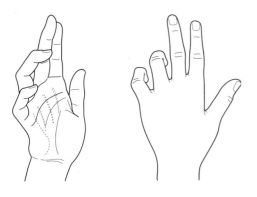

Fig. 10.5 Clawing of the hand due to ulnar nerve palsy.

Clinical features

Patients develop pain and/or paraesthesiae in the medial side of the elbow, which radiates to the medial forearm and the ulnar nerve distribution in the hand (see Fig. 10.2). The pain is often exacerbated by elbow flexion.

Examination usually reveals reduced sensation in the ulnar nerve distribution. Palpation of the nerve behind the medial epicondyle may provoke the symptoms. Motor dysfunction may result in atrophy of the hypothenar eminence. Abduction and adduction of the fingers are weak. There may be clawing of the hand due to weakness of the intrinsic muscles (Fig. 10.5).

Investigations

Nerve conduction studies confirm the diagnosis and establish the site of compression.

Management

Ulnar nerve compression due to elbow synovitis may respond to corticosteroid injection of the elbow. Surgical decompression should be performed if sensory symptoms cannot be tolerated or if there is muscle weakness or wasting.

RADIAL NERVE INJURIES

Aetiology

Radial nerve compression at the axilla is typically seen in a drunk person who falls asleep with an arm hanging over the back of a chair ('Saturday night palsy'). The radial nerve may also be injured by fractures of the humeral shaft.

Clinical features

The wrist extensors are paralysed, resulting in wrist drop. Grip strength is dramatically reduced, as the finger flexors do not function well with the wrist in a flexed position. Nerve injury in the axilla will also lead to paralysis of the triceps. Due to nerve overlap, sensory loss only affects a small area of skin on the dorsum of the hand between the first and second metacarpals.

Management

The wrist should be splinted immediately and the cause of the radial nerve palsy should be assessed. If there is no resolution, tendon transfer or nerve grafting may be indicated.

COMMON PERONEAL NERVE INJURIES

Aetiology

The common peroneal nerve winds around the neck of the fibula and is in a vulnerable position. It may be damaged by fractures of the neck of fibula or pressure from a tight bandage or plaster cast.

Clinical features

Common peroneal nerve injury results in paralysis of the ankle and foot extensors. Unopposed action of the foot flexors and inverters cause the foot to be plantar flexed and inverted. This is referred to as 'foot drop'. Patients develop a high-stepping gait, flicking the foot forwards to avoid tripping over it. There is also loss of sensibility over the anterior and lateral sides of the leg and the dorsum of the foot and toes.

Management

Pressure on the nerve should be relieved and a splint should be applied. If the foot drop does not resolve, an ankle–foot orthosis can be used to maintain some degree of dorsiflexion.

Further reading

Nashel, D.J., 2003. Entrapment neuropathies and compartment syndromes. In: Hochberg, M.C., Silman, A.J., Smolen, J.S., et al. (Eds.), Rheumatology, third ed. Mosby, London, pp. 713–724.

After reading this chapter you should be able to:
• Define and outline the pathological processes in the development of osteoarthritis (OA).
• List the causes of secondary OA.
• Describe the clinical features of OA.
• Describe the X-ray features of OA.
• Understand the basic medical and surgical treatments for OA.

DEFINITION

OA is a disorder of synovial joints characterized by articular surface degeneration, formation of new bone (attempts at repair) and secondary inflammation. It is also known as degenerative joint disease and characterized by joint pain, stiffness, swelling and deformity.

INCIDENCE

OA is the most common joint disease, with incidence and prevalence increasing with age. It affects over 80% of the population at some time in their lives. It is often asymptomatic and the true prevalence of symptomatic OA in the Western world is around 20%.

PATHOLOGY AND AETIOLOGY

Histologically, repeated microtrauma or abnormal biomechanical forces damage the weight-bearing cartilage surface which eventually wears away completely, exposing the subchondral bone (Fig. 11.1). Chondrocytes attempt repair by releasing degradative enzymes. Cysts occur because of microfracture of the articular surface and new bone is laid down (sclerosis). Disorganized new bone is produced at the margins of joints (osteophytes) and the synovial lining becomes thickened and inflamed, often producing excess synovial fluid (an effusion).

HINTS AND TIPS

These changes explain the four cardinal features seen on X-ray: joint space narrowing, sclerosis, cysts and osteophytes.

OA is described as primary where no single underlying cause is found. Risk factors are shown in Figure 11.2. Secondary OA occurs when there is a clear predisposing factor, such as trauma, congenital, developmental and metabolic diseases.

CLINICAL FEATURES

The presenting complaints of patients with OA are variable. The patient is usually systemically well and complains of burning or aching pain, localized to the joint but may be referred distally.

The history is often of gradual, asymmetric joint pain over several years, of variable severity. The pain is worse after activity and relieved by rest, and as the disease progresses night pain can be a feature. Occasionally patients present with rapidly destructive OA, which can mimic a septic or inflammatory arthritis.

HINTS AND TIPS

Classically pain in the hip can be referred to the knee.

Patients can present with single or multiple joint involvement.

Other symptoms include swelling, deformity, stiffness and weakness (usually secondary to muscle wasting). Certain recreational activities or more basic activities of daily living may be difficult (for example, patients with severe OA of the hip are unable to put on socks or cut their own toenails).

Almost any synovial joint can be affected by OA, most commonly the knee, hip, hands (often the

Early changes

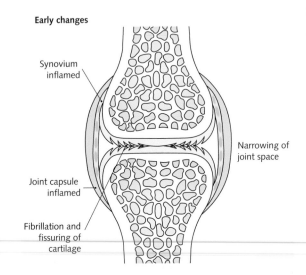

Synovium inflamed

Narrowing of joint space

Joint capsule inflamed

Fibrillation and fissuring of cartilage

Changes secondary to loss of cartilage

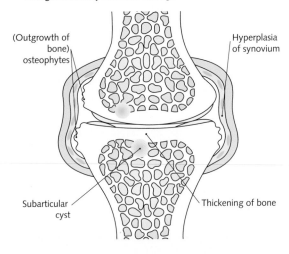

(Outgrowth of bone) osteophytes

Hyperplasia of synovium

Subarticular cyst

Thickening of bone

Fig. 11.1 Pathological changes in osteoarthritis.

Fig. 11.2 Risk factors for osteoarthritis
Obesity
Age
Female gender
Occupation
Muscle weakness
Lack of osteoporosis
Acromegaly
Calcium crystal deposition disease

first carpometacarpal joint), fingers (distal interphalangeal, proximal interphalangeal (DIP, PIP) joints) but also the spine, shoulder, elbow and wrist (Figs 11.3 and 11.4).

The examination begins as the patient enters the room:

- Look for a limp, use of a stick and how reliant the patient is on relatives for simple tasks such as undressing for examination.

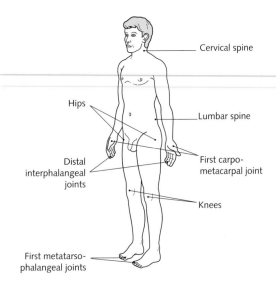

Cervical spine

Hips

Lumbar spine

Distal interphalangeal joints

First carpo-metacarpal joint

Knees

First metatarso-phalangeal joints

Fig. 11.3 Joints commonly affected by osteoarthritis.

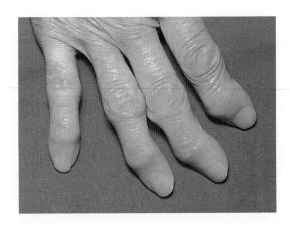

Fig. 11.4 Osteoarthritis of the hand, showing Herberden's nodes at the distal interphalangeal joints and Bouchard's nodes at the proximal interphalangeal joints. (Reproduced from Colledge NR, Walker BR, Ralston SH (eds) (2010) Davidson's Principles and Practice of Medicine, 21st edn. Edinburgh: Churchill Livingstone, with permission.)

- Deformity may be obvious but also note previous scars, redness, swelling and wasting of muscles on inspection.
- Palpate for an effusion, joint line tenderness and crepitus (crunching noise) when moving the joint.
- The joint range of movement may be diminished with fixed deformity.
- The joints above and below should be examined.

DIAGNOSIS AND INVESTIGATION

In many cases the diagnosis is clear from the history and clinical examination, and apart from a plain X-ray, further investigation may be unnecessary.

Blood tests and joint aspiration may be required to exclude septic or inflammatory arthritis in atypical cases if the treating doctor is not certain of the diagnosis.

X-rays will usually show decreased joint space, sclerosis, subchondral cysts and osteophytes (Fig. 11.5).

MANAGEMENT

There is no cure for OA and treatment is aimed at relieving pain and maintaining function. The treatment for OA is medical or surgical.

COMMUNICATION

A detailed social history is very important in patients who have OA. Ask about occupation, activities of daily living and hobbies. What is the patient's normal mobility? These types of question help to assess patients' quality of life and how their condition affects them.

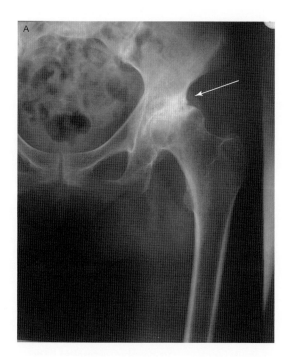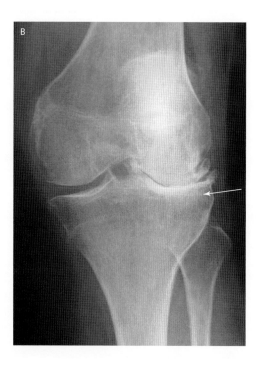

Fig. 11.5   Features of osteoarthritis on X-ray. (A) Hip joint showing sclerosis, joint space narrowing, cysts and osteophytes. (B) Knee OA affecting the lateral compartment of the femoro-tibial joint.

Fig. 11.6 Treatment of OA. COX-2, cyclooxygenase-2; NSAIDs, non-steroidal anti-inflammatory drugs; TENS, transcutaneous electrical nerve stimulation. (Reproduced from National Collaborating Centre for Chronic Conditions (2008) CG 59. Osteoarthritis: National Clinical Guideline for Care and Management in Adults. London: Royal College of Physicians, with permission).

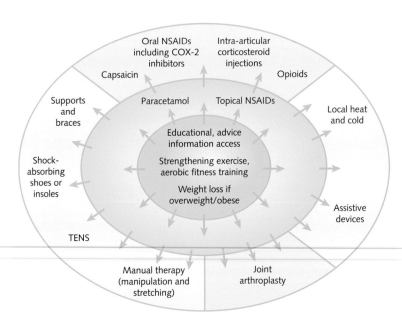

Medical

- Initially lifestyle advice, including weight loss, regular exercise and avoidance of impact loading activities, is given. Topical or oral non-steroidal anti-inflammatory drugs such as naproxen are good in the early stages, provided the patient does not have a history of peptic ulceration. Other regular analgesia such as codeine and paracetamol should be prescribed if required.
- Physiotherapy improves gait and function of an affected limb. Simple measures such as a walking stick reduce pain when mobilizing. Shoe insoles help with abnormal weight loading.
- Glucosamine is often tried, but clinical trials have shown only very marginal benefit.
- Injections of corticosteroids or hyaluronic acid derivatives are useful for temporary relief, especially in patients unfit for surgery.

The National Institute for Health and Clinical Excellence (NICE) has published guidelines on the care and management of OA in adults (Fig. 11.6).

Surgical

Surgical treatments for OA depend on age, the joint involved, level of pain and disability experienced. This is dealt with in more detail in Chapter 21.

The decision to operate can be difficult, as all surgery has risks and complications.

COMMUNICATION

Arthroplasty surgery is not risk-free and patients should be told that, although the pain should improve, the joint will never function like a normal joint. Surgery can also have serious complications, including infection and thromboembolism, which, in a small percentage of patients, may be fatal. This must be explained during the consent process.

There are generally four things a surgeon can do to a joint:

1. Joint replacement (arthroplasty). This is most commonly of the hip or knee. It gives excellent pain relief in 90% of patients for at least 10 years.
2. Joint fusion. The two sides are removed and fused together. This is most commonly used around the foot and ankle; good pain relief is achieved provided fusion occurs but obviously movement is lost.
3. Joint excision. This is less commonly used nowadays. It is still used occasionally in the first metatarsophalangeal joint and where other methods have failed (e.g. hip – Girdlestone procedure).
4. Realignment surgery. Increased load passing through a joint because of a deformity often leads to OA. The surgeon can realign the limb by cutting the bone above or below the joint, removing a wedge of bone and correcting the deformity. The most

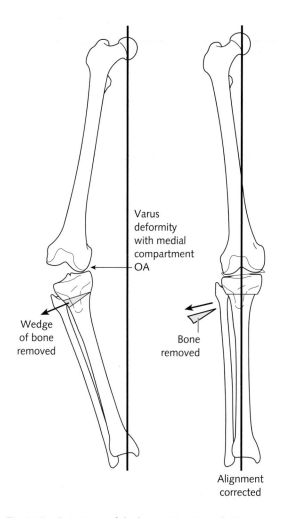

Varus deformity with medial compartment OA

Wedge of bone removed

Bone removed

Alignment corrected

Fig. 11.7 Osteotomy of the knee. OA, osteoarthritis.

common site for this procedure is the knee. The patient will usually have a varus deformity of the knee (bow legs). The tibia is realigned to redistribute the load more evenly, slowing the progression of OA (Fig. 11.7).

Further reading

da Silva, J.A.P., Woolf, A.D., 2010. Rheumatology in Practice. Springer, Philadelphia.

http://www.arthritisresearchuk.org/health-professionals-and-students/reports/reports-archives.aspx.

Miller, M.D., 2012. Review of Orthopaedics, sixth ed. Saunders.

NICE, 2008. CG 59 Osteoarthritis: NICE Guideline. Available online at: http://guidance.nice.org.uk/CG59/NICEGuidance/pdf/English.

Solomon, L., Warwick, D., Nayagan, D. (Eds.), 2010. Apley's System of Orthopaedics and Fractures, ninth ed. Hodder Arnold.

Rheumatoid arthritis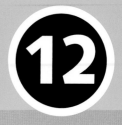

● **Objectives**

After reading this chapter you should be able to:
- Understand the role that leukocytes and cytokines play in the pathogenesis of rheumatoid arthritis (RA).
- Describe the usual distribution of joint inflammation in RA.
- Recognize the common hand deformities caused by RA.
- Understand that RA causes systemic symptoms.
- List the causes of anaemia in RA.
- Describe the four main radiological signs of RA.
- Recognize the importance of the multidisciplinary team in the care of patients with RA.
- Name some disease-modifying antirheumatic drugs (DMARDs) used in the treatment of RA.

DEFINITION

RA is a common inflammatory condition. It is characterized by a symmetrical polyarticular arthritis, usually involving the hands, follows a chronic course and can result in significant disability. RA is a multisystem disease, associated with a reduction in life expectancy.

> **HINTS AND TIPS**
>
> RA has a major impact on patients' lives. After 20 years, 80% of patients have some disability. Life expectancy is reduced by between 3 and 18 years.

INCIDENCE AND PREVALENCE

RA affects females more commonly than males. Most studies show a female-to-male excess of between two and four times. The annual incidence in the UK is 0.1–0.2/1000 in males and 0.2–0.4/1000 in females. RA prevalence in Europeans and North American Caucasians is close to 1%.

AETIOLOGY

The aetiology of RA has not been explained. It appears to be multifactorial, with both genetic and environmental factors having an important influence.

GENETIC FACTORS

Increasingly genes are being identified which predispose to RA development, with those in human leukocyte antigen (HLA) region HLA DR4 (DRβ0404 and 0401) identified as particularly important.

ENVIRONMENTAL FACTORS

Environmental influences on the development of RA are not well understood. The effects of various infections, occupations and lifestyle factors have been examined but no causal links have been found. However, there is an increased risk of RA development in smokers, who also tend to have more aggressive disease.

IMMUNOLOGICAL ABNORMALITIES

In RA, the immunological mechanisms that usually protect the body by fighting infections and destroying malignant cells target normal tissue, resulting in joint damage. T lymphocytes play a key role in the initiation of inflammation in RA (Fig. 12.1), with B cells and activated macrophages also having important roles.

A

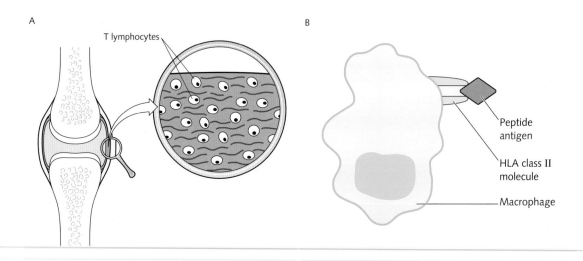

T lymphocytes

B

Peptide antigen

HLA class II molecule

Macrophage

C

Activated macrophage

Activated T lymphocyte

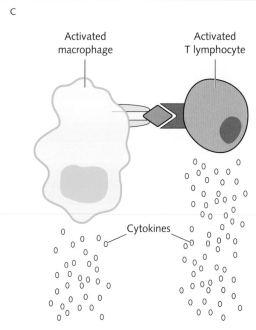

Cytokines

Fig. 12.1 (A) T lymphocytes (predominantly T-helper cells) accumulate in the synovium. (B) Synovial macrophages (antigen-presenting cells) express peptide antigens on their cell surfaces in association with human lymphocyte antigen (HLA) class II molecules. (C) T lymphocytes with appropriate receptors interact with the macrophages and both cell types become activated.

The activated cells produce cytokines (intercellular messenger proteins), e.g. tumour necrosis factor-α (TNF-α) and interleukin-1 (IL-1). These cytokines have many actions, including those shown in Figure 12.2.

Rheumatoid factor and anticitrullinated protein antibodies are produced by activated B cells in the synovium. They are found in approximately 80% of patients with RA. High levels are associated with more severe disease and the presence of extra-articular features.

PATHOLOGY

The main pathological abnormality in RA is synovitis. As inflammatory cells infiltrate the synovium, it proliferates. Macrophages and osteoclasts create chronically inflamed tissue (pannus) which extends from the joint margins and erodes the articular cartilage (Fig. 12.3). Extensive erosion of cartilage and bone leads to joint

Fig. 12.2	Actions of cytokines
Stimulation of inflammation	
Attraction of other immune cells	
Excess synovial fluid production	
Cartilage destruction	
Bone resorption	
Stimulation of B-lymphocyte differentiation and maturation	
Increased antibody production, including production of rheumatoid factor	

The clinical features of RA can be divided into:

- Articular features.
- Extra-articular features.

ARTICULAR FEATURES OF RA

The usual presenting symptoms of RA are joint pain, stiffness and swelling. Stiffness is usually noticed on waking in the morning and tends to improve as the day progresses. The duration of this early-morning stiffness is a useful marker of disease activity. RA predominantly targets small and medium joints in a symmetrical fashion (Fig. 12.4), but sometimes other patterns of joint involvement are seen.

Pain and stiffness lead to varying degrees of functional loss. Even in the early stages of the disease, patients can struggle with everyday tasks such as dressing and turning on taps because of active synovitis. In established RA, joint destruction results in further limitations.

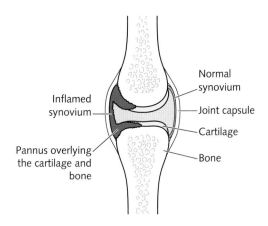

Fig. 12.3 Diagram of a synovial joint. One side is healthy; the other shows the pathological changes of rheumatoid arthritis.

deformity. Ligament insertions (entheses) are a common site of inflammation and the thickened joint capsule distends due to effusion.

CLINICAL FEATURES

RA can develop at any time of life from infancy to old age. The peak age of onset is in the fourth and fifth decades. Symptoms usually begin gradually, developing over weeks or months. However, some people experience an acute onset. Still others may initially develop a monoarthritis, or palindromic RA where temporary, flitting symptoms affect different joints.

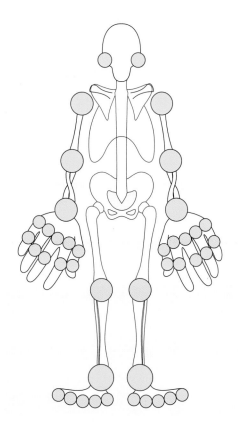

Fig. 12.4 The joints most commonly affected by rheumatoid arthritis.

Synovitis causes 'boggy' joint swelling. The skin overlying an affected joint is usually warm and red due to increased local blood flow. On palpation, the swelling is tender and has a similar consistency to that of a grape.

The effects of RA on specific joint regions

It is hoped that many of the 'classic' deformities are becoming historical because more effective therapies are being introduced earlier. Today's doctor needs to identify RA prior to deformity and refer urgently for treatment within 6 weeks of symptom onset.

The rheumatoid hand and wrist

The hands and wrists are almost always involved in RA (Fig. 12.5). Synovitis typically occurs in the wrists, metacarpophalangeal (MCP) and proximal interphalangeal (PIP) joints, sparing the distal interphalangeal (DIP) joints. This inflammation can weaken the ligaments and tendons, producing well-recognized deformities.

Ulnar deviation of the fingers results from MCP joint synovitis (Fig. 12.6). Subluxation of the MCP joints can occur, with the proximal phalanges drifting in an ulnar and volar (palmar surface) direction.

Boutonnière and swan-neck deformities of the digits are due to PIP joint synovitis and laxity and/or contractures of the extensor and flexor apparatus (Fig. 12.7). The boutonnière deformity is characterized by PIP flexion and DIP hyperextension. With swan-neck deformity there is MCP flexion, PIP hyperextension and DIP flexion.

Radial deviation of the wrist occurs partly to compensate for ulnar deviation of the fingers. Subluxation of the wrist results in prominence of the ulnar styloid.

The foot

Forefoot synovitis and damage are common in RA. The proximal phalanges sublux dorsally and the metatarsal heads become eroded and displaced towards the floor. They can be easily palpated through the sole of the foot and make weight bearing very uncomfortable. Patients

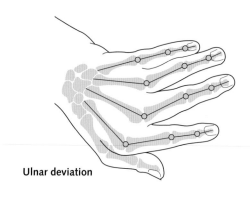

Ulnar deviation

Fig. 12.6 Ulnar deviation.

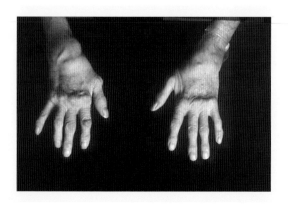

Fig. 12.5 The hands of a patient with rheumatoid arthritis. Note the swelling of the wrists, metacarpophalangeal and proximal interphalangeal joints due to synovitis.

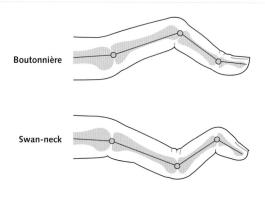

Boutonnière

Swan-neck

Fig. 12.7 Boutonnière and swan-neck deformities.

often feel as though they are 'walking on marbles'. Hindfoot involvement can also cause problems, with subtalar arthritis. Patients with established disease develop valgus deformities here. All these deformities result from poorly controlled synovitis. The rheumatologist's aim is to suppress synovitis, restricting damage and reducing disability using immunosuppressive drugs.

The cervical spine

Inflammation and erosive disease, affecting the first cervical vertebra and stabilizing ligaments of the first two cervical vertebrae, can result in atlantoaxial subluxation. The atlas slips forward on the axis, reducing the space around the spinal cord (Fig. 12.8). This produces neck pain that radiates to the occiput. Upper motor neuron damage resulting in a spastic quadriparesis is a rare complication. Damage to the articulation between the occiput and atlas may allow the odontoid peg to move upwards, through the foramen magnum. This can threaten the cervical cord and brainstem, sometimes resulting in sudden death after minor jolts to the head and neck. Subaxial subluxation can also occur (below the first cervical vertebra).

HINTS AND TIPS

It is important to take lateral flexion X-rays or magnetic resonance imaging (MRI) of the cervical spine in RA patients requiring a general anaesthetic. The anaesthetist must be aware of any cervical instability so that precautions can be taken during intubation.

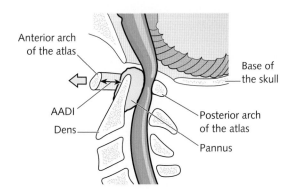

Fig. 12.8 In normal adults, the distance between the anterior arch of the atlas and the dens (anterior atlantodental interspace, or AADI) should not exceed 3 mm. The diagram shows forward subluxation of the atlas on the axis. The spinal cord is compressed between pannus around the dens and the posterior arch of the atlas.

EXTRA-ARTICULAR FEATURES OF RA

Rheumatoid nodules

Rheumatoid nodules are firm subcutaneous swellings found in up to 20% of patients. They tend to develop in areas affected by pressure or friction, such as the fingers, elbows and Achilles tendon. They are seen in patients who test positive for rheumatoid factor and are commoner in smokers. Nodules at any site can be complicated by infection. They usually accompany severe disease and are possibly due to small-vessel vasculitis. Histology reveals a central area of fibrinoid necrosis surrounded by fibroblasts.

Tenosynovitis and bursitis

Tendon sheaths and bursae are lined with synovium. This can become inflamed in RA, resulting in tenosynovitis and bursitis. The flexor tendons of the fingers are often affected by tenosynovitis, which can result in tendon rupture. The olecranon and subacromial bursae are common sites of bursitis.

Carpal tunnel syndrome

Synovitis can cause entrapment of peripheral nerves. Median nerve compression resulting in carpal tunnel syndrome is common (see Ch. 10).

SYSTEMIC FEATURES OF RA

As well as causing joint pain and swelling, active RA makes people feel generally unwell. The inflammation can result in systemic symptoms such as fever, weight loss and lethargy. These can be prominent, particularly in people with acute-onset RA, in whom infection and malignancy are important differential diagnoses.

COMMUNICATION

When patients with RA first present, they may have felt fatigued for several months. They find it reassuring to hear that systemic symptoms are common and may improve when the joint inflammation is treated.

THE EFFECTS OF RA ON DISTANT ORGANS

RA can affect many body systems (Fig. 12.9). Extra-articular disease can be serious and is associated with an increase in mortality.

Fig. 12.9 Extra-articular manifestations of rheumatoid arthritis.

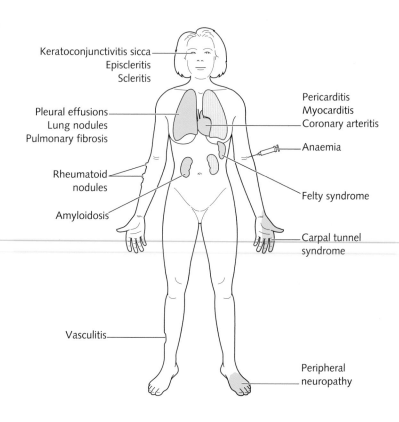

Keratoconjunctivitis sicca
Episcleritis
Scleritis

Pericarditis
Myocarditis
Coronary arteritis

Pleural effusions
Lung nodules
Pulmonary fibrosis

Anaemia

Rheumatoid nodules

Felty syndrome

Amyloidosis

Carpal tunnel syndrome

Vasculitis

Peripheral neuropathy

Anaemia

Anaemia of RA can be due to:

- Anaemia of chronic disease.
- Autoimmune haemolysis.
- Felty syndrome.
- Non-steroidal anti-inflammatory drugs (NSAIDs) can cause iron deficiency as a result of chronic blood loss from gastrointestinal inflammation.
- DMARDs sometimes produce anaemia via bone marrow suppression.

Felty syndrome

Felty syndrome is the association of RA with splenomegaly and leukopenia. It usually occurs in patients who are rheumatoid factor-positive. The leukopenia leads to bacterial infections. Lymphadenopathy, anaemia and thrombocytopenia can also occur.

Rheumatoid lung disease

Although pulmonary disease is common in RA, it does not always produce symptoms. Males are more frequently affected than females.

Pleural effusions can occur early in the disease, sometimes preceding the arthritis. Rheumatoid factor can be detected in the fluid, which is a transudate. Lung nodules are found in patients who are seropositive and usually have subcutaneous nodules. They rarely cause symptoms, but can cavitate or become infected. Pneumonitis can lead to pulmonary fibrosis, and may occur rarely with any DMARD but most frequently with methotrexate.

Additional systemic problems are highlighted in Figure 12.9.

INVESTIGATIONS

Blood tests

Full blood count may show anaemia of chronic disease, thrombocytosis secondary to inflammation or leukopenia of Felty syndrome.

Erythrocyte sedimentation rate and C-reactive protein are usually raised in the presence of synovitis and they are useful markers of response to treatment.

Rheumatoid factor is found in the serum of 70–90% of RA patients. Those patients who lack the antibodies are sometimes described as having 'seronegative rheumatoid arthritis'. It is important to remember that rheumatoid factor is also found in at least 5% of the normal population, and in higher percentages in the elderly. Patients with positive rheumatoid factor are more likely to have systemic involvement and have a worse prognosis.

Another serological test is now available to help with the diagnosis of RA. Anticyclic citrullinated peptide antibodies can be present in patients who are rheumatoid factor-negative and are felt to indicate a worse prognosis. They are not associated with systemic features, but have a higher specificity for RA.

RADIOLOGICAL INVESTIGATIONS

Plain X-rays should be obtained to look for radiological evidence of RA (Fig. 12.10). These tend to be seen first in the small joints of the hands and feet (Fig. 12.11).

Radiological changes are often not apparent when patients first present with RA. In patients with normal X-rays, but persistent symptoms, musculoskeletal ultrasound has a role in early detection of erosions and synovitis. MRI can also help where the diagnosis is in doubt, but is time-consuming and expensive (Fig. 12.12).

MANAGEMENT

Patients with RA should be cared for by a multidisciplinary team. Figure 12.13 lists the professionals involved in the care of RA patients and gives details of the roles they play.

Figure 21.9 (p. 157) lists operations which might be required where joint damage is extensive. It is anticipated that, as medical therapy improves, the requirement for surgery will lessen.

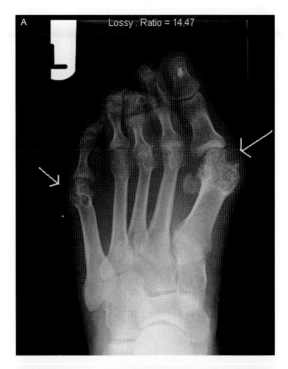
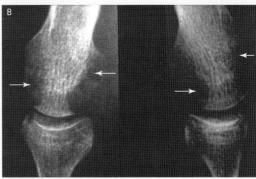

Fig. 12.11 (A) Periarticular osteopenia and erosions of the metatarsophalangeal (MTP) joints. (B) Large erosions of two metacarpophalangeal joints.

Fig. 12.10 The four main radiological signs of rheumatoid arthritis
Soft-tissue swelling
Periarticular osteoporosis
Juxta-articular erosions
Narrowing of joint space

DRUG TREATMENT

There are two main aims of drug treatment in RA:
1. Reduction of symptoms.
2. Prevention of damage by control of disease.

Non-steroidal anti-inflammatory drugs

NSAIDs can improve joint pain and stiffness, but have no effect on disease activity or progression. If a patient does not respond to one NSAID, it is worth trying another.

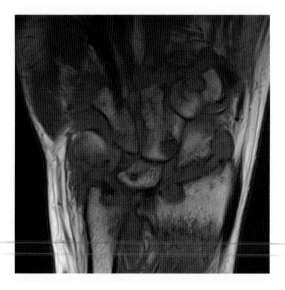

Fig. 12.12 Magnetic resonance imaging of erosions in rheumatoid arthritis.

Disease-modifying antirheumatic drugs

DMARDs suppress disease activity and slow progression of erosive joint damage. They are the mainstay of RA therapy and should be commenced by 6 weeks of disease onset. Some DMARDs suppress the immune system; others inhibit cell replication. However, for many of these drugs, the mechanism of action is not completely understood.

DMARDs are slow-acting and take several weeks to produce a clinical effect. If a patient does not respond adequately to one DMARD, a second can be added or substituted. In patients with poor prognostic markers, several DMARDS may be commenced at diagnosis.

Like many drugs, DMARDs can cause minor side-effects, including nausea, headache and rashes (Fig. 12.14). More serious complications, such as bone marrow suppression, abnormal liver function and renal impairment, are rarer, but well recognized. It is therefore important to monitor patients receiving DMARD

Fig. 12.14 Some disease-modifying drugs and their potential side-effects

DMARD	Possible side-effects
Methotrexate	Gastrointestinal upset Oral ulcers Raised liver enzymes Pneumonitis Bone marrow suppression
Sulfasalazine	Gastrointestinal upset Raised liver enzymes Bone marrow suppression
Hydroxychloroquine	Retinal damage
Leflunomide	Hypertension Gastrointestinal upset Bone marrow suppression
Gold	Rash Proteinuria Bone marrow suppression

DMARD, disease-modifying antirheumatic drug.

Fig. 12.13 Professionals involved in the care of rheumatoid arthritis patients and the roles they play

Professional	Role
Rheumatologist	Monitoring of disease activity. Prescription and monitoring of drug therapy. Identification and management of complications. Referral to other specialists when necessary. Coordination of team. Diagnosis.
Specialist nurse	Patient education. DMARD monitoring. Biologic administration and advice. Joint injections
Orthopaedic surgeon	Replacement of damaged joints. Surgical synovectomy. Tendon repairs
Physiotherapist	Use of physical therapies to combat inflammation. Prescription of exercises to maintain and improve muscular strength and range of joint movement
Occupational therapist	Splinting of acutely inflamed joints Advice on how to function whilst putting as little stress as possible on the joints (joint protection) Provision of aids and appliances to assist with activities of daily living
Podiatrist	Assessment of footwear and advice on choosing suitable shoes Provision of insoles to improve the mechanics of deformed feet Prevention and treatment of skin lesions, such as calluses and ulcers

DMARD, disease-modifying antirheumatic drug.

therapy. The monitoring protocol depends on the drug prescribed. For example, a patient taking methotrexate should have a full blood count and tests of liver and renal function performed at intervals of 4–8 weeks.

Corticosteroids

Corticosteroids can swiftly improve pain and swelling in RA. Low doses of oral prednisolone can be used to control symptoms early in the disease before DMARDs (see below) become effective. Corticosteroids can be given intra-articularly to treat local synovitis and are sometimes given via the intramuscular or intravenous route for a generalized flare of RA.

Biological therapies

Biological therapies that target inflammatory mediators in RA are now widely used. Five agents that are currently available inhibit TNF-α. Etanercept is a soluble TNF-α receptor, and infliximab, certolizumab, golimumab and adalimumab are monoclonal antibodies against TNF-α. These drugs produce excellent clinical results but are expensive and carry an increased risk of infection. The National Institute for Health and Clinical Excellence (NICE) has issued guidelines for their use in the UK. Disease activity scoring systems are employed for patient selection and to demonstrate good clinical response. There is some evidence to suggest that patients who do not respond, or have side effects with one anti-TNF agent, may respond if they are switched to another.

Other therapies licenced for use include rituximab, a monoclonal antibody against B cells which is used in the treatment of RA when one anti-TNF therapy has failed. Abatacept is a T-cell co-stimulation modulator, and tocilizumab blocks IL-6 to supress the acute-phase response of inflammation (Fig. 12.15).

Societal impact

A person's engagement with wider society is impacted by a diagnosis of RA. For example, at 3 years, 25% of RA patients are no longer in work. Personal loss of income, government loss of taxation income, drug costs, social care requirements and hospital admissions all contribute to the financial cost of the disease.

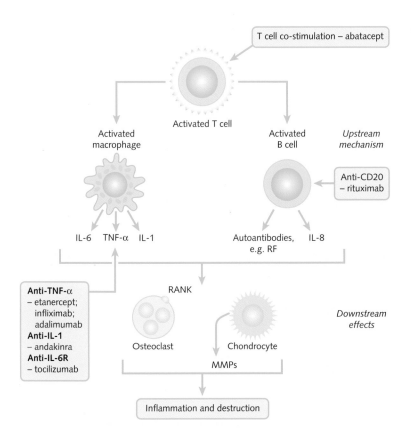

Fig. 12.15 Target sites of biologic therapies in rheumatoid arthritis.

Further reading

McInnes, I.B., Schett, G., 2011. The pathogenesis of rheumatoid arthritis. N. Engl. J. Med. 365, 2205–2219.

National Institute for Health and Clinical Excellence: CG79 Rheumatoid arthritis. Available online at: http://www.nice.org.uk/CG79.

National Rheumatoid Arthritis Society, www.nras.org.uk.

Scott, D.L., Wolfe, F., Huizinga, T.W., 2010. Rheumatoid arthritis. Lancet 376, 1094–1108.

SIGN, 2012. Mangagement of early rheumatoid arthritis. Available online at: http://www.sign.ac.uk/pdf/sign123.pdf.

Spondyloarthropathies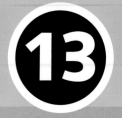

After reading this chapter you should be able to:
- Recognize the skeletal features of the spondyloarthropathies (SPAs).
- Understand how to differentiate between mechanical and inflammatory back pain on history.
- Understand treatments used for the SPAs.
- Recognize the different patterns of joint involvement in psoriatic arthritis.
- Understand the differences between reactive arthritis and septic arthritis.

Definition

The term 'spondyloarthropathy' describes a group of related and often overlapping inflammatory joint disorders (Fig. 13.1). SPA is characterized by enthesitis (inflammation at the insertion of a tendon, ligament or capsule into bone) as well as synovitis, and occurs in patients who are sero-negative for rheumatoid factor. For this reason, they are sometimes referred to as 'sero-negative spondyloarthropathy'.

Aetiology

All types of SPA are genetically associated with human leukocyte antigen (HLA) B27, a major histocompatibility complex class 1 antigen. HLA B27 is more closely linked with some SPAs than others (Fig. 13.1).

The true aetiology of the SPAs is unknown. Infection is thought to be important. It is possible that bacteria trigger an immune reaction in genetically predisposed people. For example, bacterial DNA and proteins have been detected in joints affected by reactive arthritis. The association with inflammatory bowel disease (IBD) may also be explained by an increase in the permeability of the gut to pathogens.

Pathology

The entheses are the key sites of inflammation in SPA. Initial inflammation and erosions are followed by fibrosis and ossification, which can result in ankylosis of joints. In ankylosing spondylitis (AS), the outer fibres of the vertebral discs become inflamed where they attach to the corners of the vertebral bodies. Squaring of the vertebrae occurs from loss of the anterior contour, a sequela of destructive osteitis and repair. Ossification leads to formation of syndesmophytes (bony bridges). The sacroiliac joints are commonly affected and may become fused. Synovitis is another feature of SPA. Peripheral joints tend to be more commonly involved in psoriatic and reactive arthritis than in enteropathic arthritis and AS.

Pathological changes are not always confined to the musculoskeletal system and are highlighted below.

ANKYLOSING SPONDYLITIS

Clinical features

The prevalence of AS amongst Caucasians is 0.5–1%. It is three times more common in men than in women and tends to be more severe in men. It usually develops in teenage years or early adulthood, with the peak age of onset being in the mid-20s. Presentation after the age of 45 years is rare.

Clinical features can be divided into two groups:

1. Musculoskeletal.
2. Extraskeletal.

Musculoskeletal features

Most symptoms in AS are due to spinal and sacroiliac disease. The typical patient presents with a gradual onset of lower back pain and stiffness. The time taken from first symptom until diagnosis remains unacceptably long and indeed can be many years. Early identification will allow for prompt treatment and prevention of functional loss, disability and deformity. Symptoms are worse early in the morning and after long periods of rest. They usually improve with exercise. Involvement of the thoracic spine and enthesitis at the costochondral junctions may cause chest pain. Disease of the costo-vertebral joints can reduce chest expansion and restrict breathing. Features of inflammatory back pain are shown in Figure 13.2.

Fig. 13.1 The spondyloarthropathies and human leukocyte antigen (HLA) B27. Normal HLA B27 prevalence in Caucasians is 10%

Ankylosing spondylitis	92%
Psoriatic arthropathy	60%
Reactive arthritis	60–80%
Enteropathic arthritis	60%
Undifferentiated spondyloarthropathy	25%

Fig. 13.2 Modified criteria of inflammatory back pain

Chronic back pain (>3 months), with onset of first symptoms before age 45 years:
• Morning stiffness for at least 30 minutes
• Improves with exercise, but not with rest
• Back pain awakens the patient during the second half of the night
• Alternating buttock pain

Inflammatory back pain is present if two of the above four items are fulfilled.

(After Rudwaleit M, van der Heijde D, Landewé R et al. (2006) Inflammatory back pain in ankylosing spondylitis: a reassessment of the clinical history for application as classification and diagnostic criteria. Arthritis and Rheumatism 54: 569–578.)

In the early stages of the disease, patients may have few clinical signs. In addition to Regional Examination of the Musculoskeletal System (REMS), the following examinations can be helpful:

• The sacroiliac joints are often tender and pain can be reproduced by applying physical stress to the joints. This can be achieved by applying pressure on the anterior superior iliac spines whilst the patient is lying supine (sacroiliac squeeze test).
• Mobility of the lumbar spine is reduced. The Schober test is used to assess forward flexion in this region of the spine (Fig. 13.3). With a pen, a mark is made on the skin at the lumbosacral joint, level with the dimples of Venus. A second mark is made 10 cm above. The patient bends forward with the legs straight and attempts to touch the floor. The distance between the two marks should increase by at least 5 cm.
• Lateral flexion of the lumbar spine (see Ch. 2) is even more sensitive at identifying AS.

Later in the disease process and in those with severe disease, the spine becomes progressively stiffer and posture deteriorates (Fig. 13.4). The normal lumbar lordosis is lost and the thoracic and cervical spines become increasingly kyphotic. The resulting stooped posture further

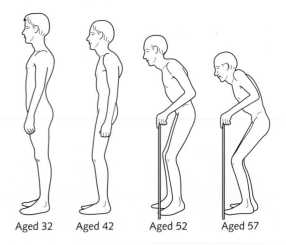

Aged 32   Aged 42   Aged 52   Aged 57

Fig. 13.4 Deterioration of posture in ankylosing spondylitis.

Fig. 13.3 The Schober test.

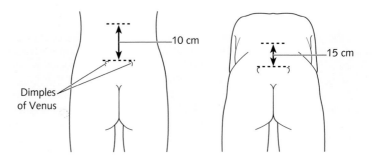

10 cm

15 cm

Dimples of Venus

restricts chest expansion and causes the abdomen to protrude. It is sometimes referred to as the 'question-mark posture'. Measurement of wall–tragus distance and chest expansion is helpful indicators of disease progression. Spinal disease can be complicated by atlantoaxial subluxation and fractures.

The peripheral joints are involved less commonly than the axial skeleton in AS. Inflammation tends to target medium and large joints such as the shoulders, hips or knees. Pain and tenderness due to enthesitis can occur at many sites. Achilles tendonitis and plantar fasciitis are common examples.

Extraskeletal features

Extraskeletal features are often referred to as the 'four As':

1. Acute anterior uveitis: acute anterior uveitis (also called iritis) occurs in approximately one-third of patients with AS. The eye becomes red and painful and vision is blurred. It requires urgent assessment by an ophthalmologist as blindness develops if left untreated. Steroid eye drops are the usual therapy.
2. Aortic incompetence/ascending aortitis.
3. Apical lung fibrosis.
4. Amyloidosis.

In addition, constitutional features such as anorexia, fever, weight loss and fatigue can occur.

> **COMMUNICATION**
>
> Patients suffering from any SPA should be warned of uveitis causing blindness and advised to seek medical help if they develop a painful red eye or visual change.

Investigations

Blood tests

- A full blood count may reveal anaemia of chronic disease.
- Erythrocyte sedimentation rate (ESR) and C-reactive protein (CRP) are often raised during active phases of the disease.
- Serological tests for rheumatoid factor are negative.
- Genotyping for HLA B27 is unnecessary for diagnosis, but useful where doubt remains.

Radiological investigations

The investigation of choice is magnetic resonance imaging (MRI). It is able to detect inflammatory back disease when X-rays may be normal in appearance. MRI also prevents X-ray exposure in the pelvis, which is particularly important in young adults. Sacroiliitis (Fig. 13.5 and

13.11) and bone oedema highlight ongoing inflammation, amenable to therapy. X-rays have a role in assessing established disease where substantial mechanical change has occurred. Views of the lumbar spine may show squaring of the vertebrae and formation of syndesmophytes (Fig. 13.6). These are due to ossification of the

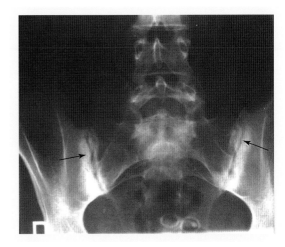

Fig. 13.5 Radiograph showing bilateral sacroiliitis (arrows).

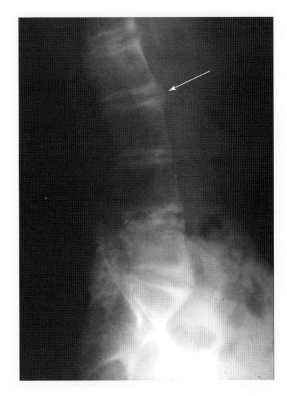

Fig. 13.6 Lateral radiograph showing syndesmophyte formation (arrow) in the lumbar spine of a patient with advanced ankylosing spondylitis.

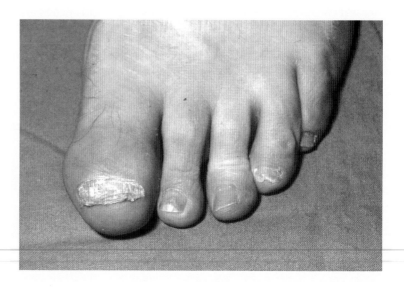

Fig. 13.7 Psoriatic nails with hyperkeratosis.

longitudinal ligaments and produce a bamboo appearance. Radiographs taken at other sites of enthesitis may show erosions, for example at the insertion of the plantar fascia or Achilles tendon.

Management

Patients with AS should be cared for by a multidisciplinary team (see Fig. 12.13).

Physiotherapy

This is an important element in the management of AS. Each patient should follow a long-term exercise programme with the aim of maintaining normal posture and physical activity. Hydrotherapy is also beneficial.

Drug treatment

Non-steroidal anti-inflammatory drugs (NSAIDs) are the mainstay of initial therapy and provide benefit for 70–80% of patients. Continuous therapy should occur in patients with evidence of ongoing inflammation. Both NSAID types cyclooxygenase-1 (Cox-1) and Cox-2 inhibitors have been shown to benefit patients and may even supress radiological progression.

Immunosuppressive drugs such as methotrexate and sulfasalazine that are used for rheumatoid arthritis are of less benefit in AS, except where a concomitant peripheral arthritis occurs.

The tumour necrosis factor (TNF) inhibitors however have excellent efficacy in treating active axial disease and preventing AS progression. Predictors of a good response include patients who are young, have elevated CRP and have shorter disease duration.

Improvements in physical function, quality of life and work disability can be expected due to reduction in spinal and sacroiliac inflammation.

PSORIATIC ARTHROPATHY

Clinical features

Psoriatic arthropathy is an inflammatory arthritis associated with psoriasis. Psoriasis occurs in 1–3% of the population, and approximately 10% of those affected develop psoriatic arthritis. It is particularly common in patients with nail involvement (Fig. 13.7) and affects men and women with a similar frequency.

Psoriatic arthritis may precede the diagnosis of psoriasis and does not correlate with the severity of the skin lesions. Different patterns of joint disease are seen (Fig. 13.8).

Patients present with joint pain, stiffness and sometimes swelling, so examination for synovitis is important. Dactylitis and enthesitis are common features. Involvement of a distal interphalangeal (DIP) joint may be associated with pitting or onycholysis of the

Fig. 13.8 Patterns of joint disease in psoriatic arthritis
Distal arthritis involving the distal interphalangeal joints
Asymmetrical oligoarthritis
Symmetrical polyarthritis indistinguishable from rheumatoid arthritis
Spondylitis
Arthritis mutilans

nail. Arthritis mutilans is extremely destructive and, fortunately, uncommon. Resorption of bone at the metacarpals and phalanges causes telescoping of the digits. They appear shortened but can be passively extended to their original length. Psoriatic spondylitis tends to cause milder symptoms than classical AS, and sacroiliitis is often asymmetrical and asymptomatic.

The diagnosis is clinical, but aided by the CASPAR criteria (Fig. 13.9).

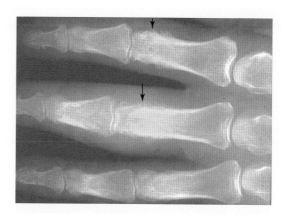

Fig. 13.10   Radiograph showing fluffy periosteal reaction and erosive changes (arrow) in the digits of a patient with psoriatic arthritis.

Investigations

Blood tests

Full blood count, ESR and CRP show a similar picture to that of AS. Rheumatoid factor is usually absent.

Radiological investigations

The radiological changes of psoriatic arthropathy are asymmetrical and target the small joints of the hands and feet, particularly the DIP joints (Fig. 13.10). X-ray changes include:

- Erosions with proliferation of adjacent bone.
- Resorption of the terminal phalanges.
- Pencil-in-cup deformities.
- Periostitis.

- Ankylosis.
- New bone formation at entheses.
- Sacroiliitis is found in up to 30% of cases and is usually asymmetrical (Fig. 13.11).

Management

- Treatment depends on the pattern of joint disease.
- Peripheral joint disease is treated with NSAIDs, methotrexate, leflunomide or sulfasalazine. Anti-TNF therapies work well in selected patients who have failed on conventional therapies.
- Axial disease is treated similarly to AS, with physiotherapy, NSAIDs and biologic therapy as the mainstay.
- All patients benefit from a multidisciplinary team approach.

Fig. 13.9 The Classification criteria for Psoriatic Arthritis (CASPAR) criteria	
Inflammatory articular disease (joint, spine or entheseal) with ≥3 points from the following:	
Evidence of current psoriasis, a personal history of psoriasis or a family history of psoriasis	2 points
Typical psoriatic nail dystrophy, including onycholysis, pitting and hyperkeratosis observed on current physical examination	1 point
A negative test result for the presence of rheumatoid factor by any method except latex	1 point
Either current dactylitis, defined as swelling of an entire digit, or a history of dactylitis recorded by a rheumatologist	1 point
Radiographic evidence of juxta-articular new bone formation appearing as ill-defined ossification near joint margins (but excluding osteophyte formation) on plain radiographs of the hand or foot	1 point
Definitions: Current psoriasis is skin or scalp disease present today as judged by a rheumatologist or dermatologist. A personal history of psoriasis is a history of psoriasis that may be obtained from a patient, family physician, dermatologist, rheumatologist or other qualified healthcare provider. A family history of psoriasis is a history of psoriasis in a first- or second-degree relative according to patient report.	
(Adapted from Taylor W, Gladman D, Helliwell P et al. 2006 Classification criteria for psoriatic arthritis: development of new criteria from a large international study. Arthritis and Rheumatism 54: 2665–2673.)	

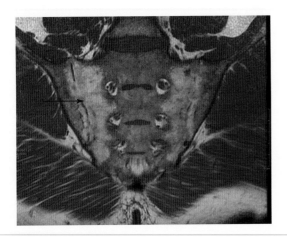

Fig. 13.11 Sacroiliitis.

Prognosis

The prognosis of psoriatic arthropathy is usually good. Joint function is well preserved in most cases, but in some, a chronic, progressive, deforming arthritis may develop.

REACTIVE ARTHRITIS

Clinical features

Reactive arthritis is an aseptic arthritis that develops after an anatomically distant infection. It mainly affects young adults and the triggering infection is usually of the gastrointestinal or genitourinary tract. Occasionally the incident infection is not found.

> **HINTS AND TIPS**
>
> Remember that *Salmonella* and *Neisseria* can cause a septic arthritis, so ensure joint cultures are negative!

Symptoms start a few days to a few weeks after the infection. The onset is sometimes acute, with fever and fatigue.

Musculoskeletal

The arthritis is typically asymmetrical and oligoarticular. It tends to target the large weight-bearing joints, fingers and toes. Dactylitis and enthesitis occur and some patients experience pain in the sacroiliac region.

Conjunctivitis

This is sterile and can be unilateral or bilateral.

Urethritis

Sterile inflammation in the urogenital tract can cause symptoms of frequency, dysuria and sometimes urethral discharge. Cervicitis or prostatitis can occur.

Reiter's syndrome

The term 'Reiter syndrome' is used to describe the triad of arthritis, urethritis and conjunctivitis in a patient following a bacterial infection.

Skin and mucosal lesions

Circinate balanitis can accompany urethritis. Some patients with reactive arthritis develop a sterile pustular rash on the palms of the hands and soles of the feet. This looks similar to pustular psoriasis and is called keratoderma blenorrhagica. Erythema nodosum is another recognized association.

> **COMMUNICATION**
>
> Enquire about the presence of genitourinary symptoms and any history of sexually transmitted infections in patients presenting with asymmetrical oligoarticular inflammatory arthritis. Patients may feel embarassed or threatened by this. It is helpful to start by explaining that joint inflammation can be triggered by genitourinary infections and that you routinely ask patients these questions.

Prognosis

The symptoms of reactive arthritis vary in severity and usually last for weeks to months. The vast majority are self-limiting. Relapses following further infective triggers can occur. At least 60% of patients have two or more attacks. Permanent joint damage can occur, but is rare.

Investigations

- Full blood count, ESR and CRP show a similar picture to that of AS.
- Serological tests, including antibodies against *Salmonella*, *Campylobacter*, *Chlamydia*, gonorrhoea and *Neisseria* may help identify the organism responsible for the infection.
- Synovial fluid from any affected joints should be examined and a Gram stain and culture performed. Cultures are negative in reactive arthritis, but it is important to exclude septic arthritis and crystal arthritis.

- A cervical/penile swab, midstream specimen of urine and stool sample should be obtained for bacterial culture to exclude ongoing infection. Partners should be offered advice where possible.
- X-rays are initially normal. Later, fluffy periostitis may be seen in the calcaneus, digits or pelvis. Plantar spurs are common, but erosions are rare. Sacroiliitis and typical AS changes develop in some patients.

Management of reactive arthritis

- Treat the causal infection with antibiotics and, in case of sexually transmitted infections, enquire about partner treatment.
- NSAIDs.
- Corticosteroid joint injections.
- Rarely, DMARD drugs may be required.

HINTS AND TIPS

Septic arthritis must be excluded before using corticosteroids.

ENTEROPATHIC ARTHRITIS

Clinical features

Arthritis occurring in association with IBD is known as enteropathic arthritis. It occurs in approximately 10–20% of patients with Crohn disease or ulcerative colitis.

Peripheral arthritis

A peripheral arthritis that is asymmetrical and mono- or oligoarticular can develop. It worsens when the severity of the bowel disease increases and improves if affected bowel is surgically removed.

Spondylitis and sacroiliitis

These are not related to the activity of the bowel inflammation and often predate the onset of Crohn disease or ulcerative colitis.

Enthesopathy

This can accompany axial or peripheral joint disease.

Examination

REMS may reveal signs of inflammation in axis, peripheral joints or enthesis.

Investigations

Most X-rays are normal. Spinal images may show similarities to AS (see p. 85). Bloods are generally unhelpful. If inflammatory bowel disease (IBD) is suspected, faecal calprotectin, inflammatory markers and referral to a gastroenterologist should be undertaken.

Management

Treatment of the IBD is the main priority and will help the arthritis. Drugs, such as corticosteroids and sulfasalazine, should improve both the bowel and joint disease. Anti-TNF therapy is licenced for IBD and, if used, can also help joint symptoms.

HINTS AND TIPS

NSAIDs often aggravate gastrointestinal symptoms in IBD. They should be used with caution and replaced with other forms of analgesia if poorly tolerated.

Further reading

Dougados, M., Baeton, D., 2011. Spondyloarthritis. Lancet 377, 2127–2137.

Perry, M., McInnes, I., 2007. Seronegative spondyloarthropathies. In: Madhok, R., Capell, H., Luthra, H.S., et al. (Eds.), The Year in Rheumatic Disorders, vol. 6. Clinical Publishing, Oxford.

Scottish Intercollegiate Guidelines Network, 2010. SIGN Guideline 121: Diagnosis and Management of Psoriasis and Psoriatic Arthritis in Adults. Available online at: http://www.sign.ac.uk/guidelines/fulltext/121/contents.html.

Extended report: European League Against Rheumatism recommendations for the management of psoriatic arthritis with pharmacological therapies. 2011. Available online at: http://ard.bmj.com/content/early/2011/09/27/annrheumdis-2011-200350.full.pdf.

Connective tissue diseases 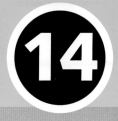14

● **Objectives**

After reading this chapter you should be able to:
- Recognize the clinical features of systemic lupus erythematosus (SLE).
- Understand the autoantibody associations with connective tissue diseases.
- Know how to recognize, investigate and treat inflammatory muscle disease.
- Understand the differences between limited and diffuse systemic sclerosis.
- Be aware of the ways in which patients with systemic vasculitis can present.

There is no strict definition of a connective tissue disease. The term is usually used to describe multisystem inflammatory diseases that are associated with immunological abnormalities. There is overlap between these disorders, which share many clinical features.

SYSTEMIC LUPUS ERYTHEMATOSUS

Definition

SLE is an inflammatory disease characterized by auto-antibody to nuclear material and can involve almost any organ or system of the body.

Prevalence

SLE has a worldwide prevalence of 10–50 per 100 000. It affects women at least 10 times more frequently than men, and is more common in Indian and Afro-Caribbean people than in Caucasians.

Aetiology

There are genetic, environmental and hormonal contributions to its aetiology. SLE can be induced by drugs, such as minocycline, oral contraceptives or hydralazine. Drug-induced lupus tends to be mild, spares the kidneys and settles when the offending drug is withdrawn. Ultraviolet light 'B' is associated with SLE development.

Pathology

Immune function in SLE is abnormal, with T- and B-cell dysfunction causing B-cell hyperactivity and impaired immune complex clearance from tissues. Dysfunction of the complement system and abberant programmed cell death mean that intracellular material is not disposed of correctly, allowing autoantibody production to develop against nuclear material. A wide variety of autoantibodies have been described, some of which are directly pathogenic (anti-Ro, anti-double-stranded DNA). The coagulation system may be abnormal and vasculopathy is frequent, resulting from clotting cascade antibodies (anti-C).

Clinical features

SLE usually develops between 15 and 40 years of age. The clinical features are diverse and the severity of the disease varies over time. Initial symptoms may be mild and rather vague, but it is the exacerbations of SLE and resultant tissue damage that cause significant ill health. Severe lupus flares can result in life-threatening problems, including renal failure and cerebral vasculitis. Factors that may trigger flares of SLE are listed in Figure 14.1.

Constitutional features

Fatigue, malaise, fever and weight loss are common in SLE. The fatigue can be quite disabling and is difficult to treat.

> **HINTS AND TIPS**
>
> Hypothyroidism is more common in SLE than in the general population and should be considered in patients with severe lethargy.

Musculoskeletal features

Approximately 90% of patients with SLE experience arthralgia, usually polyarticular. A non-erosive arthritis occurs in 25% of patients and symptoms are usually more dramatic than signs. Deformity is due to tenosynovitis and fibrosis, rather than cartilage or bone erosion (Jaccoud arthropathy).

Myalgia is a common symptom of SLE, and myositis (inflamed muscle) can occur (see myositis section, below). Avascular necrosis of bone and osteoporosis are recognized, but are usually a consequence of corticosteroid treatment and vasculopathy.

Dermatological features

There are many cutaneous manifestations of lupus. Photosensitivity is common (c. 60%) The characteristic 'butterfly' rash develops over the nose and cheeks (Fig. 14.2). Discoid lupus (demarcated, pigmented or atrophic plaques) can develop with no systemic features (Fig. 14.3).

Hair loss reflects disease activity and alopecia may develop. Mucosal ulceration may affect the nose, mouth and vagina. Cutaneous vasculitis in SLE can present with urticarial lesions, livedo reticularis, palpable purpura and splinter haemorrhages.

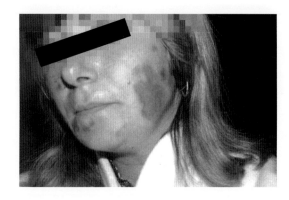

Fig. 14.3 Lesions of discoid lupus.

Cardiovascular features

Serositis is common in SLE and pericarditis is the commonest cardiac manifestation. This tends to be a sharp pain, relieved by sitting forward and associated with saddle-shaped ST elevation on an electrocardiograph.

Myocarditis may accompany myositis and can present with arrhythmias or cardiac failure. Libman–Sacks endocarditis is due to non-infective vegetations and seldom causes clinical problems.

At least one-third of patients with SLE suffer from Raynaud phenomenon: vasospasm, usually provoked by the cold, causes peripheral ischaemia. This can be seen in the digits, tip of the nose and earlobes, which become pale and numb, before turning blue. The final phase is redness and flushing due to eventual vasodilatation. Vasculitis may present with digital infarcts, skin rashes or ulcers and can rarely affect internal organs, such as the lungs and brain.

Pulmonary features

Amongst the pulmonary features of lupus, pleurisy and pleural effusions are common. Acute pneumonitis can mimic pneumonia. Chronic pneumonitis causes pulmonary fibrosis. Pulmonary hypertension is rare.

Renal features

Glomerulonephritis is the commonest cause of lupus-related death in patients with SLE. Nephritis does not cause clinical symptoms until there is significant renal damage. It is therefore important to monitor patients' blood pressure and check their urine for protein and red cells, so that renal disease can be detected early.

Neurological features

SLE can involve the central nervous system, cranial and peripheral nerves, producing a wide range of clinical features. These include headaches, psychiatric

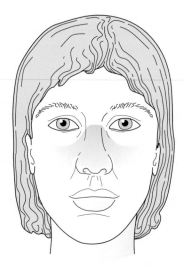

Fig. 14.2 The classic 'butterfly' rash of systemic lupus erythematosus.

problems, seizures, neuropathies and chorea. Headaches are common and often migrainous. Psychiatric symptoms such as anxiety, depression and psychosis are also well-recognized effects of lupus.

Haematological features

Lymphopenia is very common in SLE but neutropenia is also found. When patients are taking immunosuppressants it is difficult to identify drug or disease as aetiology. Anaemia can be due to chronic inflammation or to autoimmune haemolysis, which affects at least 5% of lupus sufferers. Antiphospholipid antibodies and clotting problems are discussed later in the chapter.

Gastrointestinal (GI) features

GI features tend to be rarer than other system involvement. Aseptic peritonitis can present with abdominal pain and nausea, with or without ascites. Other manifestations include mild hepatosplenomegaly from haemolysis and vasculitis affecting the mesenteric vessels.

COMMUNICATION

It is important to consider SLE as a possible cause of arthralgia, particularly in young women. Always ask about the presence of symptoms such as skin rashes, photosensitivity, oral ulcers, headaches, depression, Raynaud phenomenon and pleurisy.

Investigations

Serological tests

SLE is characterized by the presence of serum autoantibodies against nuclear components (Fig. 14.4).

Other tests

- The urine should be checked with a dipstick that detects blood and protein to look for signs of nephritis.
- Full blood count should be performed regularly to screen for anaemia, leukopenia and thrombocytopenia. Urea, creatinine and electrolyte levels should also be monitored.
- The erythrocyte sedimentation rate (ESR) will rise during a flare of SLE (Fig. 14.5), but may sometimes be high when the patient feels quite well. The C-reactive protein (CRP) tends to be normal or mildly elevated unless infection, synovitis or serositis is present.

Fig. 14.4 Autoantibodies associated with systemic lupus erythematosus (SLE)

Autoantibodies found in SLE	Comments
Antinuclear antibodies (ANA)	Detected in >95% of patients
Anti-Ro and anti-La antibodies	Associated with secondary Sjögren syndrome and pulmonary fibrosis Mothers are at risk of having babies with neonatal SLE and congenital heart block Sensitivity – SLE 25%
Anti-double-stranded DNA (dsDNA) antibodies	Present in 50% of SLE patient Very specific indicator of disease when present
Antihistone antibodies	Often positive in drug-induced SLE; sensitivity 90%
Antiphospholipid and anticardiolipin antibodies	May be positive in around 10–20% of SLE patients

Fig. 14.5 Indicators of high disease activity in systemic lupus erythematosus

Raised erythrocyte sedimentation rate (ESR)
High anti-DsDNA titres
Low C3 and C4 complement levels

- Complement levels (C3 and C4) can be depressed in active SLE.
- Coombs test will be positive in patients with autoimmune haemolytic anaemia.
- Skin biopsy shows deposition of immunoglobulin G (IgG) and complement at the dermal–epidermal junction in patients with rashes (lupus 'band' test).
- Renal biopsy is sometimes performed to aid diagnosis or to establish prognosis in patients with abnormal renal function.

HINTS AND TIPS

Consider SLE in a patient with multisystem symptoms, particularly mouth ulcers, arthralgia, Raynaud, lymphopenia, skin lesions and positive antinuclear antibody titre with a raised ESR.

Management

General measures

Education about SLE is essential. Patients are best advised to avoid factors that can precipitate lupus flares (see Fig. 14.1). They should wear long-sleeved clothes and use complete sunblock in any sunny weather. Infections should be promptly treated.

Pharmacological treatment

The choice of drug therapy in SLE depends on severity and specific organ involvement.

Mild SLE

Patients with symptoms such as arthralgia, lethargy or a faint rash may respond to non-steroidal anti-inflammatory drugs and/or antimalarial drugs, such as hydroxychloroquine.

Moderate SLE

Patients with more severe clinical features, such as serositis, severe arthritis, nephritis, autoimmune haemolytic anaemia, thrombocytopenia and neurological or psychiatric problems often require treatment with corticosteroids. Steroid-sparing agents such as azathioprine, methotrexate or mycophenolate mofetil can be used.

Severe SLE

Flares of SLE that cause severe renal, neurological or haematological problems should be treated with cytotoxic drugs combined with corticosteroids. Cyclophosphamide is very effective. Tacrolimus and mycophenolate mofetil are alternatives. The biologic drug belimumab will be available shortly for the treatment of severe lupus. It is a humanized monoclonal antibody that blocks a B-cell survival factor (Fig. 14.6). Anecdotal evidence suggests B-cell depletion (rituximab) is of value in selected patients.

Adjunctive treatment

Hypertension due to nephritis should be treated aggressively. Intravenous immunoglobulin infusions may help immune thrombocytopenia or neutropenia. Antiplatelet drugs or warfarin are required for patients with antiphospholipid antibody syndrome (see below). Anticonvulsants may be required in central nervous system disease.

Prognosis

The outlook for patients with SLE is improving. Ten-year survival is over 90%. Patients have a higher risk of vascular morbidity and mortality, especially if disease has been poorly controlled, high doses of steroids have been needed or the patient is a smoker. Malignancy and infection rates are higher.

THE ANTIPHOSPHOLIPID SYNDROME

Definition

The antiphospholipid syndrome (APS) is characterized by recurrent vascular thrombosis, fetal loss and thrombocytopenia associated with persistently elevated levels of antiphospholipid antibodies. Antiphospholipid antibody production can complicate other autoimmune diseases, especially SLE. In these circumstances, patients are said to have secondary APS.

Incidence

APS was first described 30 years ago. Incidence and prevalence are still unclear.

Fig. 14.6 B-lymphocyte-stimulating protein (BLSP) is blocked by the monoclonal antibody, belimumab, thus inhibiting B cells from producing pathogenic autoantibody.

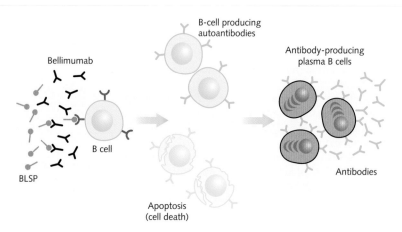

Pathology

The two main antiphospholipid antibodies are lupus anticoagulant and anticardiolipin antibodies. They have a procoagulant effect in susceptible individuals, associated impaired fibrinolysis and increased vascular tone, all contributing to clot formation and infarction.

Clinical features

The major features of APS are shown in Figure 14.7. Patients can develop additional clinical features (Fig. 14.8).

Investigations

The diagnosis is based on the detection of anticardiolipin antibodies or a positive lupus anticoagulant assay. Anticardiolipin antibodies bind to cardiolipin or β_2 glycoprotein-1. The lupus anticoagulant assay measures the ability of antiphospholipid antibodies to prolong clotting tests such as the activated partial thromboplastin time. So, although the test is for an anticoagulant, the syndrome produces clotting and thrombosis. Thrombocytopenia may occur.

Fig. 14.7 The major features of antiphospholipid syndrome

Venous thrombosis	Deep vein thrombosis and pulmonary emboli – most common Other veins can be affected (e.g. inferior vena cava, pelvic, renal, portal and hepatic veins)
Arterial thrombosis	Cerebral ischaemia (stroke, transient ischaemic attacks) Peripheral ischaemia
Fetal complications	Spontaneous abortion Premature births
Thrombocytopenia	Not severe enough to cause haemorrhage

Fig. 14.8 Associated clinical features of antiphospholipid syndrome

Livedo reticularis
Leg ulcers
Cardiac valve abnormalities (e.g. aortic and mitral regurgitation)
Chorea
Epilepsy
Migraine
Haemolytic anaemia

Management

General advice

The following steps are advisable:

- Avoidance of the oral contraceptive pill.
- Avoidance of smoking.
- Treatment of hypertension, hyperlipidaemia or diabetes mellitus.

Asymptomatic patients

Current recommendations suggest that patients who have the antibodies for anticardiolipin or antiphospholipid but have had no clinical features should not be treated. However, if they also have another autoimmune disease or significant cardiac risk factors, then aspirin can be used for primary prevention.

Venous or arterial thrombosis

Patients with APS should be anticoagulated in the usual way. However, it is recommended that anticoagulation is lifelong, because there is a risk of recurrent thrombosis. Treatment is with warfarin, aiming for an international normalized ratio of 2.5–3.5.

Recurrent fetal loss

Warfarin should be stopped before conception because it is teratogenic. Subcutaneous heparin and aspirin should be given throughout pregnancy to reduce the risk of fetal loss.

SJÖGREN SYNDROME

Definition

Sjögren syndrome is a chronic autoimmune disease, characterized by inflammation of exocrine glands. The salivary and lacrimal glands are predominantly affected, resulting in dryness of the eyes and mouth. Sjögren syndrome can be primary or secondary (associated with other autoimmune diseases). Causes of secondary Sjögren syndrome are shown in Figure 14.9.

Sicca syndrome is the presence of dry eyes or mouth as a result of non-autoimmune disease, such as smoking or drugs.

Prevalence

The prevalence of Sjögren syndrome is 1–3%. It is nine times commoner in women than men.

Fig. 14.9 Diseases associated with secondary Sjögren syndrome
Rheumatoid arthritis
Systemic lupus erythematosus
Systemic sclerosis
Polymyositis
Primary biliary cirrhosis
Chronic active hepatitis

Aetiology

The aetiology is unknown. The primary disease has a strong genetic association with human leukocyte antigen (HLA) A1 B8 DR3 haplotype. It is thought that some environmental factor (probably a virus) may trigger Sjögren syndrome in people with a genetic susceptibility.

Pathology

All organs affected by Sjögren syndrome are infiltrated by lymphocytes. In the salivary glands, this results in duct dilatation, acinar atrophy and interstitial fibrosis. There is marked activation of B cells, resulting in increased immunoglobulin production. Sicca syndrome has no immune infiltrate compared with Sjögren.

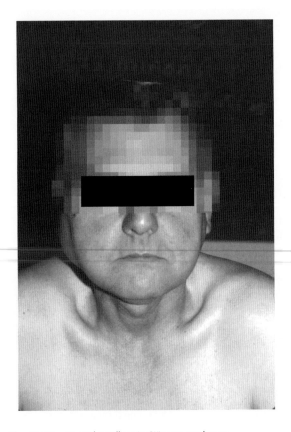

Fig. 14.10 Parotid swelling in Sjögren syndrome.

Clinical features

Sjögren syndrome predominantly affects people in their fourth and fifth decades. The main symptoms are ocular and oral.

Ocular symptoms

Reduced tear secretion results in the destruction of the corneal and conjunctival epithelium (keratoconjunctivitis sicca). Patients complain that their eyes feel dry, sore or gritty and they are usually red. Bacterial conjunctivitis is common.

Oral symptoms

Xerostomia (dryness of the mouth) leads to difficulties in swallowing dry food or talking for long periods. On examination of the oral cavity, the mucosa is dry, there is very little saliva and the tongue may be fissured. Dental caries is often seen and oral candidiasis is common. Intermittent parotid swelling affects at least half of patients with primary Sjögren syndrome (Fig. 14.10) but is less common in secondary disease.

Other symptoms of exocrine dysfunction

Secretion from other exocrine glands may be diminished, vaginal dryness leads to dyspareunia and lack of GI mucus secretion can result in oesophagitis or gastritis.

Systemic features

Primary Sjögren syndrome is a systemic disease and many patients develop extraglandular manifestations which mimic SLE:

- Constitutional features include fatigue, weight loss and fever.
- Arthritis is episodic, non-erosive and very similar to the joint disease seen in SLE.
- Circulation: Raynaud phenomenon affects up to 50% of patients. Vasculitis affects approximately 5% of patients and usually causes cutaneous lesions: purpura and ulcers.
- Respiratory: interstitial lung disease is mild and often subclinical.
- Renal: interstitial nephritis can lead to renal tubular acidosis or nephrogenic diabetes insipidus.

- Neurological features vary widely. Peripheral neuropathies result from small-vessel vasculitis. Cranial neuropathies, hemiparesis, seizures and movement disorders can also occur.
- Malignancy: lymphomas, usually B-cell, are commoner in patients with Sjögren syndrome than in the general population. They develop in the salivary glands, reticuloendothelial system, GI tract, lungs or kidneys.

Investigations

Schirmer's test

Schirmer's test is used to demonstrate reduced tear production. One end of a strip of filter paper is placed beneath the lower eyelid. Wetting the paper by less than 5 mm in 5 minutes suggests reduced secretion.

Rose Bengal staining

This is used to detect keratoconjunctivitis sicca. Rose Bengal is a dye that stains damaged cornea and conjunctiva. Ulcerated cornea is seen on slit-lamp examination in keratoconjunctivitis sicca.

Labial gland biopsy and histology

Biopsy and histology of the buccal surface of the lower lip is a very useful test. Lymphocytic infiltration can be seen.

Blood tests

- The ESR is usually raised.
- Immunoglobulin levels can be very high.
- Anti-Ro/La antibodies are a diagnostic aid, but rheumatoid factor and antinuclear antibodies are also often found.

> **HINTS AND TIPS**
>
> Do not assume that every patient with arthralgia and a positive rheumatoid factor has rheumatoid arthritis. Titres of rheumatoid factor can be very high in Sjögren syndrome and patients with primary Sjögren syndrome are often misdiagnosed as having rheumatoid arthritis.

Management

Treatment of Sjögren syndrome is topical and symptomatic. Tear substitutes such as hypromellose eye drops help to lubricate the eyes. Occlusion of the canaliculi can help to block the drainage of tears and keeps the conjunctiva moist.

Xerostomia can be treated with saliva substitutes. Pilocarpine tablets may help, but cause cholinergic side-effects such as sweating and abdominal cramps. Careful dental hygiene is essential to help prevent premature caries.

Hydroxychloroquine can help the arthritis. Corticosteroids and other immunosuppressive drugs are prescribed for serious complications like vasculitis and neurological problems.

POLYMYOSITIS AND DERMATOMYOSITIS

Definition

Polymyositis (PM) and dermatomyositis (DM) are autoimmune, inflammatory muscle diseases. DM also affects the skin.

Incidence

Both muscle diseases are rare, with a combined incidence of between 2 and 10 cases per million per year. There is a female preponderance of 2:1.

Aetiology

The aetiology of PM and DM is unknown. Family studies support a genetic predisposition. Associations with various HLA types have been reported, but are weak.

Pathology

In both conditions, muscle fibres are infiltrated by inflammatory cells and there is subsequent degeneration, necrosis and phagocytosis. The pattern of infiltration and predominant cell type allows PM to be distinguished from DM. Skin biopsy in DM shows the same histological features as in lupus.

Clinical features

Inflammatory muscle disease can affect people of any age, but the peak age of onset is 40–60 years.

Myositis

PM and DM are characterized by symmetrical proximal muscle weakness that develops over weeks to months. Patients find certain tasks increasingly difficult, such as rising from a chair, climbing the stairs or reaching for things above head height.

Involvement of the intercostal muscles and diaphragm can affect ventilation and lead to type 2 respiratory failure. Dysphagia and regurgitation of food result from weakness of the pharyngeal muscles and upper third of the oesophagus. Patients may complain of muscle pain and tenderness. Muscle bulk and tendon reflexes appear normal, except in advanced disease.

Cutaneous manifestations

The skin rashes of DM usually precede the weakness. Typical lesions are:

- Gottron's papules – erythematous, scaly papules or plaques over the metacarpophalangeal and proximal interphalangeal joints and also over the extensor surfaces of the knees and elbows.
- A heliotrope rash develops on the skin over the eyelids; lilac discoloration is often accompanied by periorbital oedema.
- A macular erythematous rash may develop on the face, neck, chest, shoulders and hands.
- Calcinosis – this occurs more commonly in juvenile DM.
- Cutaneous vasculitis can cause ulceration.
- Periungual telangiectasia may be seen and the cuticles are often thickened and irregular.

Extramuscular features of PM and DM

Constitutional features
Fatigue, malaise, weight loss and fever are common.

Skeletal features
Many patients develop polyarthralgia as well as myalgia.

Pulmonary features
Interstitial lung disease occurs in up to 30% of cases. Ventilatory failure can result from weakness of the intercostal muscles and diaphragm. Aspiration pneumonia is a risk in patients with dysphagia.

Cardiovascular features
Myocarditis can present with cardiac failure or arrhythmias, but most cases are asymptomatic. Raynaud phenomenon and vasculitis can accompany myositis.

GI features
Vasculitis that can result in intestinal haemorrhage or perforation is particularly common in juvenile DM.

Malignancy
Approximately 5–15% of adults with inflammatory muscle disease have an underlying malignancy. The association is thought to be much stronger for DM than for PM. Common sites of malignancies reported in association with DM include:

- Lung.
- GI tract – oesophagus and colon.
- Endocrine – breast and ovary.

Investigations

Serum levels of muscle enzymes

Serum levels of muscle enzymes (e.g. creatinine kinase) are elevated due to myositis.

Erythrocyte sedimentation rate

The ESR is usually raised, but does not correlate well with disease activity.

Autoantibodies

Anti-Jo-1 is anti hystidyl t-RNA synthetase but antibodies can be made against other tRNA synthetase enzymes in PM and DM. Anti-Jo-1 is an anticytoplasmic antibody and is associated with interstitial lung disease, arthralgia and Raynaud phenomenon (antisynthetase syndrome).

Muscle biopsy

This is the most definitive investigation. Histology shows the typical inflammatory cell infiltration of either PM or DM.

Electromyography and nerve conduction studies

Electromyography and nerve conduction studies can show that the weakness is due to a myopathic process, but do not give a specific diagnosis.

Magnetic resonance imaging

MRI can identify areas of muscle oedema, but again is non-specific.

Management

Although the muscle enzymes respond quickly to treatment, the improvement in muscle strength is usually much slower. Physiotherapy plays an extremely important role in the rehabilitation of patients with inflammatory muscle disease.

Most patients with PM or DM require immunosuppressive therapy. Corticosteroids are used to control myositis. They are initially prescribed at high doses. Serum creatine kinase is monitored and, as it falls, the corticosteroid dose is gradually reduced. Methotrexate and azathioprine are commonly used. Cyclophosphamide may be prescribed for patients with severe interstitial lung disease. If an underlying malignancy is found, it should be treated appropriately.

Steroid myopathy is a common complication of treatment. It may be difficult to distinguish from active myositis, but should be considered in patients with normal creatine kinase levels whose muscle strength is deteriorating. Biopsy may help differentiate.

Prognosis

The 5-year survival rate of patients with PM and DM has improved and is currently over 80%. However, many patients are left with significant persisting symptoms as a result of their disease or therapy.

SYSTEMIC SCLEROSIS

Definition

The term 'scleroderma' means hardening of the skin. It can occur as a condition confined to skin (cutaneous scleroderma) or involve other organs (systemic sclerosis) (Fig. 14.11). The systemic form is subdivided into limited and diffuse disease, the former having less extensive skin involvement than the latter.

Incidence and prevalence

These are rare conditions. The incidence of scleroderma is 0.6–1.9 per million per year. The UK prevalence is approximately 100 per million. Women are affected four times as often as men.

Aetiology

In most patients, the aetiology is unknown.

Pathology

The two main pathological processes in systemic sclerosis are fibrosis and microvascular occlusion. Overactive fibroblasts produce excessive extracellular matrix

Fig. 14.11 Classification of systemic sclerosis and related conditions
Localized cutaneous scleroderma
Morphoea Linear scleroderma
Systemic sclerosis
Limited cutaneous systemic sclerosis Diffuse cutaneous systemic sclerosis Scleroderma *sine* scleroderma

in the dermis. Perivascular inflammatory infiltration and intimal proliferation lead to narrowing of arteries and arterioles and obliteration of capillaries. There is immune activation and release of cytokines.

Clinical features

Skin manifestations

Scleroderma begins with an inflammatory phase. The skin becomes puffy and feels tight and sometimes itchy. These symptoms typically affect the forearms, hands and feet initially. Over several months, skin thickening and induration develop. Common features found on examination are:

- Sclerodactyly (Fig. 14.12).
- Microstomia (Fig. 14.13).
- Furrowing of skin around the lips (Fig. 14.13).
- Loss of normal skin creases.
- Tethering of skin to underlying structures.

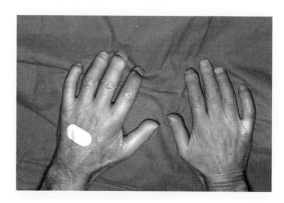

Fig. 14.12 Sclerodactyly.

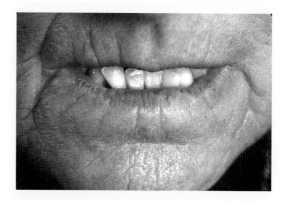

Fig. 14.13 This patient with systemic sclerosis has microstomia and furrowing of the skin around her mouth.

Fig. 14.14 A comparison of skin disease between limited and diffuse systemic sclerosis

	Limited systemic sclerosis	Diffuse systemic sclerosis
Distribution of skin fibrosis	Hands* and feet Over the face and neck	Limbs, face, neck and trunk
Skin tethering to underlying structures	Common	Less common
Inflammatory features	Mild	Swelling and pruritus prominent
Telangiectasia	Commonly occurs on the face and digits	Less common
Calcinosis	Cutaneous and subcutaneous Calcification common	Less common

*Scleroderma affecting the fingers is often referred to as 'sclerodactyly'.

- Skin hypo- or hyperpigmentation.
- Flexion contractures of joints.
- Thinning and atrophy (late stage).

The skin changes differ between diffuse and limited cutaneous systemic sclerosis. The main differences are outlined in Figure 14.14.

The effects of systemic sclerosis on other body systems

In addition to causing disfiguring skin changes, systemic sclerosis can have profound effects on many other organs. Limited disease is twice as common as diffuse and is sometimes referred to as CREST syndrome (**CREST**= calcinosis, **R**aynaud phenomenon, **o**esophageal disease, sclerodactyly and telangiectasia). Symptoms develop most commonly in the fifth decade of life.

Involvement of internal organs is more frequent in diffuse than in limited disease.

Cardiovascular manifestations

Raynaud phenomenon
This occurs in nearly every person with systemic sclerosis. Severe disease may cause ischaemic changes in the fingertips and possibly gangrene. The toes, ears, nose and nipples can also be involved.

Cardiac disease
- Myocardial fibrosis can cause cardiac failure and arrhythmias.
- Pericarditis can be silent.

Pulmonary disease

Pulmonary disease is the most frequent cause of death in systemic sclerosis.

Interstitial lung disease
This affects approximately 25% of patients with limited disease and up to 40% of those with the diffuse cutaneous form.

Pulmonary hypertension
This affects 10–12% of patients and now represents a major cause of death in scleroderma patients.

Primary pulmonary hypertension is more common in limited cutaneous systemic sclerosis, and is not associated with other lung pathology. Secondary pulmonary hypertension is more common in diffuse cutaneous systemic sclerosis and is caused by interstitial lung disease.

Renal disease

Scleroderma renal crisis
This implies rapidly progressive renal failure, usually with accelerated hypertension. It tends to occur in patients with diffuse cutaneous disease within 5 years of onset and is often preceded by deterioration of skin disease. Patients present acutely with headaches, visual disturbance and sometimes seizures. Left ventricular failure can occur and death from renal failure is likely without rapid intervention.

> **HINTS AND TIPS**
>
> Scleroderma renal crisis is a life-threatening medical emergency that needs urgent treatment.

GI manifestations

Scleroderma can affect any part of the GI tract, but oesophageal problems are particularly common. Reflux oesophagitis and oesophageal dysmotility cause heartburn and dysphagia. Hypomotility can lead to bacterial overgrowth in the small bowel and constipation in the large bowel.

Musculoskeletal complications

Most patients suffer with arthralgia and joint stiffness at some time in their disease. Flexion contractures of the interphalangeal joints are common.

Neurological complications

Both central and peripheral neuropathy can occur, and overlap myositis/myopathy is well recognized.

Investigations

The diagnosis of scleroderma is clinical. It is important to establish whether patients with systemic sclerosis have diffuse cutaneous or limited cutaneous disease, as this determines prognosis.

Serological tests

Antinuclear antibodies are found in most patients. The presence or absence of other autoantibodies can help predict complications and prognosis. For example:

- Anticentromere antibodies are associated with limited disease and a relatively good prognosis. They signify a risk of pulmonary hypertension, but not pulmonary fibrosis.
- Antitopoisomerase-1 (Scl-70) antibodies are associated with diffuse disease, higher risk of lung fibrosis, renal involvement and mortality.

Management

Treatment

To date, no definitive treatment exists. Symptoms should be treated on an organ by organ basis (Fig. 14.15).

Screening for complications

Monitoring pulmonary function tests, echocardiography, blood pressure and renal function help control long-term lung and systemic complications.

Prognosis

The survival of patients with systemic sclerosis is improving. This probably reflects better management of complications and proactive cardiovascular risk assessment. Five-year survival rate is around 90% for limited disease, but much worse for the diffuse variant.

THE VASCULITIDES

Vasculitis is inflammation of blood vessels. It is a feature of many illnesses and can be primary or secondary. The primary vasculitides are uncommon diseases in which vasculitis is the predominant feature. Secondary vasculitis complicates other established diseases, such as rheumatoid arthritis and SLE. In addition vasculitis

Fig. 14.15 Treatment of organ disease in systemic sclerosis	
Complication	**Intervention**
Raynaud phenomenon	Hand warmers Vasodilators • Calcium-channel blockers • ACE inhibitors • Intravenous prostacyclin (iloprost) for severe ischaemia Digital sympathectomy is useful for ischaemia of one or two digits
Pulmonary fibrosis	Prednisolone, with or without cyclophosphamide
Pulmonary hypertension	Anticoagulation Vasodilators • Calcium-channel blockers • Bosentan • Sildenafil • Prostacyclins Diuretics for right ventricular failure, if present
Gastrointestinal problems	Proton pump inhibitor for gastro-oesophageal reflux Antibiotics for small-bowel overgrowth Bulk-forming agents for constipation
Renal crisis	Antihypertensives – give immediately • ACE inhibitors • Calcium-channel blockers • Temporary dialysis may be required
Cardiac problems	Diuretics and ACE inhibitors for cardiac failure Antiarrhythmics if necessary Corticosteroids for myocarditis

ACE, angiotensin-converting enzyme.

may be caused by drugs, infection and malignancy. Only primary vasculitis will be discussed here.

Pathology

Vasculitis is characterized by inflammatory cell infiltration of the blood vessel wall, resulting in fibrinoid necrosis. For this reason, the term 'necrotizing vasculitis' is sometimes used. There is often associated granuloma formation. Vascular inflammation can have severe consequences:

- Aneurysm formation can lead to rupture of vessels and haemorrhage.
- Vessel stenosis or occlusion can lead to distal infarction.

Anti-neutrophil cytoplasmic antibodies (ANCAs) are particularly specific for vasculitis and are helpful for diagnosis and classification. They are antibodies that bind to enzymes in the cytoplasm of neutrophils. There are two types of ANCA:

- Proteinase-3 (PR-3) is found throughout the neutrophil cytoplasm and anti-PR-3 antibodies were called cytoplasmic (c) ANCA. It is found in patients with Wegener granulomatosis and is highly specific.
- Myeloperoxidase (MPO) is found in a peri-nuclear distribution in neutrophils and anti-MPO antibodies were called perinuclear (p) ANCA. It is found in polyarteritis nodosa, microscopic polyangiitis and Churg–Strauss syndrome.

Classification of primary vasculitis

The vasculitides are commonly classified on the basis of the size of the vessels they affect (Fig. 14.16).

Clinical features

Although vasculitis is rare, it can affect any system of the body and may be life-threatening. Awareness of the general effects it can cause is important (Fig. 14.17), but detailed knowledge of specific diseases is beyond the scope of this book.

Giant cell (temporal) arteritis (GCA) and polymyalgia rheumatica (PMR)

Clinical features
GCA is a large-vessel vasculitis. It often coexists with PMR (a non-vasculitic illness), which is why they are discussed together here. They have an incidence of approximately 1–5 in 10 000. They both affect people over 60 years of age and are twice as common in females as in males. About

Fig. 14.16   Classification of primary vasculitis
Large-vessel vasculitis
Giant cell (temporal) arteritis and polymyalgia rheumatica Takayasu arteritis
Medium-vessel vasculitis
Polyarteritis nodosa Kawasaki disease
Small-vessel vasculitis
Wegener granulomatosis* Churg–Strauss syndrome* Microscopic polyangiitis* Henoch–Schönlein purpura Essential cryoglobulinaemic vasculitis
*Vasculitides most commonly associated with antineutrophil cytoplasmic antibodies.

Fig. 14.17 The effects that vasculitis can have on different body systems	
Body system or organ	**Manifestations of vasculitis**
Constitutional	Fatigue, anorexia, weight loss, fever
Skin	Rashes Palpable purpura Ulceration Ischaemia (Fig. 14.18)
Joints	Arthralgia Arthritis
Kidneys	Glomerulonephritis
Gastrointestinal tract	Ischaemia
Nervous system	Neuropathies Stroke
Lungs	Pulmonary haemorrhage

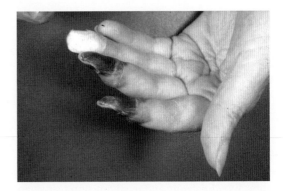

Fig. 14.18   Ischaemic changes in the fingers of a patient with vasculitis.

50% of patients with GCA have symptoms of PMR and 20–50% of patients with PMR have GCA symptoms.

Giant cell arteritis
Most symptoms are due to inflammation of the carotid artery or its branches, although other large arteries can be involved. The onset of GCA can be insidious or abrupt, with symptoms often appearing overnight. Patients complain of:

- Headache/scalp tenderness from skin ischaemia.
- Pain on chewing food (jaw claudication from masseter muscle ischaemia).
- The temporal artery is thickened and tender on examination, sometimes with absent pulsation.
- Visual change – optic artery ischaemia, which may be preceded by transient change, such as amaurosis fugax.

Blindness can occur. This is due to ischaemic optic neuritis, caused by arteritis of the posterior ciliary artery and branches of the ophthalmic arteries. Patients may experience transient disturbance of vision first. Stroke is another serious potential complication.

Polymyalgia rheumatica

Patients present with symmetrical pain and stiffness in the shoulder and pelvic girdles. Proximal muscles may be tender. Peripheral synovitis affecting medium-sized joints can occur.

Investigations

The diagnosis of PMR is clinical. It is important to exclude mimics such as malignancy and other connective tissue diseases.

Temporal artery biopsy is the investigation of choice for GCA, but it is not always helpful. The arteritis is patchy and, if a 'skip lesion' is biopsied, histology will be normal. Inflammatory cell infiltration, giant cells and granulomata should be seen.

The ESR is usually raised in both conditions. However, a normal ESR does not exclude the diagnosis. Anaemia is common.

Management

Both GCA and PMR should be treated with corticosteroids. Prednisolone at a dose of 15–20 mg is usually prescribed for PMR. Higher doses are required for GCA (1 mg/kg prednisolone), particularly in patients with visual symptoms. They should be started promptly to reduce the risk of blindness.

There is usually a dramatic response to corticosteroid therapy, with symptoms improving within a few days. Once the disease activity has been suppressed, the corticosteroid dose can be gradually tapered. Ninety-five per cent of patients should be off steroid therapy by 2 years. Azathioprine and methotrexate are sometimes used as steroid-sparing agents if weaning off prednisolone is proving difficult.

Takayasu arteritis

This is a rare disease that predominantly affects young women. The arteritis affects the aortic arch and its branches. Symptoms are due to vascular ischaemia and include claudication, dizziness, visual loss and stroke. Differences in blood pressure between arms may occur, as well as subclavian bruits. Imaging with computed tomography, magnetic resonance imaging or positron emission tomography may help confirm the diagnosis. Steroids are the mainstay of treatment but vascular surgery may be required to bypass obliterated vessels.

Polyarteritis nodosa

Polyarteritis nodosa is a necrotizing arteritis that leads to aneurysm formation. It affects men more frequently than it does women. It is associated with hepatitis B infection. Clinical features include skin ulceration and rashes, peripheral neuropathy, renal disease and gut infarction, which presents with bleeding and abdominal pain. Angiography may show microaneurysms, which are usually found in renal arteries and the coeliac axis. Renal, rectal or sural nerve biopsies can be diagnostic.

Polyarteritis nodosa is treated with corticosteroids and, in more severe patients, cyclophosphamide is used, with improved prognosis.

Kawasaki disease (mucocutaneous lymph node syndrome)

This vasculitis predominantly affects children under the age of 5 years but occurs rarely in adults. Features include desquamation of the skin of the hands and feet, conjunctival congestion, cervical lymphadenopathy, arthritis and coronary artery aneurysms, which can lead to acute myocardial infarction and heart failure. Treatment is with low-dose aspirin.

Wegener granulomatosis

Wegener granulomatosis is a granulomatous disorder associated with necrotizing vasculitis. It is strongly linked with the presence of PR3 ANCA. The peak age of onset is in the fourth and fifth decades. Many systems can be affected (Fig. 14.19), but it is respiratory and renal complications that are the most serious: renal failure and pulmonary haemorrhage. Survival in Wegener granulomatosis has improved dramatically since the introduction of cyclophosphamide therapy, which is usually given in conjunction with corticosteroids. Rituximab (B cell depletion therapy) has recently been shown to have equivalence with cyclophosphamide and is licensed for treatment. Some patients with

Fig. 14.19 Clinical features of Wegener granulomatosis

Body system or organ affected	Clinical features
Upper and lower respiratory tracts	Subglottic stenosis Lung nodules ± cavitation Pulmonary haemorrhage Pulmonary infiltrates
Kidneys	Glomerulonephritis (often rapidly progressive)
Ear, nose and throat	Sensorineural deafness Nasal discharge, crusting and epistaxis 'Saddling' of the nose due to destruction of the septal cartilage (Fig. 14.20)
Joints	Arthralgia Arthritis
Skin	Rashes Palpable purpura Livedo reticularis
Nervous system	Cranial nerve palsies Peripheral neuropathy Granulomatous meningitis

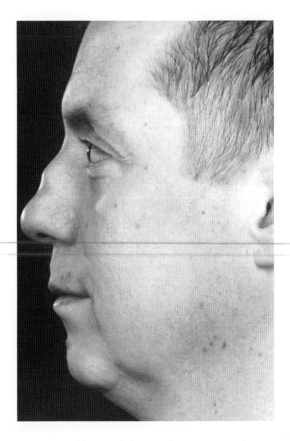

Fig. 14.20 Saddle nose deformity of Wegener granulomatosis (late complication).

limited, non-life-threatening Wegener granulomatosis can be treated less aggressively with drugs such as mycophenolate, methotrexate or azathioprine.

Other types of vasculitis include:

- Churg–Strauss syndrome: eosinophilia and wheeze.
- Microscopic polyangiitis: renal failure and rash.
- Henoch–Schönlein purpura: childhood tendency, lower-limb rash and abdominal pain from GI involvement.
- Cryoglobulinaemic vasculitis: leg ulcers from vasculitic rash, arthralgia, renal failure.

Further reading

Berden, A., Goceroglu, A., Jayne, D., et al., 2012. Diagnosis and management of ANCA associated vasculitis. Br. Med. J. 344, e26.

Gabrielli, A., Awedimento, E.V., Krieg, T., et al., 2009. Scleroderma. N. Engl. J. Med. 360, 1989–2003.

Salvarani, C., Cantini, F., Hunder, G.G., 2008. Polymyalgia and giant-cell arteritis. Lancet 372, 234–245.

Tsokos, G.C., 2011. Systemic lupus erythematosus. N. Engl. J. Med. 365, 2110–2121.

Metabolic bone disease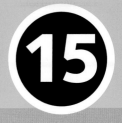

Objectives

After reading this chapter you should be able to:
- Understand the risk factors and problems associated with the development of osteoporosis.
- Know the common fractures that occur in osteoporotic patients.
- Be aware of strategies for fracture prevention in osteoporosis.
- Understand the clinical features and potential complications of Paget disease.
- Know the pathways of vitamin D metabolism.
- Recognize the differences between rickets and osteomalacia.

OSTEOPOROSIS

Because of the ageing population, fractures resulting from osteoporosis put enormous pressure on hospital services and incur vast costs.

Definition

Osteoporosis is a skeletal disorder characterized by decreased bone mass, leading to reduced bone strength and increased risk of fracture. Bone mineral density (BMD) is used as a measure of bone strength and expressed as a T-score. This is the number of standard deviations by which the BMD varies in relation to the mean value for young normal adults. The World Health Organization defines osteoporosis as a T-score of less than −2.5. Osteopenia is defined as a T-score of between −1 and −2.5.

Aetiology and pathology

Peak bone mass is usually attained by the age of 30 and thereafter declines (Fig. 15.1). Bone loss is accelerated in osteoporosis due to an imbalance between the rates of bone resorption and formation, which are governed by activity of osteoclasts and osteoblasts respectively (Fig. 15.2). Risk factors for osteoporosis can be modifiable or non-modifiable (Fig. 15.3).

Osteoporosis is divided into primary (idiopathic or age-related) and secondary (resulting from another disease process). The causes of secondary osteoporosis are shown in Figure 15.4.

Clinical features

Patients present with pain, deformity or immobility due to fractures, or they are detected by screening measurements of their BMD. Osteoporotic fractures are usually provoked by low-energy injuries.

COMMUNICATION

Osteoporosis is often asymptomatic, so the importance of treatment to prevent fractures in the future must be emphasized to patients.

Vertebral fractures

Vertebral compression (or wedge) fractures (Fig. 15.5) usually present with thoracic back pain after a minor fall. They are frequently multiple and result in loss of height and a kyphotic deformity. Some patients do not experience pain, but complain that they are shrinking or becoming 'round-shouldered'.

These are stable fractures and treatment is aimed at controlling symptoms with analgesia. Newer treatments for controlling pain include vertebroplasty and kyphoplasty. Both involve the injection of cement into the fractured vertebra.

Other common fractures include those of the hip and wrist and these are discussed in more detail in Chapter 18.

Diagnosis and investigation

Plain X-ray cannot be used to diagnose osteoporosis but osteopenic appearances may indicate the need for further investigation. The usual screening test is dual X-ray absorptiometry (DEXA). DEXA is used in most departments to measure BMD at the lumbar spine and hip. Two photon beams are generated by the X-ray machine, which allows a difference between soft tissue and bone to be appreciated (Fig. 15.6).

A full history and examination should be performed when assessing a patient with low BMD. It is important to enquire about risk factors for osteoporosis and to

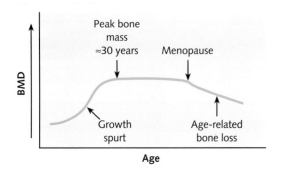

Fig. 15.1 'Lifeline' of bone mineral density (BMD).

Fig. 15.3 Risk factors for osteoporosis

Non-modifiable	Modifiable
Age Race (Caucasian, Asian) Female sex Early menopause Small size Positive family history	Poor calcium and vitamin D intake Lack of exercise Smoking Alcohol excess

thyroid-stimulating hormone and parathyroid hormone. Serum testosterone should be measured in men.

Management

The aim is to reduce the risk of fractures. This can be achieved by the following methods.

Modification of risk factors

Patients should change any modifiable risk factors for osteoporosis (see Fig. 15.3), for example, by stopping smoking and increasing weight-bearing exercise.

consider the presence of any underlying illnesses, such as those listed in Figure 15.4. Osteoporosis in males and young people is more likely to be due to a secondary cause.

Investigations to exclude a secondary cause will be necessary in some patients. These should include full blood count, erythrocyte sedimentation rate, serum calcium, alkaline phosphatase, creatinine, electrophoresis,

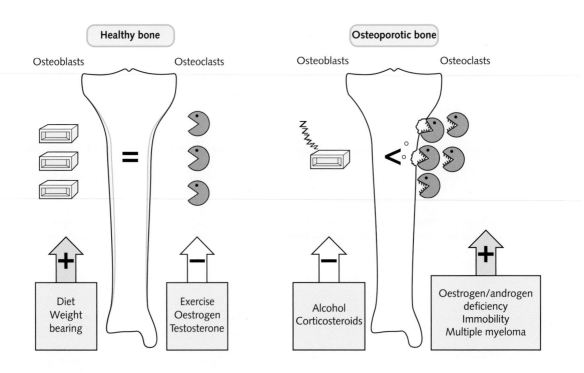

Fig. 15.2 Cell interactions in normal and osteoporotic bone.

Fig. 15.4   Causes of secondary osteoporosis

Hyperthyroidism
Hyperparathyroidism
Hypogonadism
Cushing syndrome
Rheumatoid arthritis
Inflammatory bowel disease
Coeliac disease and malabsorption states
Renal failure
Multiple myeloma
Anorexia nervosa
Medications:
• Corticosteroids
• Anticonvulsants
• Heparin

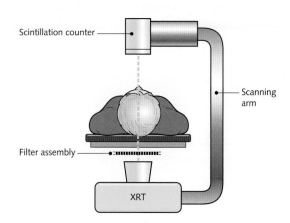

Fig. 15.6   Dual X-ray absorptiometry (DEXA) apparatus. The patient lies with the X-ray tube (XRT) below. The filter allows two different beams to be produced, which are narrow to reduce scattered radiation. These beams are detected by the scintillation counter which then generates an image.

Denosumab

This is a new humanized monoclonal antibody against RANK ligand that reduces osteoclastogenesis. It has been shown to improve BMD and reduce fractures in postmenopausal women.

Strontium

This can be used as a second-line agent or when bisphosphonates are not tolerated. It probably works to remodel the bone structure, with both antiresorptive and bone formation effects.

Other agents for the treatment of osteoporosis include calcitonin and parathyroid hormone.

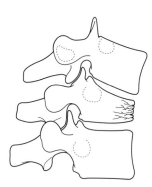

Fig. 15.5   Compression fracture of a thoracic vertebra.

Drug therapy to increase bone mass

Bisphosphonates

First-line therapy is usually with a bisphosphonate in combination with calcium and vitamin D supplements. Bisphosphonates are antiresorptive and work by inhibiting osteoclasts. Daily, weekly, monthly and yearly preparations are available and have good efficacy. Gastrointestinal intolerance can be a problem in some patients.

Raloxifene

Selective oestrogen receptor modulators (e.g. raloxifine) can be used in postmenopausal women. Patients should be advised regarding cardiovascular outcomes and malignancy risk.

Prevention of falls

The majority of osteoporotic fractures occur as a result of falls. These are more common in the elderly for a number of reasons:

1. Intrinsic factors:
   • Ageing process – leads to slower reaction times (patients unable to stop falling).
   • Poor mobility – patients often have other conditions, such as osteoarthritis.
   • Poor eyesight.
   • Medical comorbidity, e.g. syncope/cardiac arrhythmia.
2. Extrinsic factors:
   • Lack of social services.
   • Inadequate housing/unsafe local environment.

Falls can be reduced by various interventions, such as the avoidance of drugs that have a sedative effect or cause hypotension, the use of walking aids for people with poor mobility and the removal of obstacles in the home. These is also some evidence that replacing vitamin D improves balance and prevents falls.

PAGET DISEASE

Definition

Paget disease is a disorder of bone remodelling.

Incidence

The incidence varies widely across the globe. In the UK, approximately 3% of the population over the age of 40 years are affected by the disease.

Aetiology

The cause of Paget disease is unknown, but clustering of cases within families has been observed, suggesting a strong genetic contribution. Another hypothesis suggests that it is triggered by a viral infection.

Pathology

There is a dramatic increase in bone resorption, mediated by large multinucleated osteoclasts. Osteoblasts then respond by producing weak, disorganized bone. Repeated cycles of this activity lead to areas of bone becoming abnormally large and deformed with increased vascularity (Fig. 15.7).

Clinical features

Only one-third of patients are symptomatic. They present with bone pain, deformity or fracture. Paget disease can affect a single part of the skeleton or multiple sites. The commonest sites are the pelvis, lumbar spine, femur, skull and tibia. The affected area may be tender and warm due to increased blood flow.

Paget disease is usually diagnosed in asymptomatic patients when an X-ray is performed for another reason. For example, pagetic changes may be noticed in the pelvis on an abdominal X-ray.

Figure 15.8 demonstrates some of the possible complications of Paget disease. Many of these are due to bone overgrowth, which can cause localized problems, such as deafness due to auditory nerve entrapment. Osteosarcomas can occur in pagetic bone, but are rare.

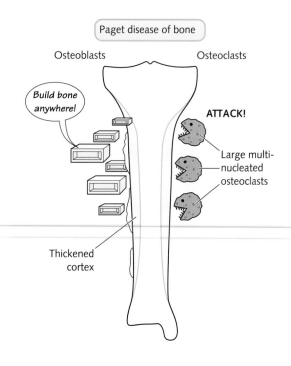

Fig. 15.7 Cell interactions in Paget disease of bone.

Diagnosis and investigation

- Serum alkaline phosphatase levels are elevated and correlate with the extent of skeletal involvement.
- Plain radiographs show disorganized patterns of affected bone with areas of lysis and sclerosis. The cortex is usually thickened.
- Isotope bone scans will show areas of focal increased uptake and are the most sensitive test in identifying pagetic lesions.

Treatment

Bisphosphonates are very effective at inhibiting bone resorption and reducing symptoms of Paget disease. Calcitonin is sometimes used, but is less well tolerated.

Asymptomatic disease may not require treatment. Determining if lesions are active is key to deciding if treatment should commence.

Surgical treatment is reserved for complications of:

- Fracture – needs surgical stabilization.
- Deformity – osteotomy is rarely performed.
- Osteosarcoma – these tumours are highly aggressive with a poor prognosis. If the appendicular skeleton is involved, resection or amputation is required, followed by chemotherapy.

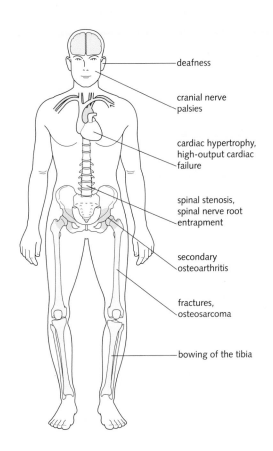

Fig. 15.8   Potential complications of Paget disease.

Pagetic bone is very vascular and bleeds a lot during surgery. Blood should be cross-matched in advance.

RICKETS AND OSTEOMALACIA

Both of these conditions are the result of failure of mineralization of bone. Rickets affects the growing skeleton in children and is a disorder of defective mineralization of cartilage in the epiphyseal growth plates of children. Osteomalacia occurs in adults.

Aetiology

Vitamin D deficiency is the commonest cause of both conditions. Hypophosphataemia is a much rarer cause. Figure 15.9 illustrates the pathways of vitamin D metabolism. The causes of vitamin D deficiency are shown in Figure 15.10.

Pathology

Histological examination of bone biopsies in both conditions shows an increased amount of osteoid with deficient mineralization.

Clinical features

The main clinical features of rickets and osteomalacia are:

- Bone pain.
- Skeletal deformity.
- Muscle weakness.
- Fracture.

Tetany or convulsions due to hypocalcaemia can occur, but are rare.

Rickets

The growth of children with rickets is impaired. The clinical manifestations depend on the age of the child. Those under 12 months of age may have softening

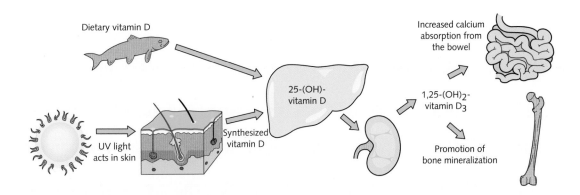

Fig. 15.9   Pathways of vitamin D metabolism. UV, ultraviolet.

Fig. 15.10 Causes of vitamin D deficiency
Low dietary intake plus inadequate sunlight exposure
Intestinal malabsorption (coeliac disease, gastric surgery)
Liver disease
Renal disease
Drugs that affect vitamin D metabolism (anticonvulsants)

and frontal bossing of the skull. There may be swelling of the epiphyses of the wrists and at the costochondral junctions (the 'rickety rosary'). Older children develop bowing of the long bones and valgus or varus deformities at the knee.

The following radiological changes are seen in rickets:

- Delayed opacification of the epiphyses.
- Widened growth plates.
- Thin cortices.

Osteomalacia

Osteomalacia tends to present with vague bone pain, especially in the long bones and pelvis. Severe, localized pain may be due to fracture. The myopathy is usually proximal.

Diagnosis and investigation

The following laboratory abnormalities are usually found:

- Low or low/normal serum calcium.
- Low or low/normal serum phosphate.
- Raised serum alkaline phosphatase.
- Low serum vitamin D.
- Raised parathyroid hormone.
- Low urinary calcium excretion.

In osteomalacia, the characteristic appearance on X-ray is of Looser's zones, which are spontaneous incomplete fractures.

Treatment

Both rickets and osteomalacia can be treated with vitamin D supplementation. The underlying cause of vitamin D deficiency should be addressed.

Further reading

Rachner, T.D., Khosla, S., Hofbauer, L.C., 2011. Osteoporosis: now and the future. Lancet 377, 1276–1287.

Ralston, S.H., Langston, A.L., Reid, I.R., 2008. Pathogenesis and management of Paget's disease of bone. Lancet 372, 155–163.

World Health Organization, 2004. WHO scientific group on the assessment of osteoporosis at primary health care level. Available online at: http://www.who.int/chp/topics/Osteoporosis.pdf.

Gout and pseudogout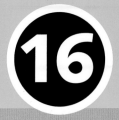

Objectives

After reading this chapter you should be able to:
- Understand the many risk factors for gout.
- Recognize the clinical features of acute and chronic gout.
- Know how to investigate and manage gout.
- Recognize the articular manifestations of calcium pyrophosphate dihydrate disease (CPPD).

GOUT

Definition

Gout is a consequence of hyperuricaemia and uric acid crystal formation. Clinical features include:

- Arthritis.
- Crystal deposition in the soft tissues (tophi).
- Renal disease.
- Urolithiasis.

Prevalence

Gout affects 1.4% of people in the Western world. It is commoner in men but the incidence in women is increasing.

Aetiology

Gout is caused by a sustained increase in serum uric acid levels. Uric acid is derived from the breakdown of purine bases, which are components of nucleic acids. It is present in two forms in the body: uric acid and monosodium urate. Synthesis mainly occurs in the liver (Fig. 16.1).

Daily turnover of uric acid is high and approximately two-thirds is renally excreted. Serum levels are related to age, sex, body mass, diet and genetic factors. They are higher in males than in females from puberty until the menopause, when the difference lessens.

Hyperuricaemia is usually due to reduced renal urate excretion, rather than increased production. The risk factors for developing gout are in Figure 16.2.

COMMUNICATION

It is important to take a detailed drug and alcohol history from patients presenting with gout.

Pathology

Prolonged hyperuricaemia leads to the formation of urate crystals. These are deposited in the synovium, other connective tissues and the kidney. Joint inflammation occurs when crystals are shed from deposits within the joint and phagocytosed by polymorphonuclear leukocytes. Urate deposition in the kidney can cause interstitial nephritis, renal stones and acute tubular damage.

Clinical features

Acute gout

Acute gout is extremely painful. It typically presents as a rapidly accelerating monoarthritis. Symptoms often develop overnight and include severe pain and swelling. The skin overlying the joint is usually shiny, warm and red and the joint is extremely tender. Attacks subside spontaneously within a few days to a couple of weeks.

The first metatarsophalangeal joint is the commonest to be affected, but the ankle, knee, elbow, wrist and hand joints can also be involved. Oligoarticular presentations are also common. Acute gout can also affect bursae and is a common cause of olecranon bursitis. Initially, acute attacks resolve, leaving the patient free of symptoms. Some people have no further problems, but most will have further attacks within a year. Without treatment, acute attacks become more frequent and erosive bone damage occurs.

HINTS AND TIPS

Asymptomatic hyperuricaemia is common but should not be treated.

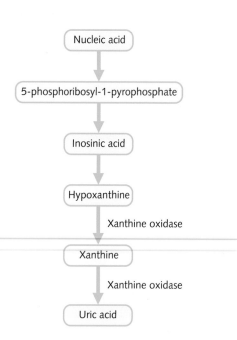

Fig. 16.1   The steps in the synthesis of uric acid.

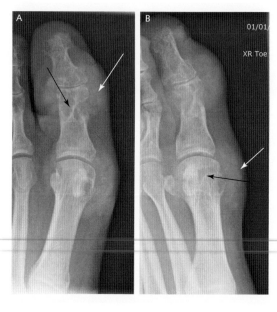

Fig. 16.3   (A and B) X-rays showing tophus formation (white arrows) and joint destruction (black arrows) in gout.

Fig. 16.2   Risk factors for gout
Alcohol (especially beer) Obesity Diet – high-protein: red meats, shellfish, high-fructose drinks Diuretic use Male gender Hypertension and renal disease Cancer Psoriasis

Investigations

Synovial fluid analysis

This is the single most important test in the diagnosis of suspected gout. Synovial fluid should be obtained by needle aspiration of symptomatic joints and examined with a microscope under polarized light. Monosodium urate crystals are needle-shaped and show strong negative birefringence (Fig. 16.4). This means that crystals parallel to the plane of light appear yellow, whereas those at right angles are blue. Aspirated material from tophi can be examined in a similar way. Synovial fluid

Chronic gout

Musculoskeletal features

Chronic gout occurs in patients with uncontrolled hyperuricaemia, who have had recurrent attacks of acute gout for years. It is characterized by tophus formation and joint destruction. Tophi are soft-tissue deposits of urate. They commonly develop in the digits, bursae and tendon sheaths. They can interfere with function and sometimes ulcerate, discharging chalky white material. Cartilage destruction and bony erosion in chronic gout can lead to deformities (Fig. 16.3).

Renal disease

Urate deposition in the renal interstitium and collecting tubules can cause a nephropathy. Uric acid stones can also form in the urinary tract.

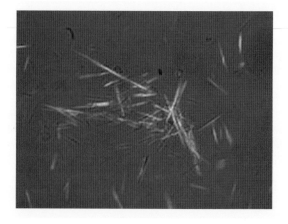

Fig. 16.4   Needle-shaped crystals of gout viewed by polarized light microscopy.

Gram stain and culture should be performed to exclude infection.

Blood tests

Serum uric acid is usually elevated, but one-third of patients have normal levels during an acute flare. The erythrocyte sedimentation rate and C-reactive protein are usually raised in acute gout and a full blood count may reveal a polymorphonuclear leukocytosis.

Radiology

Radiological changes do not usually appear until years of recurrent gouty attacks have elapsed. Radiographs show soft-tissue swelling and opacities due to tophi. Erosions may be seen (see Fig. 16.3) in juxta-articular regions and, unlike in rheumatoid arthritis, the surrounding bone is sclerotic.

Management

Management of acute gout

Acute gout should be treated promptly for a short period of time with one of the following drugs:

- Non-steroidal anti-inflammatory drugs (NSAIDs) are used most commonly, and should be continued until the pain and inflammation subside.
- Colchicine should be used in those with a contraindication to NSAIDs, such as previous peptic ulcer and asthma, and at a dose of 500 µg twice or thrice daily, as higher doses often cause diarrhoea.
- Corticosteroids are a useful therapy for patients who are unable to tolerate NSAIDs or colchicine. They should not be used for long-term treatment. Steroid joint injections are highly successful.

Prophylactic therapy

Drugs that lower serum urate can be used to prevent attacks of gout: indications for prophylactic treatment are listed in Figure 16.5. Allopurinol should be used first-line. It reduces uric acid synthesis by inhibiting the enzyme xanthine oxidase. The dose should be increased regularly until the patient's serum uric acid level is <0.36 µg (Fig. 16.6). Care should be taken in the elderly and those with impaired renal function.

Febuxostat is another xanthine oxidase inhibitor which is highly successful. Newer drugs such as

Fig. 16.5 Indications for prophylactic treatment of gout
Recurrent attacks
Tophi
Radiological damage
Renal disease

Fig. 16.6 Timetable of urate-lowering therapy in gout	
Weeks following acute flare	**Treatment**
0–4	NSAID/colchicine/prednisolone
4–26	Allopurinol NSAID/colchicine/prednisolone
26 onward	Allopurinol (target serum urate level 36 µmol/L)
NSAID, non-steroidal anti-inflammatory drug.	

PEG-uricase and rasburicase may have value in severe tophitic disease. These drugs use the enzyme uricase to catalyse purine breakdown via alternative pathways. Yet other drugs work by increasing renal urate excretion.

Changes in the serum urate can precipitate episodes of gout. Urate-lowering therapy should not be commenced until an acute attack has settled completely and NSAIDs or colchicine should be co-prescribed for the first few weeks or months.

Correction of risk factors

Attempts should be made to identify each patient's risk factors for gout. The factors listed in Figure 16.7 that are known to precipitate acute attacks should be avoided if possible.

Vascular risk

Gout is an independent risk factor for vascular disease and gout patients are twice as likely to have a

Fig. 16.7 Factors that can precipitate attacks of gout
Trauma
Intercurrent illness
Surgery
Excess alcohol intake
Starvation
Initiation of drugs that alter urate levels

myocardial infarction. Modifiable risk factors should be addressed.

CALCIUM PYROPHOSPHATE DIHYDRATE DISEASE

Definition

CPPD is an arthropathy associated with the deposition of calcium pyrophosphate dihydrate crystals. It tends to present as an acute synovitis, often referred to as 'pseudogout'.

Prevalence

CPPD is less common than gout, but estimates of prevalence vary greatly. It is predominantly a disease of the elderly and has a slight female preponderance.

Aetiology

The cause of CPPD deposition is unknown. Associations with osteoarthritis and various metabolic diseases are recognized (Fig. 16.8), but not well understood. Predisposing factors include dehydration and intercurrent infections.

Pathology

CPPD crystals are deposited mainly in cartilage, but also in the synovium, joint capsule and tendons.

Clinical features

The two main clinical presentations of CPPD are:

1. Acute synovitis (pseudogout).
2. Chronic arthritis (pyrophosphate arthropathy).

Fig. 16.8 Metabolic diseases predisposing to calcium pyrophosphate dihydrate deposition
Hypothyroidism
Hyperparathyroidism
Haemochromatosis
Acromegaly
Gout

Pseudogout

This is the commonest cause of acute monoarthritis in the elderly. Patients present with an acute onset of joint pain, stiffness and swelling, sometimes accompanied by fever. The knee and wrist are the commonest sites, but the ankle, elbow and shoulder are also targets. Attacks unusually affect more than one joint at a time. As with gout, examination reveals a swollen, erythematous and tender joint. Attacks usually resolve within a few weeks.

Chronic pyrophosphate arthropathy

This has many similarities to osteoarthritis. Onset is gradual and symptoms include pain, stiffness and loss of function. Commonly affected joints are knees, hips, shoulders, elbows, wrists and metacarpophalangeals (particularly the second and third). Some patients develop acute attacks of synovitis. Examination reveals signs of osteoarthritis, at times with synovitis. Pyrophosphate arthropathy may be indistinguishable from inflammatory osteoarthritis.

Investigations

Synovial fluid examination

Synovial fluid examination with polarized light microscopy is the key to the diagnosis. The CPPD crystals are either rhomboid or rod-shaped and show weak positive birefringence. They are intracellular. Gram stain and culture of synovial fluid should be performed to exclude infection.

Radiology

CPPD causes the following radiographic signs:

- Chondrocalcinosis.
- Osteoarthritis-like changes.

Calcification of cartilage (chondrocalcinosis) is often seen in the menisci of the knee (Fig. 16.9A), triangular cartilage of the wrist (Fig. 16.9B) and the symphysis pubis. The cartilage loss, sclerosis, cysts and osteophytes seen in osteoarthritis all occur in pyrophosphate arthropathy.

Other investigations

A serum calcium should be checked in all patients. CPPD deposition in younger patients is unusual and should be investigated by screening for the underlying associated metabolic disorders (see Fig. 16.8).

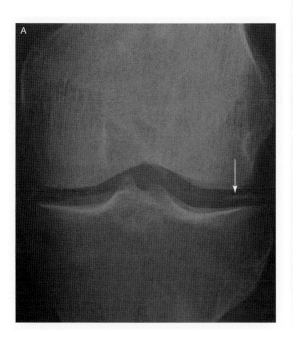
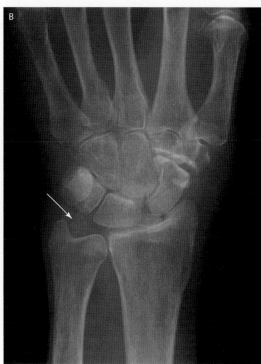

Fig. 16.9   (A) Chondrocalcinosis in the menisci of the knee. (B) Calcification of the triangular cartilage in the wrist.

Management

Attacks of pseudogout should be treated with analgesics. Joint aspiration and corticosteroid injection often produce rapid relief of symptoms, and colchicine can also be effective. Unlike gout, there is no specific prophylactic treatment for chronic pyrophosphate arthropathy. It should be managed in a similar way to osteoarthritis, with emphasis on weight reduction, physiotherapy, pain control and, when necessary, joint replacement. Episodes of synovitis can be improved by intra-articular corticosteroid injection.

Further reading

Jordan, K.M., Cameron, J.S., Smith, M., et al., 2007. British Society for Rheumatology and British Health Professionals in Rheumatology Guideline for the Management of Gout. Available online at: http://www.rheumatology.org.uk/ includes/documents/cm_docs/2009/m/management_of_ gout.pdf.

Perry, M.E., Madhok, R., 2010. Treatment failure gout: failure to treat? Rheumatology 49, 2233–2234.

Richette, P., Bardin, T., 2010. Gout. Lancet 375, 318–328.

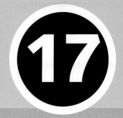
After reading this chapter you should be able to:
- Describe normal variations of gait and joints commonly referred to paediatric clinics.
- Recognize the clinical features of developmental dysplasia of the hip (DDH) and know how to investigate and treat it.
- Recognize and describe features of Perthes disease and a slipped upper femoral epiphysis (SUFE).
- Describe the different ages that the three childhood hip conditions usually present and know how to treat these conditions.
- Recognize the clinical features of clubfoot.
- Describe the features and management of osteogenesis imperfecta (OI).
- Understand the common causes of knee pain in children, including Osgood–Schlatter disease and osteochondritis dissecans.
- Know the orthopaedic problems associated with cerebral palsy.

Of all the joint disorders affecting children the most important to the orthopaedic surgeon are those affecting the hip. Many of these children will require hip replacement surgery in adult life, with the most severely affected having such surgery in their 20s or 30s.

NORMAL VARIANTS

The majority of referrals to paediatric orthopaedic surgeons are for normal variations in growth of a healthy child brought in by anxious parents. The single most reassuring feature is the symmetrical appearance of the limb. If the child has only one side affected then the condition is much more likely to be pathological.

Examples of normal conditions commonly referred include the following.

Flat feet

This condition is usually physiological, painless and may be associated with laxity of ligaments. Simple advice only is required as even the use of insoles is questionable and most children develop normally regardless. Pain or fixed deformity suggests an underlying pathological condition.

Toe walkers

Often a child who is beginning to walk does so on tiptoes. Usually the child 'grows out' of this but examination is required to exclude a tight Achilles tendon or an underlying condition such as cerebral palsy.

In-toeing gait

Causes of in-toeing are at three levels: the hip, the tibia and the foot.

Persistent femoral torsion leaves the patient with an excessive internal rotation and the child often sits in a W position rather than cross-legged (Fig. 17.1). The natural history of this condition is of spontaneous resolution as the child grows, but a small number require femoral osteotomy.

Internal tibial torsion also results in in-toeing but almost always resolves with no treatment.

In the foot, metatarsus adductus (inwardly pointing forefoot) is the cause of in-toeing and again this usually resolves over time.

Bow legs (genu varum)

It is normal for toddlers to have bow legs and they almost always grow out of this over time. Very rarely, pathological conditions such as rickets can cause bowing but the child is usually older and the disease is on one side only.

Knock knees (genu valgum)

Older children 3–8 years old gradually become more valgus as they grow normally, and again the majority straighten spontaneously. Pathological genu valgum is rare, usually asymmetrical, severe and progressive.

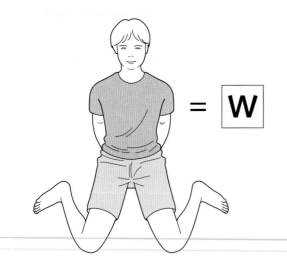

Fig. 17.1 Child sitting in the W position in excessive femoral anteversion.

PAEDIATRIC HIP DISORDERS

Developmental dysplasia of the hip

Introduction

Previously called congenital dislocation of the hip (CDH), this disorder is due to failure of normal development of the acetabulum resulting in abnormal hip anatomy. This disorder encompasses the spectrum of disease from a frankly dislocated hip to acetabular dysplasia (in which the slope of the roof of the acetabulum is too steep).

Incidence

The incidence is approximately 5–20 per 1000 live births; however the majority of these settle, stabilize and develop normally without treatment. Only 1–2 per 1000 live births will require intervention.

Aetiology and pathology

The condition is seven times more common in females. It is also more common in certain races (northern Italy and North American indigenous population).
DDH is associated with:

- Breech presentation.
- Family history.
- Other congenital deformities.

The left side is more commonly affected but the condition is bilateral in 20%.
The acetabulum relies on the presence of the femoral head for normal development. In DDH there is excessive laxity of the joint with a shallow acetabulum (socket) (Fig. 17.2). This allows the femoral head to develop out of the socket, in severe cases forming a false acetabulum (located above the normal one).

Clinical features

The majority are picked up on routine baby check and referred appropriately.
Late-presenting DDH can occur as the child begins to walk. The child will have a limp and shortness of one leg (if unilateral).
The clinical findings of DDH include:

- Loss of abduction.
- Leg length discrepancy.
- Asymmetrical posterior skin crease.

Fig. 17.2 Anatomy of the hip showing (A) normal and (B) pathological hip development. DDH, developmental dysplasia of the hip.

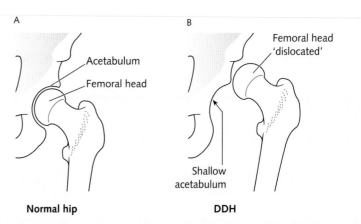

Normal hip

DDH

The special tests for dysplastic hips are called Barlow's and Ortolani's tests.

Barlow's test

This is an attempt to dislocate a reduced hip.

The examiner holds the child's thigh so that the thumb is on the medial aspect of the thigh with the middle finger on the trochanter. Then with the child's hip and knee flexed to 90°, the hip is slightly adducted and a gentle downward force applied to try to dislocate the hip. A clunk is felt if positive (Fig. 17.3).

Ortolani's test

This is an attempt to reduce a dislocated hip.

Both hips are examined together. The hand is placed in a similar position and the hip is flexed to 90° and then gently abducted. The test is positive if the hip reduces with a clunk.

Diagnosis and investigation

All babies are screened clinically by examination at birth but unfortunately this is unreliable. At-risk babies with the factors listed above are screened with ultrasound. If there is doubt this investigation can be repeated.

An older child should be investigated with X-rays, which once the femoral head has ossified should clearly show if there is a dislocation (Fig. 17.4).

Management

This depends on whether the hip is dislocated and, if so, whether the hip is easily reducible.

Conservative

An abduction splint is used to hold the hip in abducted and stable position, keeping the hip in joint. An example of splintage is the Pavlik harness.

Surgical

If the hip is not reduced, closed or open, reduction is performed.

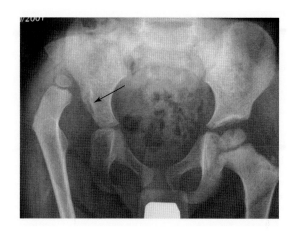

Fig. 17.4 X-ray showing developmental dysplasia of the hip (arrow).

A variety of surgical osteotomies to the pelvis or femur can be used to correct anatomy and maintain reduction.

Prognosis

The outcome depends upon the degree of dysplasia, duration of dislocation, and whether or not complications such as osteonecrosis develop. Secondary osteoarthritis is common in this group of patients.

Perthes disease

Introduction

This is a rare disease, of unknown aetiology, in which blood supply to the femoral head is interrupted, causing segmental avascular necrosis and collapse of the femoral head. It is often referred to as Legg–Calve–Perthes disease.

Epidemiology

Approximately 1 in 1000 are affected. Perthes disease is four times more common in boys and is bilateral in 15%. It usually presents between the ages of 4 and 8. It is more common in Caucasians than other ethnic groups.

The condition is associated with:

- Family history.
- Lower socioeconomic groups.
- Low-birthweight children.
- Delayed bone age.

Variable amounts of the head are involved and this has an effect on outcome. In severe cases of collapse the femoral head migrates out of the joint (subluxation).

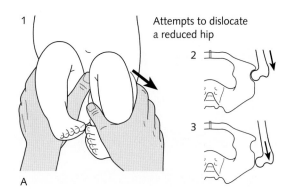

Fig. 17.3 Barlow's test: attempts to dislocate a reduced hip.

Clinical features

The child (usually a boy) presents with a gradual history of hip or knee pain associated with a limp. Clinical features will show loss of hip motion, particularly abduction and internal rotation, and there may be fixed deformity. Complete loss of abduction is a worrying sign and may signify subluxation of the hip.

Diagnosis and investigation

Perthes disease in an acutely presenting child could be confused with septic arthritis and therefore inflammatory markers should be checked – they are normal in Perthes disease.

A plain X-ray (Fig. 17.5) is the mainstay of diagnosis. The features of Perthes on X-ray are:

- Loss of epiphyseal height.
- Increased density of the femoral epiphysis.
- Subchondral fracture, partial collapse and fragmentation of the head.
- Abnormal shape and size of femoral head.
- Subluxation. Magnetic resonance imaging (MRI) is very sensitive for diagnosis and staging.

Treatment

This depends upon the age of the patient and the extent of the disease.

Conservative

In all, 75% of children require no treatment and will have a good long-term outcome. Young patients with less than 50% involvement of the femoral head have a good prognosis.

Surgical

Older patients and female patients (closer to skeletal maturity) and patients with greater than 50% involvement have a poor prognosis, and significant early osteoarthritis is likely. These children may require containment of the femoral head with surgery, e.g. a pelvic or femoral osteotomy.

Slipped upper femoral epiphysis

This condition is a disorder in which there is structural failure through the growth plate of an immature hip.

Incidence

Approximately 3 per 100 000 children are affected.

It is more common in boys than in girls, usually occurring during the early adolescence growth spurt between 11 and 14 years of age. Approximately 60% are bilateral.

Aetiology and pathology

Two groups are affected: athletic children of either sex or overweight boys with delayed puberty.

The exact cause is not known but may relate to failure of the epiphyseal cartilage to mature as the child grows. Some hormonal conditions are associated, e.g. hypothyroidism, diabetes mellitus.

The slip results in the epiphysis lying posterior and inferior to the femoral neck.

Clinical features

The child presents with groin or knee pain (or both) and a limp. The history can be acute, or gradual.

Examination findings reveal an external rotation deformity with limitation of most movements. There may be a slight leg length discrepancy. Check for evidence of hypogonadism, hypopituitarism and hypothyroidism.

Diagnosis and investigation

Diagnosis is based on X-ray changes. An anteroposterior (AP) X-ray is taken, but it is the frog lateral which most clearly demonstrates the pathology (Fig. 17.6).

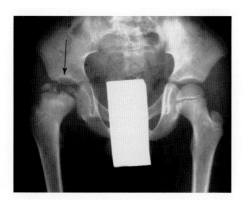

Fig. 17.5   X-ray of Perthes disease (arrow).

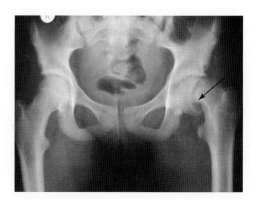

Fig. 17.6   X-ray of slipped upper femoral epiphysis (arrow).

Management

Surgical

Once diagnosed the epiphysis should be pinned in situ to prevent further displacement as soon as possible; consideration should be given to prophylactically fixing the other hip.

Attempts to reduce severe slips are associated with avascular necrosis.

Prognosis

There is a high incidence of secondary degenerative osteoarthritis.

CONGENITAL TALIPES EQUINOVARUS (CLUBFOOT)

Congenital talipes equinovarus encompasses a deformity of the lower limb with calf wasting and the classical inwardly pointing foot.

Incidence

The incidence is approximately 1 per 1000 live births. Males are affected twice as often as females.

Aetiology and pathology

The exact aetiology is not known but arrest of normal limb bud development in utero may be the cause. Genetic factors play a role, with family history being important.

The basic pathology is at the level of the subtalar joint with a cavus deformity (high arch) and metatarsus adductus (Fig. 17.7). The Achilles tendon is also tight, resulting in an equinus deformity.

Associated soft-tissue contractures occur on the medial side.

Clinical features

The condition is easily noted at birth as a fixed varus and equinus deformity of the foot. The calf is underdeveloped when compared with the normal side.

The baby should be examined for associated syndromes or conditions (such as spina bifiida or DDH).

Diagnosis and investigation

The diagnosis is a clinical one and X-rays are usually taken after initial treatment or surgery.

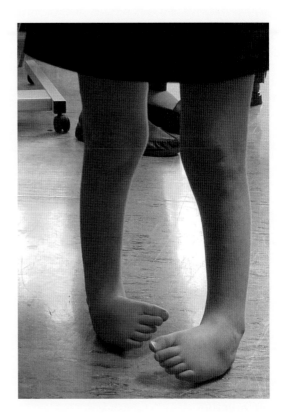

Fig. 17.7 Untreated talipes.

Management

Conservative

Initial treatment is with serial casting changed weekly for up to 3 months.

Surgical

Surgery is reserved for those cases that fail to correct fully or for later recurrence.

Prognosis

The foot and limb will never be normal in terms of appearance but most patients lead a normal life.

OSTEOGENESIS IMPERFECTA

Also known as brittle bone disease, this disorder predisposes to multiple fractures.

Incidence

The condition is rare.

Aetiology and pathology

OI is usually inherited as an autosomal dominant condition, although sporadic and recessive cases can occur.

There are four different types of OI. The primary abnormality is a defect in the synthesis of type 1 collagen.

Clinical features

The child may present with a low-energy fracture and the diagnosis is made subsequently, following examination and investigation.

Blue sclerae are pathognomonic but not always present. Children are usually small with bony deformities (including scoliosis) and joint abnormalities. Associated features include deafness and joint laxity.

Diagnosis and investigation

X-rays may show:

- Multiple fractures.
- Deformity.
- Thin-looking cortex.

Treatment

Conservative

Gentle handling is needed to prevent fractures.

Bisphosphonates such as pamidronate can be given intravenously to try to improve bone strength.

Surgical

Sheffield intramedullary telescoping rods are the mainstay of treatment for the prevention of deformity and further fracture.

Established deformity is treated with osteotomy.

Prognosis

The outcome depends on the type of OI; some are incompatible with life.

CEREBRAL PALSY

Definition

This is a non-progressive neuromuscular disorder that results from injury to an immature brain.

Incidence

Incidence is 2 per 1000 births.

Aetiology and pathology

The cause is often unknown, but can include prematurity, perinatal anoxia, perinatal infection, including meningitis, and kernicterus.

Clinical features

There is a mixture of muscle weakness and spasticity. This leads to characteristic joint deformities (Fig. 17.8). There may be athetosis and ataxia. This can be associated with varying degrees of cognitive impairment and emotional disturbance. Children may also develop seizures.

Diagnosis and investigation

Cerebral palsy is a clinical diagnosis which is based on a thorough birth and developmental history and is normally apparent within the first 2 years of life. MRI of the brain may show periventricular leukomalacia.

Management

Conservative

Depending upon the severity of the disease, children will benefit from physiotherapy, occupational therapy, speech and language therapy and other forms of special needs care.

Surgical

In children who have not developed fixed contractures, intramuscular botulinum injections can temporarily reduce spasticity. For fixed deformity, soft-tissue release or tendon lengthening is required to improve function. Severe muscle imbalance can result in bone deformity, sometimes requiring corrective osteotomy.

NON-ACCIDENTAL INJURY

Non-accidental injury (NAI) is becoming increasingly recognized and is often diagnosed late but it is important as the child may die.

Fig. 17.8 Characteristic joint deformities associated with cerebral palsy
Flexion at elbows and wrists with clasped fingers
Adductor spasticity of the hips, resulting in a 'scissors' stance
Flexion at the hips and knees
Equinus deformity of the feet

Clinical features

The history is often vague, inappropriate or changes each time it is told. In young children (<2 years) it is rare for accidental fractures to occur, particularly in long bones. Delayed presentation is often a feature of NAI.

The child may have external features of abuse such as bruising in other areas of the body away from the fracture. The child may be withdrawn, particularly when the parents are present.

Diagnosis and investigation

In suspected cases a skeletal survey or bone scan is performed to look for occult fractures. Certain fractures such as of the rib or tibial metaphysis are typical of NAI.

Conditions such as OI can be confused with NAI.

Management

The child should be admitted for protection if NAI is strongly suspected and the fracture should be treated in the usual way.

Paediatricians and social workers should be involved from early on.

Prognosis

A child left in an abusing environment has a 5% risk of death.

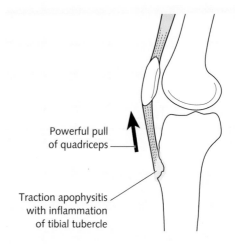

Powerful pull
of quadriceps —

Traction apophysitis
with inflammation
of tibial tubercle

Fig. 17.9 Osgood–Schlatter disease.

Clinical features

The patient complains of localized pain over the tubercle. The pain is usually made worse by activity and relieved by rest.

Clinically a tender swollen tuberosity is found.

Diagnosis and investigation

Fragmentation and sclerosis of the tibial tuberosity are present.

Sometimes a visible ossicle remains.

Management

Conservative

Treatment is with rest if the knee is very inflamed, with simple analgesia and modification of activities.

Parents are usually very worried and need reassurance.

The child may choose to 'put up' with the pain and continue sporting activities and this has no detrimental effect and will not prolong the natural history of the disease process.

Surgical

Surgery is used only for a painful ossicle.

Prognosis

The natural history is complete resolution of symptoms after 2 years.

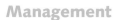

PAEDIATRIC KNEE CONDITIONS

Osgood–Schlatter disease

Definition

Osgood–Schlatter disease is traction apophysitis of the tibial tuberosity.

Incidence

The condition is very common, usually in adolescent boys.

Aetiology and pathology

It occurs during a period of rapid growth and is related to the pulling force of the patellar ligament on the tibial tuberosity (Fig. 17.9).

It is more common in athletic individuals.

Osteochondritis dissecans

Definition

Osteochondritis dissecans is a small area of avascular bone on an articular surface, usually of the knee.

Incidence

The incidence is 4 per 1000.

Presentation is between 10 and 20 years of age and is more common in boys.

Aetiology and pathology

The condition is most common in the knee (medial femoral condyle) but can affect other joints.

It is thought to be due to repeated trauma in a susceptible patient.

Clinical features

The patient has intermittent ache, swelling and 'catching' in the knee. The patient may complain of the knee giving way owing to acute sharp episodes of pain.

Diagnosis and investigation

X-rays show a variably sized lesion on the medial femoral condyle, which is fragmented in the child but in mature adults the lesion shows as a clear, demarcated sclerotic zone. The lesion can be attached or may be a loose body.

An MRI scan further defines the lesion. An isotope bone scan confirms the presence of activity and hence healing potential.

Management

Conservative

Activity modification with avoidance of sporting activity is adequate to allow small well-fixed lesions to heal.

Surgical

Lesions that become detached or give significant persistent symptoms require surgical stabilization. If the fragment becomes a loose body, removal may be the only option.

JUVENILE IDIOPATHIC ARTHRITIS

Definition

Juvenile idiopathic arthritis (JIA) is a chronic inflammatory condition in children which primarily involves synovial joints. It does not include 'specific' diseases

Fig. 17.10   The subtypes of juvenile idiopathic arthritis
Oligoarticular disease
Extended oligoarticular disease
Polyarticular disease – rheumatoid factor-negative
Polyarticular disease – rheumatoid factor-positive
Systemic-onset disease
Enthesitis-related arthritis
Psoriatic arthritis

such as systemic lupus erythematosus, or the arthritis of inflammatory bowel disease.

JIA has been classified into seven subtypes (Fig. 17.10). This classification is based partly on the number of joints involved 3 months into the disease process. It is useful as it gives a guide to prognosis.

Incidence and prevalence

Incidence is approximately 1 per 10 000 and prevalence is 10 per 10 000 children.

Clinical features

Joint disease

Children develop symptoms and signs of joint inflammation similar to those in adults, including joint pain, stiffness and swelling. Presentation depends on the joints affected and the age of the child. A 12-year-old with knee synovitis will complain of pain, whereas a 2-year-old may just be irritable and reluctant to mobilize. Paediatric Gait Arms Legs Spine (p-GALS) is a useful screening tool for examination of children.

Eye disease

Some forms of JIA can be associated with anterior uveitis. Acute anterior uveitis presents with pain and redness of the eye. Chronic anterior uveitis, however, is more insidious and can cause significant visual loss. All children with JIA need regular eye checks.

Constitutional symptoms

Fatigue, malaise and other systemic symptoms affect JIA patients, in particular those with systemic-onset disease. Growth retardation is an important consequence of prolonged inflammation in childhood.

JIA subtypes

Oligoarticular disease

Between one and four joints are affected, commonly in the lower limb. The prognosis is good; many children 'grow out of it'. This group of patients has the greatest risk of developing chronic anterior uveitis.

Extended oligoarticular disease

Initially fewer than four joints are involved, but these patients gradually develop a polyarthritis after the first 3 months. The outcome is often poor.

Polyarticular disease

More than four joints are affected from an early stage. There are two types. Rheumatoid factor-negative arthritis targets small and large joints and tends to persist into adult life. Rheumatoid factor-positive arthritis is the equivalent of adult RA. It is seen mainly in teenage girls and frequently has a poor outcome.

Systemic-onset disease

This arthritis is characterized by prominent systemic symptoms. It was previously known as Still disease. Patients present with a swinging fever, plus any of the following features:

- Evanescent rash.
- Hepatomegaly.
- Splenomegaly.
- Anaemia.
- Lymphadenopathy.
- Serositis, especially pericarditis.

The differential diagnosis includes infection and malignancy. Joint involvement may be mild or absent initially.

Enthesitis-related arthritis

Inflammation of entheses, e.g. Achilles tendonitis, is a prominent feature. Enthesitis-related arthritis encompasses juvenile ankylosing spondylitis. A positive family history of ankylosing spondylitis or related diseases is common and patients are often HLA B27-positive.

Psoriatic arthritis

This is usually oligoarticular and often involves weight-bearing joints. A personal or family history of psoriasis is common.

Investigations

The diagnosis of JIA is clinical. X-rays are helpful in excluding other causes of joint pain, such as malignancy, but are usually normal in early JIA.

Blood tests are useful, but not diagnostic. Full blood count may reveal anaemia or thrombocytosis and the erythrocyte sedimentation rate and C-reactive protein are usually elevated. Serum rheumatoid factor should be measured. It is also important to know if the patient has positive antinuclear antibodies, as they are associated with an increased risk of uveitis.

Management

> **HINTS AND TIPS**
>
> All children with JIA should be seen by a specialist.

Physiotherapy

This is vital to maintain mobility and function. Hydrotherapy is commonly used and is popular with children. Splinting is sometimes required to prevent deformity.

Drug treatment

Initial treatment is with non-steroidal anti-inflammatory drugs and corticosteroid joint injections. Disease-modifying therapy with drugs such as methotrexate is used. Corticosteroids may be necessary in severe or systemic-onset disease. Biological agents, such as the antitumour necrosis factor drugs, are indicated for children with persistent major synovitis or unresolving systemic features.

Eye screening

Children should have their eyes examined regularly by an ophthalmologist.

> **HINTS AND TIPS**
>
> Eye screening is particularly important in young children with JIA, as they do not reliably report visual disturbance to their parents.

Further reading

Cassidy, J.T., Petty, R.E., 2001. Textbook of Pediatric Rheumatology. Saunders, Philadelphia.

Orthoteers website: http://www.orthoteers.co.uk.

Prakken, B., Albani, S., Martini, A., 2011. Juvenile idiopathic arthritis. Lancet 377, 2138–2149.

Prince, F.N., Otten, M.H., van Suijlekom-Smit, L.W., 2010. Diagnosis and management of juvenile idiopathic arthritis. Br. Med. J. 341, 6434.

Solomon, L., Warwick, D., Nayagan, D. (Eds.), 2001. Apley's System of Orthopaedics and Fractures, eighth ed. Hodder Arnold, London.

Woo, P., Laxer, R.M., Sherry, D.D., 2007. Paediatric Rheumatology in Clinical Practice. Springer, London.

Objectives

After reading this chapter you should be able to:
- Understand the terms 'fracture' and 'pathological fracture'.
- Classify and describe fractures.
- Recognize the clinical features of a broken bone and know how to investigate this.
- Understand the basic principles of fracture management.
- Describe some of the common methods of surgical fixation of fractures.
- Describe the complications of fractures.
- Explain the difference between Colles and Smith fractures of the wrist.
- Understand the difference between intra- and extracapsular neck of femur fractures, and their differing management.
- Describe ankle fractures.

In this chapter we will discuss the basic principles of managing fractures, and describe the issues surrounding common fractures: wrist, hip and ankle fractures.

Advanced Trauma Life Support and the management of a multiply injured patient are covered in Chapter 19.

INCIDENCE

Fractures are very common and most of us will have at least one during a lifetime. They occur in peaks during childhood, young adult life and again in the elderly when osteoporosis has weakened bony structure (see Ch. 15).

DEFINITIONS

The following are the terms used to describe fractures (Fig. 18.1):

- Fracture: loss of continuity of the cortex of a bone.
- Pathological fracture: a fracture through bone weakened by a pre-existing pathological process.
- Simple: a bone fractured into two pieces.
- Comminuted: a bone in three or more pieces.
- Segmental: fractures at two levels of the same bone.
- Closed: a fracture with intact skin overlying it.
- Open: a fracture with a skin breach over it (formerly known as a compound fracture).
- Extra-articular: a fracture that leaves the adjacent joint entirely undamaged.
- Intra-articular: a fracture that involves a joint.

- Undisplaced: a fractured bone with its anatomy entirely unchanged.
- Displaced: a fracture whose components are no longer in their original anatomical position. Displacement describes the position of the distal fragment in relation to the proximal fragment. A displaced fracture may involve translation, angulation, rotation or distraction/compression.
- Fracture pattern: may be transverse, oblique or spiral.

The causes of pathological fractures are shown in Figure 18.2.

In children the fracture may occur through the growth plate (physis), and these injuries are classified as shown in Figure 18.3.

When concentrating on the bone it is easy to forget the soft tissues surrounding the bone. Soft-tissue integrity is vital, as it is the soft tissues that will eventually provide a healing environment to the injured bone via the blood supply from soft tissues. As a result a fracture can be thought of as a soft-tissue injury with a broken bone inside.

CLINICAL FEATURES

The patient almost always gives a clear history of an injury. Difficulty can arise if the patient cannot give a history – because of dementia in the elderly, intoxication or coma in major trauma. In cases where the history cannot be directly elicited, information must be obtained from a third person such as a carer, witness to the accident or ambulance personnel.

Fig. 18.1 Fracture patterns.

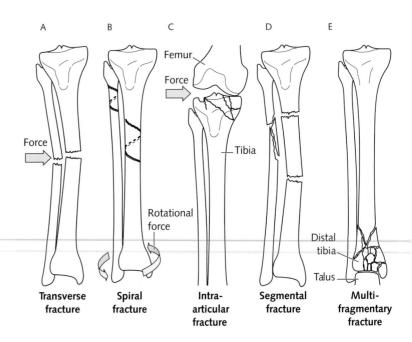

A	B	C	D	E
Transverse fracture	Spiral fracture	Intra-articular fracture	Segmental fracture	Multi-fragmentary fracture

Labels in figure: Femur, Force, Tibia, Rotational force, Distal tibia, Talus, Force

Fig. 18.2 Underlying causes in pathological fractures
Tumours

• Benign
• Malignant:
  • Metastasis (most common by far)
  • Primary

Paget disease
Metabolic bone disease
• Osteomalacia/rickets • Hyperparathyroidism • Osteogenesis imperfecta
Other malignancy
• Lymphoma • Myeloma
Rheumatoid arthritis
Infection

Patients will complain of pain. They may have noticed a deformity (e.g. 'my ankle pointed the wrong way, doctor').

The patient should be examined as a whole for associated injuries and then the injured limb.

The affected limb will be swollen and bruised with significant tenderness to palpation. The bone ends may be heard grating together (crepitus) but eliciting this is cruel and unnecessary (and may further damage soft tissues, or result in an open fracture).

It is very important to note and document:

- Skin condition (i.e. open or closed, but also note blisters, abrasions and swelling).
- Peripheral nerve function – any weakness or numbness of the hand or foot.
- Distal vascular status – assess peripheral pulse and capillary refill.

Compare the abnormal with the normal limb.

The patient may also have a clinical deformity associated with a particular fracture, such as angulation, shortening or a 'dinner fork' deformity in Colles fracture.

Patients with suspected spinal injuries need to be log-rolled, to avoid any further neurological injury, for examination and a full peripheral nervous system examination performed.

DIAGNOSIS AND INVESTIGATION

X-rays should be taken in two orthogonal planes (90° to each other) – usually anteroposterior (AP) and lateral – and include both ends of the injured bone. The anatomical area in question should be in the centre of the X-ray (Fig. 18.4). Special views are taken for certain fractures (e.g. scaphoid views).

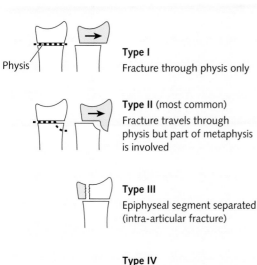

Type I
Fracture through physis only

Type II (most common)
Fracture travels through physis but part of metaphysis is involved

Type III
Epiphyseal segment separated (intra-articular fracture)

Type IV
Fracture crosses physis and involves joint interface
Requires accurate reduction to prevent growth problems leading to deformity

Type V
Crush injury
Difficult to diagnose initially becomes obvious later when growth arrest occurs

Fig. 18.3 The Salter–Harris classification of fractures of the growth plate (physeal fractures).

Computed tomography (CT) scans are helpful to diagnose and categorize complex fractures and to plan surgery.

Magnetic resonance imaging (MRI) or isotope bone scans are occasionally used to diagnose a fracture where doubt exists or to assess associated soft-tissue injuries.

Describing X-rays

This is something that requires a systematic approach and practice.

When asked to comment on an X-ray, state:

- Name and age of patient, and date of X-ray.

- What anatomical region is shown- e.g. AP X-ray of pelvis, lateral X-ray of a wrist.
- Remember ABC:
  - A is for adequacy and alignment (is the film rotated? of acceptable quality, i.e. too light or too dark?).
  - B is for bone:
    - State which bone is fractured, e.g. tibia.
    - State where in the bone the fracture is, i.e. metaphysis/diaphysis/epiphysis.
    - State whether the fracture is simple or comminuted.
    - Fracture pattern; transverse, oblique, spiral, segmental.
    - Displacement of the fracture (Fig. 18.5).
    - Joint: intra-articular, dislocation.
  - C is for covering soft tissues: look for air (may indicate an open fracture), foreign material, swelling or joint fluid – haemarthrosis or lipohaemarthrosis.

> **COMMUNICATION**
>
> When describing a fracture, remember to add important clinical features:
> - General condition of patient.
> - Skin (open or closed) (Fig. 18.6).
> - Neurovascular status.

MANAGEMENT

Initial management

Ensure the patient's general condition is optimized: airway, breathing, circulation, fluid management, oxygenation. Then:

- Control any external bleeding by direct pressure.
- For open fractures cover any wounds with sterile dressings. Ensure antibiotic cover and tetanus prophylaxis.
- Immobilize the fractured bone: plaster, splint, brace, sling.
- Give adequate and appropriate analgesia: often this will require intravenous opiates.
- Arrange investigations and form a management plan.

Definitive management

The basic principles for the treatment of any fracture are:

- Reduction of any deformity (displacement, angulation, rotation), i.e. put the bones back into the correct place.
- Stabilization (maintain reduction until healing occurs).

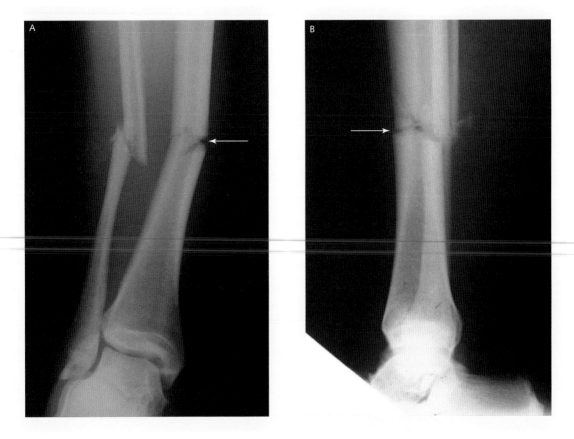

Fig. 18.4 Fracture of the tibia: (A) anteroposterior view showing angulation; (B) lateral view.

Fig. 18.5 Deformity associated with fractures.

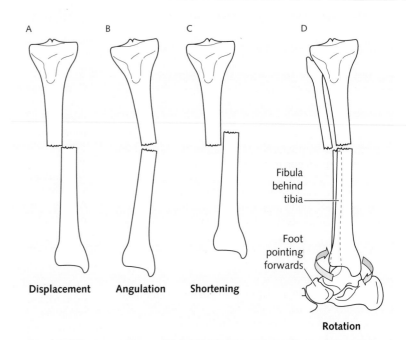

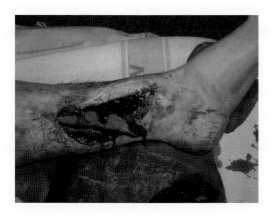

Fig. 18.6 An open tibial fracture.

- Rehabilitation (rehabilitate the limb and the person back to normality).

Reduction

Reduction can be performed open or closed.

- Closed reduction is performed by manipulating the fracture into position. This can be done under sedation or a general anaesthetic.
- Open reduction is performed in the operating theatre and involves a surgical procedure to open up the fracture site and accurately reduce the bones under direct vision. It is usually accompanied by operative stabilization.

Intra-articular fractures are treated with open reduction so that the joint can be accurately reduced, minimizing the risk of secondary osteoarthritis.

Stabilization

This can be achieved by external splintage ,e.g. plaster cast, without an operation. Intraoperative fixation can be with percutaneous pinning with wires, plates and screws, intramedullary nail for long-bone fractures or external frame fixation (Fig. 18.7).

Rehabilitation

Following healing, or if the fracture is stable, the limb can be mobilized and range-of-movement exercises begun. One of the principles of operative stabilization is to allow early mobilization. The physiotherapist may need to instruct the patient in the use of crutches for restricted weight bearing.

Rehabilitation of the limb may often take as much time as the fracture took to heal.

Following a hip fracture elderly patients require intensive input from physiotherapy, occupational therapy and social workers in order to become self-caring and safe prior to discharge.

COMPLICATIONS OF FRACTURES

Any complication can be local or general, and immediate, early or late.

Fig. 18.7 Methods of surgical stabilization of fractures.

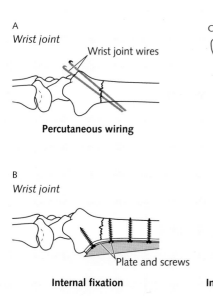

A
Wrist joint

Wrist joint wires

Percutaneous wiring

B
Wrist joint

Plate and screws

Internal fixation

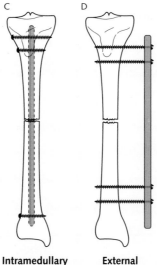

C

Intramedullary nail

D

External fixation

Immediate

Local

Initial displacement can cause the skin to tear, resulting in an open fracture. Fracture fragments may press on nerves, producing a nerve palsy (common in the humerus, resulting in radial nerve palsy) or blood vessels, producing ischaemia (e.g. femur – popliteal vessels).

Very occasionally nerves and blood vessels are completely torn and repair is needed.

General

Haemorrhage from fractures can be excessive, especially from femoral, pelvis, open or multiple fractures. Hypovolaemic shock may result (see Ch. 21).

Early

Local

Compartment syndrome

This is a true emergency in orthopaedics. It results from excessive pressure developing in a closed fascial muscle compartment; the forearm and lower leg are the commonest sites. Whilst uncommon, if left untreated the condition can be limb- or even life-threatening. Following an injury (within a few hours usually), swelling can cause the blood supply to the muscle to be impaired, causing muscle ischaemia. This occurs at the level of small vessels, and peripheral pulses are usually still present. The patient will complain of extreme pain (much more than normal) and increased pain on passive stretching of the muscles in the compartment. Paraesthesia and pulselessness are late signs; irreparable damage has already occurred. The diagnosis is clinical (it is possible to confirm it with pressure monitoring). Immediate treatment is by removal of any circumferential bandage or splint. If the pain does not settle within 15 minutes surgical decompression (fasciotomy) is required at once.

Infection

This can occur early or late following operative stabilization or open fracture. See Chapter 21.

Complex regional pain syndrome

This unusual condition can occur after any injury or operation. The exact cause is not known but is thought to relate to the sympathetic nervous system.

Usually the upper limb, or foot and ankle, is affected. The patient has red, swollen shiny fingers with excessive joint stiffness. Atypical pain is a feature. Referral to a multidisciplinary pain management team is indicated.

General

Thromboembolism

Deep vein thrombosis can occur after any lower-limb injury. Prevention in the form of mechanical (foot pumps, graduated compression stockings) or chemical agents is routinely used.

The limb will be swollen and may be painful because of the injury. If in doubt obtain a duplex scan or venogram. Some at-risk patients are treated prophylactically with anticoagulation. Pulmonary embolism is a rare, but potentially fatal, complication.

Fat embolus

This condition may occur after long-bone fractures (particularly of the femur) and occurs due to fat entering the circulation and embolizing to the lungs. The condition occurs because the medullary canal of long bones contains fat. Early stabilization of fractures reduces the risk.

The patient presents with shortness of breath, petechial haemorrhages and sometimes confusion from low circulating P_{O_2} usually 2–3 days after injury.

This condition is potentially very serious and may lead on to acute adult respiratory distress syndrome, which can be fatal.

Treatment is supportive with oxygen and fluids. Transfer to a high-dependency unit is advised.

Late

Delayed union/non-union

Some fractures are slow to unite or fail to do so despite adequate treatment. Certain fractures (e.g. of the tibia) are more prone to this and it is more likely if the initial injury was high-energy or complicated by compartment syndrome. Further surgery may be required to encourage the bone to heal.

Malunion

The fracture heals but in an abnormal position. This is usually due to inadequate reduction or stabilization of the fracture. The resulting deformity may reduce movement in an associated joint and predisposes to late arthritis.

Osteoarthritis

Osteoarthritis, which is discussed in Chapter 11, is more common after intra-articular fractures.

Stiffness

Prolonged immobilization can result in severe joint stiffness. The joint may be held in a flexed positon from ligament and capsular contracture.

Growth disturbance

Fractures occurring through the growth plate in children can stop growth. Growth arrest can be partial (i.e. one side of the limb grows, the other does not), leading to deformity, or complete, leading to shortness of the limb. Treatment of such problems is complex.

COMMON FRACTURES

Any bone can be fractured and the patterns and treatment options are extensive. It is beyond the realms of this book to cover all of them. Consequently we have picked three common fractures to discuss: distal radial, hip and ankle.

Distal radial fractures

These are common at all stages of life, from greenstick fractures in children to osteoporotic fractures in the elderly. They are usually the result of a fall on to an outstretched hand.

Clinical features

The patient will present with a grossly swollen and frequently deformed wrist (the deformity will depend upon the type of fracture). Pain will be the main complaint. The patient will have a markedly reduced range of motion at the wrist. The patient may complain of altered sensation in the hand due to compression of the median nerve. The commonest fracture is dorsally translated and dorsally and radially angulated. This is commonly called a Colles fracture. A distal radius fracture that is volarly translated and angulated in known as a Smith fracture (Fig. 18.8).

Investigations

Wrist fractures are diagnosed with plain film X-ray. Heavily comminuted or intra-articular fractures may require a CT scan, for planning prior to theatre.

Treatment

The fracture pattern and the age, comorbidity and function of the patient will influence treatment.

Undisplaced fractures of the wrist, minimally angulated fractures and angulated fractures in the elderly may only require immobilization in a cast for 4–6 weeks. Very comminuted and intra-articular fractures, and angulated fractures in young and high-demand patients will require open reduction and internal fixation.

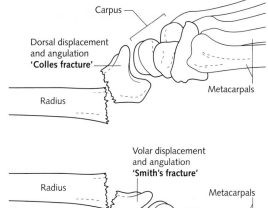
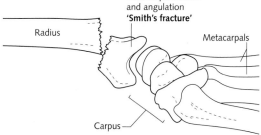

Fig. 18.8 Common distal radial fractures (lateral view).

Whatever treatment option is used the wrist will often be stiff afterwards and require physiotherapy to restore movement.

Hip fractures

Hip fractures, or femoral neck fractures, are very common. They particularly occur in elderly patients with osteoporosis. Femoral neck fractures can also occur as pathological fractures related to metastatic malignancy. They are rare in young patients when they occur after high-energy trauma and are subject to different considerations. Hip fractures in the elderly place a huge impact on health resources, as well as having major implications to the patient with regard to mortality, disability and loss of independence. Approximately one-third of patients with a hip fracture will die within a year of injury.

Hip fractures can be broadly divided (Fig. 18.9) into:

- Intracapsular fractures.
- Extracapsular fractures (intertochanteric, subtrochanteric).

The blood supply to the femoral head orginitates predominantly from the medial femoral circumflex artery via the ascending cervical arteries. These travel from the capsular attachment along the intertrochanteric line to the femoral head and are closely attached to the posterior femoral neck. Consequently:

- In an intracapsular fracture (Fig. 18.10A), the fracture line is between the blood supply and the head, potentially severing the blood supply to the head. This leads to a risk of avascular necrosis and non-union.

- In an extracapsular fracture (Fig. 18.10B), the head is in continuity with its blood supply and therefore the head does not have a risk of avascular necrosis.

Aetiology

Most hip fractures are the result of a simple fall from standing height.

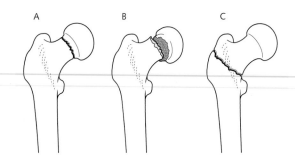

Fig. 18.9 Fractures of the femoral neck: (A) undisplaced intracapsular fracture; (B) displaced intracapsular fracture; (C) extracapsular trochanteric fracture.

Clinical features

The patient will complain of severe pain around the affected hip or in the groin. This pain will be exacerabated by any attempt to move the leg. The patient will usually be unable to weight bear.

Classically patients will have a shortened and externally rotated leg on the affected side. They will be unable to straight-leg raise because of pain in the hip or groin. The patient may demonstrate tenderness on palpation over the greater trochanter or in the groin.

Diagnosis

Femoral neck fractures are usually diagnosed with plain film X-rays (AP pelvis, and lateral hip views). However sometimes occult fractures may not show up on X-ray, and further imaging may be required – MRI or isotope bone scan.

Treatment

Non-operative treatrment with immobilization carries a very high mortality and morbidity rate. In the vast majority of cases, femoral neck fractures are treated surgically. Postoperative patients are mobilized early to minimize these complications. Even when faced with a bed-bound nursing home resident, surgeons still usually operate to provide pain relief.

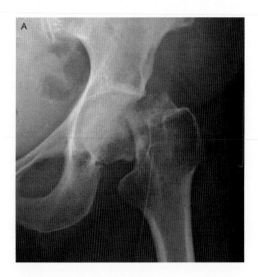
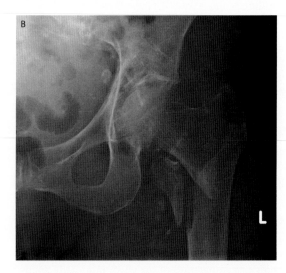

Fig. 18.10 (A) Intracapsular fracture with the fracture line potentially severing the blood supply to the head. (B) Extracapsular fracture with blood supply intact.

Intracapsular fractures can be divided into undisplaced and displaced.

- Undisplaced fractures have a low chance of disruption to their blood supply, and can be treated with internal fixation. However a third will develop avascular necrosis or a non-union and must be followed closely.
- Displaced fractures (Fig. 18.11) are normally treated with hemiarthroplasty; the femoral head is removed, leaving the artificial head articulating with the normal acetabulum. A total hip replacement may be more appropriate in younger or more active patients.

Extracapsular fractures are trochanteric or subtrochanteric and are treated with internal fixation with either a dynamic hip screw or an intramedullary nail.

HINTS AND TIPS

The subtrochanteric region is a common place for metastatic deposits. Be suspicious of a fracture in this region and consider getting preoperative imaging ± biopsy.

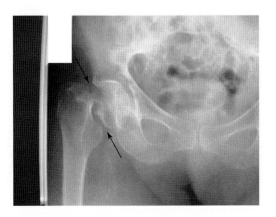

Fig. 18.11 Displaced intracapsular hip fracture (arrows).

Ankle fractures

The tibia and fibula form a 'mortice' in which the talar dome sits, supported by ligaments. Damage to the bones or ligaments can lead to instability.

Clinical features

The patient will describe pain and swelling around the ankle, and may be unable to weight bear. The ankle may be obviously deformed. There will be tenderness over fracture or ligaments. The fibula can fracture anywhere along its length in some fractures – palpate for tenderness along its length; a high fibular fracture results in an unstable ankle – a Maisonneuve fracture. It is important to check the neurological and vascular status of the foot.

Diagnosis

Diagnosis is once again made by X-ray. However you should not wait for an X-ray before you reduce an obviously deformed ankle. If no fracture can be seen at the ankle on the background significant ankle injury, or there is proximal fibular tenderness, a full-length tibia and fibula X-ray is required.

Management

Fracture patterns thought to be stable can be managed conservatively with external splintage. Unstable ankle fractures – usually injuries that involve both the medial and lateral sides of the ankle – require surgical stabilization.

Further reading

Charnley, J., 1999. The closed treatment of common fractures, new Golden Jubilee edition. Colt Books, Cambridge (*gives an excellent practical account of plaster and traction techniques*).

McRae, R., 2008. Practical Fracture Treatment. Churchill Livingstone.

Orthoteers website: http://www.orthoteers.co.uk.

Wheeless' Textbook of Orthopaedics. Available online at: http://www.wheelessonline.com.

After reading this chapter you should be able to:
- Understand the principles of Advanced Trauma Life Support (ATLS).
- Define and understand the management of open fractures.
- Understand basic spine anatomy and recognize structures that can be injured.
- Understand the signs and consequences of pelvic trauma.

DEFINITION

Trauma can refer to any bodily injury but in the context of surgery normally refers to a patient with major isolated or multiple injuries.

INCIDENCE

Trauma is the leading cause of death in the first four decades of life, the majority from road traffic accidents.

CLINICAL FEATURES

The Advanced Trauma Life Support programme and the Golden Hour

ATLS prioritzes examination and intervention by system, so that the most immediately life-threatening injuries are treated first: this is known as the primary survey. This can be remembered simply as 'ABCDE' and is summarized in Figure 19.1. It is important to reassess the patient continually.

Airway

Lack of oxygenated blood delivered to the brain and other major organs causes rapid death in the injured patient. A protected, unobstructed airway is a priority in order to avoid hypoxia. A patient's airway can be compromised with:

- A decreased level of consciousness (head injury, hypoxia, hypovolaemia, drugs).
- Facial trauma.
- Neck trauma.
- Aspiration of vomit or teeth.

- Swelling of subcutaneous tissues associated with burns or smoke inhalation.

Assessment of airway patency should be rapid (Fig. 19.2). All trauma patients should receive oxygen initially.

Cervival spine control

All trauma patients should be assumed to have unstable neck injuries until proven otherwise, especially in those with an altered conscious level or with injuries above the level of the clavicle. The cervical spine can be immobilized manually or with an appropriately sized hard collar, sandbags and tape across the patient's forehead. The patient should remain immobilized until the cervical spine can be cleared both clinically and radiologically.

Breathing

Adequate ventilation is required in order to oxygenate blood and therefore major organs such as the brain. Causes of ventilatory compromise include:

- Central nervous system depression (head injury, alcohol, drugs, cervical spine injury).
- Tension pneumothorax (needs immediate decompression *before* a chest X-ray).
- Open pneumothorax.
- Rib fractures.
- Haemothorax.
- Flail chest.

Figure 19.2 shows some signs of airway and ventilatory compromise.

Circulation

Shock is defined as inadequate organ perfusion and tissue oxygenation. The most common cause of this in the trauma patient is hypovolaemia secondary to haemorrhage.

Fig. 19.1	Priorities for Advanced Trauma Life Support
A	Airway with cervical spine control
B	Breathing
C	Circulation with haemorrhage control
D	Disability/neurological evaluation
E	Exposure and environment

Fig. 19.3	Neurological assessment using AVPU
A	*Alert*
V	Responds to *verbal* stimuli
P	Responds to *pain*
U	*Unresponsive*

It is important to recognize hypovolaemic shock so that treatment is not delayed. The patient should have pulse rate, blood pressure, capillary refill, urinary output and conscious level closely monitored. Clinical findings allow the doctor to estimate the circulating blood volume (approximately 5 L in adults). Blood pressure can be normal with up to 30% blood loss, but, as the patient decompensates, there is tachycardia, hypotension and confusion.

There are five areas to consider for potential blood loss – chest, abdomen, pelvis, long bones … and on the floor (at the scene of the accident as well as in hospital). Intravenous access should be gained as soon as possible and appropriate fluid resusitation commenced.

Disability/neurological status

This is based on the Glasgow Coma Scale and ranges from 3 to 15. This should be monitored regularly to observe for deterioration in the patient's condition. A simpler method to determine conscious level is AVPU (Fig. 19.3).

Exposure and secondary survey

Look from head to toe for other injuries. This includes log-rolling the patient (with cervical spine control) to assess for trauma to the back and spine.

The secondary survey involves a full history and examination of all systems. It is important that the secondary survey does not begin untill the primary survey is complete and initial management has begun.

COMMUNICATION

When taking a history from a multiply injured patient, the assessment should be rapid to avoid delays in diagnosis of life-threatening conditions. Specifically ask about allergies, drug history, past medical history, the last time the patient ate or drank and the events surrounding the injury. Seek a collateral history from others such as paramedics or people at the scene for clues about the mechanism (e.g. damage to the car) and to gain an idea of the patient's initial condition.

INVESTIGATIONS

A trauma series of X-rays (performed in the resuscitation area) should include at least chest and pelvis films, and, if indicated, cervical spine films. Blood tests include full blood count, urea and creatinine, clotting and blood should be grouped and saved in case the patient needs a blood transfusion.

Fig. 19.2	Signs and symptoms of airway and breathing compromise	
Signs	**Airway compromise**	**Inadequate ventilation**
Look	Poor respiratory effort Agitation (hypoxia) Cyanosis Decreased consciousness (unable to protect airway) Tongue, loose teeth, vomit or blood	Asymmetrical rise of chest wall (flail chest, pneumothorax) Laboured breathing Increased respiratory rate Visible penetrating wounds Low oxygen saturations
Listen	Stridor (upper-airway obstruction causing inspiratory noise) Hoarse voice (burns)	Decreased/unequal air entry (haemopneumothorax)
Feel	Remove visible obstructions	Trachea deviation (tension pneumothorax) Tenderness or crepitus (rib fractures) Unequal chest expansion Percussion (hyperresonant = pneumothorax; dull = haemothorax)

TREATMENT

Treat life-threatening conditions in order, using ABCDE. It is then important to identify all other injuries through the secondary survey so that they can be managed by the relevant surgical specialties.

OPEN FRACTURES

Definition

This is when there is an external wound leading to the fracture site potentially allowing contamination with bacteria (see Fig. 18.6). They were formerly called compound fractures.

Incidence

Incidence of open fracture is approximately 23 per 100 000 patients per year.

Aetiology and pathology

Most open fractures are the result of high-energy trauma, and are associated with significant damage to soft tissues. They can also occur when the fracture is grossly angulated or displaced, and the sharp fracture end exits through the skin. The greatest risk to the bone is infection and the development of chronic osteomyelitis.

Clinical features

Check ABCDE. Assess the fractured limb for deformity and neurovascular status. Any wound around the fracture site should be assumed to communicate with the bone. Also assess for evidence of compartment syndrome (still possible in open fractures).

Management

The wound should be photographed then irrigated, and dressed with saline-soaked swabs. Splint the limb and start intravenous antibiotics as soon as possible. Give tetanus prophylaxis if immunizations are not up to date. The wound should be aggressively debrided in theatre as soon as possible (without putting the patient's health at risk), to minimize bacterial infection of the fracture. The fracture can then be stabilized with a suitable method of internal or external fixation.

SPINAL INJURIES

Definition

Spinal injuries include fractures and subluxations/dislocations of vertebrae. They also include damage to the spinal cord, even in the absence of a fracture.

Incidence

This is a common injury in the trauma patient. In all, 10–20% of patients with a spinal fracture will have a second spinal fracture at another level.

Aetiology and pathology

Spinal injuries most often occur after road traffic accidents. Other examples include neck injuries from diving into a shallow pool, thoracic injuries from hyperflexion and lumbar injuries, which commonly occur from falls from a height. Thoracolumbar injuries classically occurred as a result of wearing a lap belt in a road traffic accident. In elderly patients with osteoporosis, low-energy trauma can result in simple wedge fractures (see Ch. 15).

The stability of the spine depends on the bony structures and the integrity of strong ligaments. It can be thought of as two columns (Fig. 19.4). Fractures involving one column only, such as anterior wedge fractures, are stable (see Fig. 15.5) and can be treated conservatively. Fractures involving both columns, such as a high-energy burst fracture (Fig. 19.5), are often unstable. Injuries may involve the bony structures only, both ligaments and bones or purely ligaments. This means that even if the X-ray is normal, you cannot assume the spine is stable as *all* the ligaments may be torn!

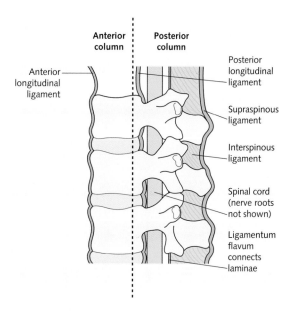

Fig. 19.4 Anatomy of the spine divided into anterior and posterior columns.

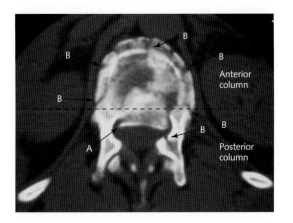

Fig. 19.5 Axial computed tomography scan showing an unstable two-column burst fracture (arrows B) with retropulsion of a bone fragment (arrow A) into the spinal canal.

Clinical features

Check ABCDE. The conscious patient will complain of pain at the level of injury (beware in patients with decreased conscious level).

Clinical examination may reveal tenderness, a boggy swelling, bony step or a gibbus. The patient should be log-rolled with cervical spine control in order to examine the thoracic and lumbar spine. Check limbs for abnormal neurology. A full neurological examination should include a rectal examination for anal tone and sensation (sacral nerves). Knowledge of dermatomes and myotomes will guide the doctor to the level of spinal cord injury if present.

Remember that spinal injury may cause bradycardia and hypotension (spinal shock). These patients should receive intravenous fluids cautiously.

Diagnosis and investigation

Neck – anteroposterior, lateral (to at least T1) and odontoid peg views.

Thoracic and lumbar spine – anteroposterior and lateral views if indicated.

X-rays can be normal, even with spinal cord trauma.

Further imaging may be required – CT in the case of equivocal or inadequate X-rays; magnetic resonance imaging to look for ligament and spinal cord damage.

Treatment

This depends on the stability of the fracture.

Stable fractures can be mobilized.

Unstable fractures require immobilization (e.g. halo vest), bracing or possibly internal fixation.

Prognosis

The patients with spinal cord damage have the worst prognosis and often require extensive rehabilitation on a spinal unit.

PELVIC FRACTURES

These are high-energy injuries commonly associated with massive bleeding, urethral, bladder and abdominal injuries.

Incidence

Pelvic fractures are rare injuries but careful assessment of the polytraumatized patient is necessary to avoid missing them. Most deaths in polytrauma patients occur as a result of pelvic fractures.

Aetiology

The pelvis can be thought of as a stable ring formed from the sacrum, ilium and pubis bones held together by strong ligaments. The basic mechanisms of injury are anteroposterior compression (blow from the front: Fig. 19.6), lateral compression (side impact), vertical shear forces (usually fall from height) or a combination of all three.

Clinical features

Once again check ABCDE. The patient will have pain and may be shocked due to blood loss.

Clinical examination may reveal asymmetery to the pelvis or lower limbs, and bruisng and swelling around the pelvis itself. There may be blood at the urethral meatus (urethral tear) and bruising in the scrotal region.

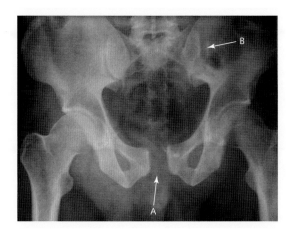

Fig. 19.6 X-ray of an open-book pelvic fracture. There is widening at the symphysis pubis (arrow A) and the left sacroiliac joint (arrow B).

Rectal examination may reveal blood or a boggy, high-riding prostate (urethral tear). Bone fragments may be palpable. Do *not* assess pelvic stability by bimanual compression of the iliac wings ('springing' the pelvis) as this may displace a clot and cause rebleeding.

Diagnosis and investigation

An anteroposterior X-ray of the pelvis should be checked for fractures, symmetry and normal contours. Once stable, a CT scan more accurately defines the fracture.

Emergency treatment

The patient should be managed according to ATLS protocol and resuscitated with intravenous fluids. Those patients who either transiently respond or do not respond are likely to have ongoing bleeding. There is haemorrhage from bones, the pelvic venous plexus and, rarely, arteries.

Bleeding can be reduced by stabilizing the pelvis. This can be done immediately by tying a bed sheet around the pelvis, or applying a pelvic binder – this closes the pelvic ring and reduces its volume. If this fails, angiography and embolization of bleeding vessels or laparotomy may be required.

Stable fractures require pain relief and mobilization. Unstable fracture patterns require surgical fixation.

Prognosis

Mortality can be high, especially when the patient has associated head, chest or abdominal injuries. Complications such as urethral tears, sciatic nerve damage or persistent sacroiliac pain can affect quality of life in the long term.

Further reading

Committee on Trauma, American College of Surgeons, 2008. Advanced Trauma Life Support for Doctors, eighth ed. American College of Surgeons, Chicago, IL.
Orthoteers website: http://www.orthoteers.co.uk.

Infection of bones and joints 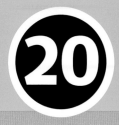20

● Objectives

After reading this chapter you should be able to:
- List the common organisms associated with osteomyelitis.
- Know how osteomyelitis develops and understand the terms 'sequestrum' and 'involucrum'.
- Recognize the clinical features of septic arthritis in children and adults.
- Describe the treatment and complications of septic arthritis.
- Know useful investigations for the diagnosis of bone and joint sepsis.
- Describe the features of tuberculosis (TB) and how these differ from other orthopaedic infections.

Introduction

Bone and joint infection has thankfully become much less common in western society over the last century. This is explained by increasing use of antibiotics and the general improvement in nutrition and health of the population as a whole.

Infection does still occur and needs to be recognized and treated promptly to avoid serious or potentially fatal complications.

In this chapter we will discuss osteomyelitis (infection in bone) and septic arthritis (infection in a joint).

OSTEOMYELITIS

Infection of bone can be caused by direct inoculation (exogenous) or blood-borne bacteria (haematogenous).

In childhood or adolescence osteomyelitis is usually caused by haematogenous spread of bacteria. In adults the source is more likely to be exogenous, most commonly due to infection developing after surgery or after injury (particularly in the case of an open fracture).

Incidence

Osteomyelitis is now uncommon.

Aetiology and pathology

In children there is often a history of preceding trauma, which may predispose the limb to infection. The most common infecting organism overall is *Staphylococcus aureus*; other pathogens are shown in Figure 20.1. If unusual organisms are present, consider specific predisposing factors, as listed in Figure 20.2; for example,

patients with acquired immunodeficiency syndrome (AIDS) can get fungal infections.

The three most common causes of osteomyelitis are:

1. Posttrauma osteomyelitis.
2. Postsurgery osteomyelitis.
3. Acute haematogenous osteomyelitis.

Posttrauma osteomyelitis

An open fracture means the skin is broken, allowing bacteria direct access to the bony surfaces. Large dirty wounds associated with high-energy injuries are more likely to result in posttrauma osteomyelitis. Urgent surgical debridement and lavage are required in order to remove contaminated material and dead bone, and reduce the risk of subsequent osteomyelitis. Inadequate or delayed surgery will lead to osteomyelitis due to bacteria being harboured within dead bone. In these circumstances the fracture will often fail to heal – an infected non-union.

Postsurgery osteomyelitis

Many surgical procedures in orthopaedics involve using implants such as joint prostheses or plates and screws. These 'foreign bodies' can harbour infection if bacteria are introduced at the time of surgery. Due to the lack of blood supply to the implants, eradication is almost impossible without surgery. For this reason orthopaedic surgeons are fastidious about aseptic techniques in the operating theatre, and routinely use antibiotics as prophylaxis. Despite this, infection does still occur and may spread around the implant, devitalizing bone.

Acute haematogenous osteomyelitis

This form of osteomyelitis is usually seen in children and may develop spontaneously, but frequently may

Fig. 20.1 Common pathogens in osteomyelitis

Patient age	Common organisms
Newborns (younger than 6 months)	*Staphylococcus aureus, Streptococcus* (group A and B), *Enterobacter*
Children (6 months to adult)	*Staphylococcus aureus, Haemophilus influenzae, Streptococcus, Enterobacter*
Adult	*Staphylococcus aureus, Streptococcus, Enterobacter*
Immunocompromised	*Pseudomonas, Mycobacterium tuberculosis,* fungal infection

Fig. 20.2 Conditions associated with osteomyelitis

Congenital	Acquired
Sickle cell disease Haemophilia	Diabetes Renal failure Intravenous drug use Malnutrition Immunosuppression Human immunodeficiency virus (HIV)/acquired immunodeficiency syndrome (AIDS)

be precipitated by trauma. Blood supply to bone is from the endosteum and periosteum.

The pathogenesis of acute haematogenous osteomyelitis is as follows (Fig. 20.3):

1. A bacteraemia that settles in the metaphysis of a long bone.
2. Inflammation and pus formation within the bone.
3. Pus escapes through the haversian canals to form a subperiosteal abscess.
4. Pus is now present on both sides of the bone, causing this part of the bone to die.
5. Dead bone, now called the sequestrum, harbours infection.
6. Periosteal new bone, called involucrum, forms around the sequestrum as the body tries to fight the infection.

Acute osteomyelitis can easily become chronic if the sequestrum is neglected or not completely excised at surgery.

Other conditions associated with osteomyelitis

The above three causes of osteomyelitis are the most common but it also occurs in the other conditions listed in Figure 20.2.

Fig. 20.3 Sequence of events in osteomyelitis. The primary focus of infection (A) has spread through bone, causing the death of cortical bone and formation of a subperiosteal abscess (B). Infection can spread into the joint (C), causing septic arthritis. Death of a segment of bone (sequestrum) occurs (D), and the area is surrounded by new subperiosteal bone (involucrum).

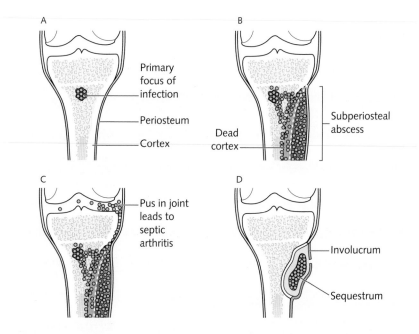

Sadly we are now seeing more and more cases of bone and joint infection in intravenous drug users. When you consider that these patients are often malnourished, immunosuppressed (possibly human immunodeficiency virus (HIV)-positive), frequently inject themselves deeply with dirty needles and often neglect small abscesses, it is not difficult to understand why. Consequently these patients are at risk of oppurtunistic infections.

Clinical features

Acute osteomyelitis causes pain, fever and loss of funtion (often a limp if the lower limb is involved).

It is more common in the tibia and femur. The limb will be tender to palpate, erythematous and possibly swollen.

At the extremes of age (neonate, infant or elderly) the symptoms and signs are often non-specific (such as general malaise). These patients can be seriously ill and it can be extremely difficult to pinpoint the exact site of the problem.

Occasionally a patient presents with multiple sites affected or there may be another focus of infection which has then spread from or to bone, for example infective endocarditis. This is called seeding of infection.

In postsurgery and posttrauma osteomyelitis, the wound will be painful, red and inflamed. Normally, once postoperative pain has settled, patients are comfortable and can mobilize without pain. If pain persists or increases, infection is a possible cause. Wounds will continue to leak, and eventually break down or there will be dehiscence. If left untreated a sinus will result.

A limb with chronic osteomyelitis will be swollen and have thickened 'woody' skin. Here the focus of infection remains within the bone as a sequestrum and the infection remains quiet for a period of time (can be many years) and then flares up unexpectedly, often producing an abscess. A chronic discharging sinus can result.

Diagnosis and investigation

The diagnosis may be obvious on clinical features, particularly if the history reveals a clear predisposing factor.

A raised white cell count (WCC), erythrocyte sedimentation rate (ESR) and C-reactive protein (CRP) will be present on blood tests.

Initially X-rays will be normal, but after 10 days, features of lysis, periosteal elevation and new bone formation are seen. Later the sequestrum may be seen as a sclerotic area. A Brodie's abscess may be seen in the distal femur (Fig. 20.4).

Early osteomyelitis can be detected before X-ray changes, using a bone scan or white cell-labelled scan (shows increased uptake) or magnetic resonance imaging.

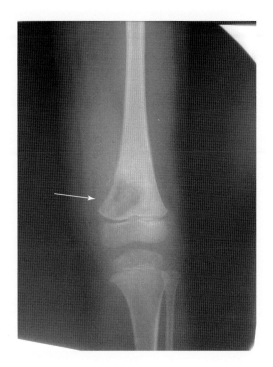

Fig. 20.4 Brodie's abscess (arrow).

It is very important to send microbiology specimens such as blood cultures prior to starting antibiotics.

Management

Conservative

The patient needs adequate analgesia, splintage of the affected limb and appropriate antibiotics. Most hospitals or health boards will have an antibiotic policy; however, consultation with the microbiologist is advisable.

As the majority of infections are with *Staphylococcus aureus*, flucloxacillin is the first-line antibiotic, usually in combination with fusidic acid or rifampacin. The course is given initially intravenously for 6 weeks, with further oral antibiotics if necessary.

Antibiotic-resistant strains such as meticillin-resistant *Staphylococcus aureus* (MRSA) are becoming more prevalent and, if suspected, then vancomycin or teicoplanin can be used instead after consultation with a microbiologist.

Provided the patient does not have an abscess or dead bone present, then antibiotics will suffice.

Surgical

If an abscess is present this should be drained surgically. Dead bone, the sequestrum, needs to be removed, otherwise irradication is impossible.

In a chronic case if the patient and surgeon decide to attempt to cure the infection, extensive surgery is required to remove all infected bone, and implants if presents. Techniques for doing this vary depending on the extent of involvement and the site.

It is possible simply to treat the 'flare-ups' and suppress the infection with antibiotics when required – particularly in patients not fit for major surgery.

Complications

Complications occur if:

- Osteomyelitis persists.
- The physis is damaged, leading to growth disturbance and deformity.
- The infection spreads to the joint, causing septic arthritis.

Prognosis

For acute osteomyelitis the outcome is good and the majority make a full recovery provided none of the above complications occur. In chronic cases following surgery or trauma many surgical procedures are often required and amputation is not an uncommon outcome.

HINTS AND TIPS

Chronic osteomyelitis is very difficult to treat. It may remain dormant for many years and then flare up intermittently, causing pain and loss of function. These flare-ups are often managed simply with antibiotics. Some people cannot tolerate long-term loss of function of the limb, in which case amputation may be indicated.

SEPTIC ARTHRITIS

Septic arthritis is infection within a synovial joint.

Incidence

The condition is uncommon, but is seen more often in children, young adults and the elderly. It is more common in the developing world and in patients with a predisposing factor. In children, it is less common than osteomyelitis.

Aetiology and pathology

Infection reaches a joint via the haematogenous route, direct spread from the metaphysis or penetrating trauma/surgery. Associated conditions are similar to those for acute osteomyelitis (see Fig. 20.2), with the addition of rheumatoid arthritis and crystal arthropathy.

Certain organisms are more common at different ages. *Haemophilus influenzae* used to be the most common infecting organism in infants prior to the introduction of the vaccination programme. In young sexually active adults the most likely infecting organism is *Neisseria gonorrhoeae*.

In haematogenous septic arthritis the bacterium settles in the synovium, which may be inflamed due to trauma or disease. Proliferation of bacteria causes an inflammatory response by the host with numerous leukocytes migrating into the joint. The variety of enzymes and breakdown products produced damages the delicate articular cartilage very quickly (within hours) and, if left unchecked, permanent damage will ensue (Fig. 20.5).

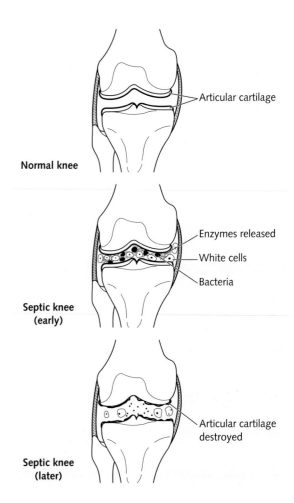

Fig. 20.5 Sequence of events in septic arthritis.

Clinical features

The patient will have an acutely hot swollen joint with a fever and be systemically unwell. An infant or young child will be distressed, unwell and difficult to assess. There may be a history of recent systemic infection such as otitis media.

Septic arthritis is more common in the hip and knee but can present in any synovial joint.

Any movement at all causes intense pain, and weight bearing will not be tolerated. If the joint is superficial an effusion is palpable.

In neonates and infants the diagnosis may be less obvious, particularly if the joint is deeply situated, such as the hip. These patients may be seriously unwell, and systemically compromised.

HINTS AND TIPS

Patients with an infected joint will not let you put the joint through a passive range of movement. It is too painful!

Diagnosis and investigation

- WCC, CRP and ESR will be raised.
- X-rays will be normal initially and show joint destruction late.
- If available, ultrasound scanning is useful to see if there is a joint effusion where the hip is the suspicious joint.
- Any joint suspected of infection must be aspirated and sent for urgent Gram stain, culture and examination for crystals.

Management

Conservative

Relieve pain by giving analgesia and splinting the limb. Aspiration should be performed at the earliest oppurtunity, preferably before the commencement of antibiotics. Give appropriate antibiotics as directed by the microbiologist, depending on the age of the patient and any predisposing illness.

Surgical

Unlike in osteomyelitis, the treatment of septic arthritis is always surgical drainage. This should be done as an emergency to limit the damage to the joint cartilage.

Complications

- Seeding of infection can occur to the spine or other organs.
- Recurrence of infection.
- Joint destruction with long-term arthritis or even anklyosis (bony fusion across the joint).
- Avascular necrosis (particularly in the hip).

Prognosis

If treated promptly, prognosis is good, but if joint destruction occurs it is very poor. Septic arthritis, if missed or left untreated, can be fatal.

TUBERCULOSIS

Incidence

TB is common in global terms and causes significant morbidity and mortality in Africa and Asia.

TB is making a 'comeback' in the UK, with over 10 000 cases per year, most of which are in the Asian community or immunocompromised patients.

Aetiology and pathology

TB is due to *Mycobacterium tuberculosis* or *M. bovis* infection.

Histologically the classical appearance is of granulating caseating necrosis.

Musculoskeletal TB results when primary TB (lung) becomes widespread or when later reactivation or re-infection occurs (immunosuppressed patients).

Clinical features

Patients have general symptoms of ill health, such as malaise, weight loss, cough and loss of appetite. The most common musculoskeletal sites affected by TB are the spine, hip and knee.

Unlike other orthopaedic infections, TB presents with gradual symptoms of pain and may be initially diagnosed as osteoarthritis or inflammatory arthritis.

Diagnosis and investigation

The two commonest tests for TB exposure are the Mantoux and Heaf tests, which are skin hypersensitivity tests.

For confirmation, large samples of bone or synovial fluid are required which need to be cultured (Löwenstein–Jensen medium) for a prolonged period (6 weeks).

If mycobacterial infection is suspected, samples should be submitted to a Ziehl–Neelsen stain and looking for acid/alcohol-fast bacilli. Remember to ask for this specifically when requesting a Gram stain.

X-rays show variable amounts of joint destruction with periarticular osteopenia.

In the spine, vertebra plana may be found with almost complete collapse of the vertebral body (see Fig. 9.11).

Treatment

Drugs commonly used are rifampicin, isoniazid and ethambutol, and multidrug therapy is required.

A spinal abscess may need drainage with stabilization of the spine.

Ankylosed joints from old treated TB can be replaced (usually the hip).

Further reading

Orthoteers website: http://www.orthoteers.co.uk.

Solomon, L., Warwick, D., Nayagan, D. (Eds.), 2001. Apley's System of Orthopaedics and Fractures, eighth ed. Hodder Arnold, London.

Principles of orthopaedic surgery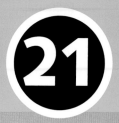

After reading this chapter you should be able to:
- Understand the purpose of preoperative assessment and think of examples of important conditions that may be discovered at this stage.
- Understand the basic principles of joint surgery for osteoarthritis and rheumatoid arthritis.
- Outline basic postoperative care.
- Classify complications of surgery.
- List ways to prevent complications from orthopaedic surgery.

Most doctors will be exposed to orthopaedic patients undergoing surgery during their career. However the surgical procedure is only a very small part of the overall surgical process. This chapter aims to take you through the patient's journey, starting with the preoperative period, through the basics of orthopaedic surgery to postoperative management.

PREOPERATIVE ASSESSMENT

Elective patients are seen a few weeks before surgery in the preoperative assessment clinic. It is important that concurrent medical problems are stabilized and new conditions identified, investigated and treated appropriately.

General

The following should be recorded:
- Observations (blood pressure, pulse, temperature): the patient may have undiagnosed atrial fibrillation or hypertension.
- History, including past medical history and drug history: the patient may be on warfarin and will need this to be stopped prior to surgery and may need admission for intravenous heparin.
- Detailed systemic enquiry: the patient may have shortness of breath on exertion and chest pain (angina). Such a patient following investigation may even go on to have coronary bypass surgery prior to the orthopaedic operation.
- Examination: e.g. the patient may have a heart murmur.
- Blood tests (unnecessary in young, fit patients for simple surgery): full blood count (FBC), glucose,

urea and electrolytes (U&E), liver function tests and clotting screen. Patients of Afro-Caribbean origin should have a sickle cell test. Arterial blood gases may be required if the patient has chest disease.
- Blood can be grouped and saved and cross-matched if significant blood loss is expected.
- Urinalysis for diabetes mellitus or urinary tract infection (UTI). If a patient has an UTI, it should be treated prior to any orthopaedic operation.
- Electrocardiogram (ECG) and chest X-ray (if indicated).
- Further investigations should be ordered if required, e.g. cardiac echo in aortic stenosis.

COMMUNICATION

Informed consent should be taken by a surgeon capable of performing the operation so that particular risks and expectations can be explained to the patient. This means the foundation programme doctor is not the best person for the job! The limb to be operated on should be clearly marked on the day of surgery.

Local

The patient should be asked if the limb is still painful because the surgery may be unnecessary.

The limb is examined.

Note skin condition (there may be a rash or skin breakdown over the operation site), pulses and range of movement and look for any distal infection. For example, a knee replacement procedure should not be carried out in a patient with an infected ingrowing toenail.

IMMEDIATE PREOPERATIVE CARE

Additional monitoring such as an arterial line and central venous line can be inserted in the anaesthetic room for patients expected to have a complicated anaesthetic.

A urinary catheter is important to assess fluid balance in patients who may lose significant amounts of blood.

Intravenous antibiotics and deep vein thrombosis (DVT) prophylaxis (chemical and/or mechanical) are also given if necessary.

SURGERY

There are several things a surgeon can do for a painful joint.

Joint debridement

A diseased joint can be debrided surgically in an attempt to improve range of movement or to reduce symptoms such as pain and swelling.

Debridement means removing diseased tissue. Osteophytes are often removed in osteoarthritis but debriding a joint does not cure or stop the progression of the disease process.

Examples of joints where debridement is performed include the first metatarsophalangeal (MTP) joint in hallux rigidus (Fig. 21.1).

Arthroscopy

Keyhole surgery techniques have become routine in recent years.

In the past, arthroscopy was seen as a diagnostic procedure but now a number of operations are possible by purely arthroscopic means. Examples are stabilization or rotator cuff repair in the shoulder, and meniscal repair or anterior cruciate ligament reconstruction in the knee.

It is now commonplace for many joints to be arthroscoped, including the shoulder, ankle, hip and wrist.

Joint excision (excision arthroplasty)

This operation has been mostly superseded by joint replacement. It is still occasionally performed for severe arthritis of the first MTP joint (Keller procedure) and also in the hip (Girdlestone procedure) if the patient has had an infected joint (Fig. 21.2).

The operation leaves the joint unstable and it may still be painful.

First metatarsophalangeal joint arthritis

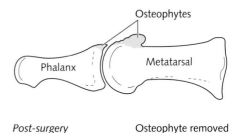

Osteophytes

Phalanx

Metatarsal

Post-surgery

Osteophyte removed

Allows more movement

Fig. 21.1 Joint debridement.

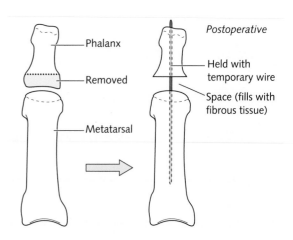

Phalanx

Removed

Metatarsal

Postoperative

Held with temporary wire

Space (fills with fibrous tissue)

Fig. 21.2 Excision of a joint.

Joint arthrodesis

Arthrodesis or fusion is performed to make the bones 'heal' together across a joint. Movement is obviously lost but if the fusion is sound then the joint will be strong and pain free.

Bones are most commonly fused around the foot and ankle or hand and wrist, usually in patients with rheumatoid arthritis. Examples include ankle fusion, subtalar fusion and wrist fusion.

Fusion can be achieved by different means, such as:

- Internal fixation (screws, staples, plates) (Fig. 21.3A).
- Intramedullary nail (Fig. 21.3B).
- External fixation.

A bone graft may be used to encourage union.

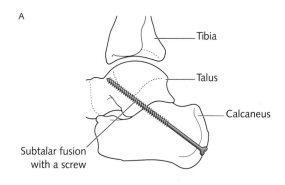

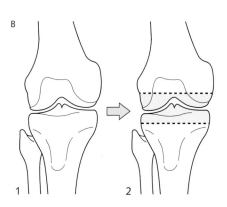

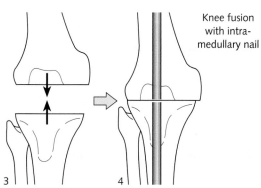

Fig. 21.3 Joint fusion. (A) Internal fixation. (B) Intramedullary nail.

Joint arthroplasty

Almost any joint can now be replaced. The primary reason to replace a joint is pain.

The advantage of replacement over fusion is that movement is maintained and therefore function can return to near normality.

Implants are usually made from metal; however the actual bearing surfaces can be made from a combination of a metal, high-density polyethylene or ceramic. The joint surfaces are highly polished for low friction.

The joint components are either cemented in place or uncemented.

Joint replacements are available for almost any joint, although the most commonly performed are:

- Knee (Fig. 21.4).
- Hip (Fig. 21.5).
- Shoulder.
- Elbow.

The majority of replacements should last over 15 years, but this is partly dependent on the patient. A young patient is more likely to wear out a prosthesis due to higher demand.

The most common reasons for failure of an implant are loosening, infection and fracture (Fig. 21.6).

Osteotomy/deformity correction

An osteotomy is an operation to cut a bone and realign the joint or deformity.

The most common place for this to occur is the first ray of the foot, in the case of hallux valgus. Osteotomies are also performed at the knee to offload arthritic compartments in younger patients, reducing pain and postponing the need for arthroplasty.

Deformity can occur for other reasons: malunion of fractures (tibia and femur) and congenital deformity (e.g. clubfoot); and correction of such deformity is an important part of orthopaedic surgery.

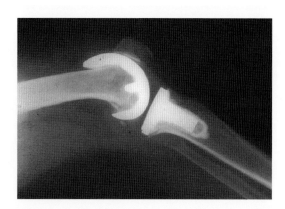

Fig. 21.4 Total knee replacement.

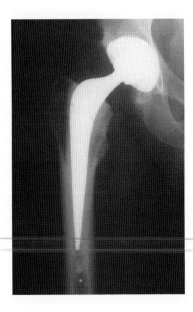

Fig. 21.5 Total hip replacement.

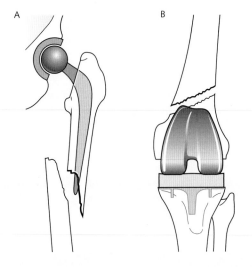

Fig. 21.6 Periprosthetic fracture of the femur: (A) at the hip; (B) at the knee.

It is also possible to lengthen bones gradually with external fixation, usually in the form of circular frames with a variety of hinges and movable rods (Fig. 21.7).

Synovectomy

In the case of inlammatory arthritides a synovectomy may be performed. The aim of this operation is to remove the synovial lining of the diseased joint or the tenosynovium around tendons. The procedure needs to be performed early and has three possible beneficial effects:

1. Reduction of swelling.
2. Slowing of disease progression.
3. Prevention of tendon rupture.

Unfortunately it is impossible to remove the whole synovium with synovectomy, and symptoms often return. This procedure is usually performed around the wrist.

POSTOPERATIVE CARE

General

Patients are taken to recovery until fully awake, then transferred to the ward. Higher risk patients may need transfer to a high-dependency unit or intensive therapy unit.

Regular recordings are made of blood pressure, pulse and oxygen saturation.

Adequate pain relief is very important.

After major surgery requiring an inpatient stay, patients will need:

- FBC and U&E checked the day after surgery.
- X-rays of the joint operated upon.

Once patients are well, every effort is made to mobilize them and encourage early safe discharge. DVT prophylaxis is continued until patients are mobile.

A multidisciplinary approach is needed to achieve this, with physiotherapy, occupational therapy, social workers, nursing staff and sometimes physicians having input.

Home modifications are required for patients having a joint arthroplasty.

Local

Elevation in a Bradford sling (for an arm) or on a Braun's frame (Fig. 21.8) is very important to reduce swelling.

Distal neurovascular observations are performed to check the perfusion and function of the limb distal to the operation.

As soon as possible, physiotherapy is encouraged, to mobilize the limb.

COMPLICATIONS

Any surgical procedure has risks and complications, and knowledge of these helps minimize and prevent them.

Patients now need to be made aware of these important complications before informed consent is obtained.

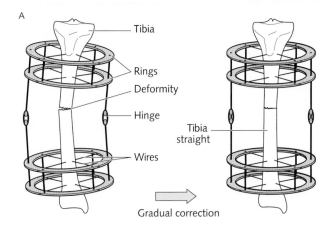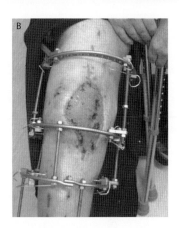

Fig. 21.7 Deformity correction with frames. (A) The use of an external fixator 'frame' to achieve gradual correction of a deformity over several weeks. Note that the frame is also bent but straightens out as the bone is corrected. (B) Ilizarov frame on a fractured tibia.

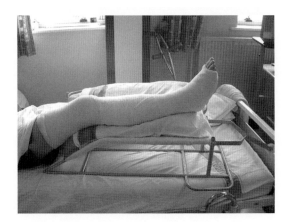

Fig. 21.8 Braun's frame used to elevate a lower limb.

Complications are divided into:

- Local (specific to that operation).
- General (common to any operation).

We further subdivide complication on the basis of the time that has elapsed after surgery into:

- Immediate (within 24 hours).
- Early (days/weeks).
- Late (months/years).

General respiratory

Chest infections

Complications affecting the respiratory system are very common postoperatively.

A chest infection typically presents early with fever and shortness of breath. Elderly patients may be confused.

There may be signs of consolidation on examination and a low Po_2.

Treatment is with physiotherapy, nebulizers and antibiotics.

Venous thromboembolism

Immobile orthopaedic patients with traumatized limbs are very susceptible to DVT. Risk is reduced by mechanical (foot pumps, graduated compression stockings) and chemical agents (heparin, clexane, aspirin, warfarin) and early mobilization.

If the clot propagates and then breaks off it travels to the lungs (a pulmonary embolus), which can be fatal. The patient becomes acutely short of breath and has pleuritic chest pain with signs of tachycardia, tachypnoea and a low Po_2. An ECG may show a sinus tachycardia, arrhythmias or the classical, but rare, S1Q3T3.

Treatment should be started immediately in the form of low-molecular-weight subcutaneous heparin if suspected and diagnosis is proven with a computed tomographic pulmonary angiogram (CTPA).

Cardiac

Myocardial infarction (MI)

MI is a relatively common postoperative complication, particularly in the elderly or those with pre-existing heart disease. Patients do not always have typical central

155

crushing chest pain radiating to the left arm associated with sweating and nausea and the cardiac event may be silent or occur during anaesthesia. This should be suspected in any patient with unexplained hypotension.

Diagnosis is made based on ECGs and raised troponin cardiac enzymes.

Treatment includes oxygen and aspirin. Further agents may be used based on an opinion from the physicians (it is usually impossible to give thrombolytic drugs to postoperative patients owing to the risk of bleeding).

Left ventricular failure

This can result from a cardiac event or from aggressive fluid management over the perioperative period. It is important not to give too much fluid, particularly to elderly patients with little physiological reserve.

These patients present with shortness of breath, and signs include a raised jugular venous pressure and bibasal crackles. Simple measures such as sitting the patient up and giving oxygen can dramatically improve the patient's condition. Further treatment includes diuretics, morphine/diamorphine and nitrates.

Blood loss and blood transfusion

Most patients do not require a blood transfusion postoperatively, even after a total hip or knee replacement. Blood transfusions are expensive (£400 per unit) and are associated with transfusion reactions, transmission of infections (hepatitis, human immunodeficiency virus (HIV), variant Creutzfeldt–Jakob disease) and immunosuppression. Therefore blood should be prescribed sparingly. Most patients can tolerate a haemoglobin of 80 g/L even if they have pre-existing ischaemic heart disease.

Gastrointestinal

Bleeding

The most important complication of the gastrointestinal (GI) system is bleeding, and the most common reason for this on the orthopaedic wards is non-steroidal anti-inflammatory drug (NSAID) therapy.

Patients with haematemesis or melaena have a suspected upper GI bleed until proven otherwise. Diagnosis is confirmed with upper GI endoscopies performed as soon as possible. Supportive measures including starting a proton pump inhibitor, cross-matching of blood, fluid resuscitation, careful observations and oxygen if required.

Referral to a gastroenterologist or surgeon is needed.

Paralytic ileus

This is a less serious complication presenting with abdominal distension and nausea. Operations or trauma to the spine predispose to ileus, which usually spontaneously corrects after a few days on intravenous fluids and a nasogastric tube.

Renal

Renal failure

Pre-existing renal impairment is common in orthopaedic patients and the additional insult of a fracture or surgery with the associated blood loss can tip the balance, causing renal failure.

Factors influencing the development of renal failure include drugs (diuretics, NSAIDs) and hypovolaemia. It is very important to keep patients well hydrated with enough fluid to prevent prerenal failure.

Careful monitoring of fluid input with hourly urine output and daily U&E measurement is important when assessing such a patient.

> **HINTS AND TIPS**
>
> Low urinary output postoperatively is almost always due to hypovolaemia and patients require fluid. It is very important to assess fluid balance carefully, so that diuretics are not given to such patients just to increase the output. This may precipitate renal failure!

Urinary tract infection

UTIs postoperatively are very common. Diagnosis is made on urinalysis and a midstream urine sample is sent to microbiology. Antibiotics are started until culture and sensitivity results are known.

Local

Figure 21.9 lists local complications, their timing, causes, signs and symptoms, and management.

INFECTION

Infection is the major concern in elective orthopaedic surgery. Deep infection in joint replacement surgery is disastrous when it occurs as simple measures such as antibiotics and abscess drainage will not eradicate the infection. The patient may be worse off than before surgery and may require lengthy hospital stays with extensive further surgery and significant risks.

Fig. 21.9 Local complications of orthopaedic surgery

Postoperative timing	Complication	Cause	Signs/symptoms	Management
Immediate–first 24 hours	Tight cast	Swelling Dressing/cast too tight	Pain, tingling in toes/fingers Poor distal perfusion Numbness Ischaemia of limb	Elevation Split cast
	Compartment syndrome	Swelling in a closed fascial compartment (usually postfracture)	Pain: pain on passive stretch, tense compartments Altered sensation	Fasciotomy
	Primary haemorrhage	Technical problem at surgical site, e.g. bleeding vessel Other risk factors include: major surgery, e.g. total hip replacement; drugs, e.g. warfarin; obesity	Haemodynamic instability Anxiety Slow capillary refill Tachycardia Hypotension Low urine output Confusion	Replace losses—fluids $\pm$ blood Reverse cause, e.g. warfarin Pressure dressing Clamp drains If heavy bleeding re-explore wound
	Nerve injury	Usually retractor, e.g. sciatic nerve in hip replacement	Pain, weakness, paraesthesia	Wait and see Usually recovers
Early–first 4 weeks	Secondary haemorrhage	Occurs at 5–10 days, usually secondary to infection	Bleeding with signs of infection	Treat infection Wound debridement and washout
	Infection (see Ch. 20)	Infection at time of surgery Can occur later with haematogenous seeding	Early: red, hot, swollen, discharging, temperature Late: persistent pain, loosening of prosthesis	Early: debridement and washout Late: removal of implant and debridement Reimplantation at second stage once infection treated
	Wound dehiscence (breakdown)	Within first week: usually due to poor surgical technique Later: invariably infection and poor healing	Wound gapes open Other features in keeping with infection may be present	Early: clean wounds are taken back to theatre for primary closure Later: treat infection as above
Late (in theory these can occur at any time)	Dislocation of total hip replacement	Patient: inappropriate patient activity, poor stem or cup position Excessive wear Infection	Severe pain, shortening External rotation (anterior) Internal rotation (posterior)	Reduce hip Abduction brace for 6 weeks if early Revision surgery if there is a problem with position of implant
	Periprosthetic fracture	Intraoperative: if a prosthesis is too big for the bone when inserted Late: loosening of the prosthesis, infection or trauma	Increased pain, deformity, unable to weight bear	Intraoperative: fixation of fracture Late: revision of prosthesis
	Heterotopic ossification	Abnormal bone formation in soft tissues: more common in head-injured patients and with hip surgery or trauma	Stiffness	Surgical excision and immediate non-steroidal anti-inflammatory drugs or radiotherapy postoperatively

Continued

Fig. 21.9 Local complications of orthopaedic surgery—cont'd

Postoperative timing	Complication	Cause	Signs/symptoms	Management
	Aseptic loosening	Loosening of prosthesis occurs because particle wear of the implant triggers macrophages. These cause osteolysis around the prosthesis	Pain, instability	Revision of the prosthesis

The risk of infection is minimized by the following preoperative, perioperative and postoperative factors.

Preoperative factors

- Cleaning the skin.
- Avoidance of concurrent infection (e.g. UTI).
- Preoperative antibiotics on induction of anaesthesia.
- A healthy, well-nourished patient.

Perioperative factors

- Clean laminar airflow theatre (air is specially filtered).
- Adequate skin preparation and impervious exclusion drapes.
- Exhaust suits (enclosed clothing with air evacuation to prevent skin contaminants falling on to the wound).
- Sterile instruments and prostheses.
- Careful surgical technique (including haemostasis).
- The use of antibiotic-loaded cement in joint arthroplasty.

Postoperative factors

- Wound dressing.
- Prophylactic antibiotics for possible bacteraemia (e.g. during catheterization).
- Postoperative antibiotics.

SHOCK

Shock is defined as an inability to maintain adequate tissue perfusion and oxygenation.

Every doctor should be able to recognize shock.

On the orthopaedic wards the most likely causes are hypovolaemic, septic and cardiogenic shock, although neurogenic shock can occur after spinal cord injury. Anaphylactic shock is less common, but possible if patients are allergic to drugs or latex.

Hypovolaemic

Haemorrhage is the most likely cause of hypovolaemic shock, which is due to inadequate circulatory volume. These patients require intravenous fluids and sometimes blood to restore blood pressure.

Cardiogenic

The heart is unable to maintain adequate cardiac output, usually because of infarction. Intravenous fluids may further overload the heart and positive inotropes such as noradrenaline (norepinephrine) may be required.

Neurogenic/spinal

This is due to peripheral vasodilatation secondary to spinal cord injury.

It is important not to overload such a patient with fluid in an attempt to raise the blood pressure (the blood pressure remains low because of loss of peripheral resistance). A sytolic blood pressure of 100 mmHg is normally acceptable in these patients.

Septic

Peripheral vasodilatation is due to bacterial endotoxins in severe infection. Patients require intravenous antibiotics, whilst receiving haemodynamic support.

Anaphylactic shock

This occurs in patients already sensitized to an allergen. There is an aggressive immune response resulting in massive histamine release from basophils. The patient may rapidly deteriorate, and develop a generalized urticaria, with stridor (upper-airway narrowing), wheeze and shortness of breath. There is massive vasodilatation and a tachycardia associated with hypotension. Treatment should be rapid, including emergency airway procedures, oxygen, nebulizers, intravenous hydrocortisone, antihistamines (chlorphenamine) and intramuscular or intravenous adrenaline (epinephrine) and fluid resuscitation.

Treatment

Basic treatment of shock should be instituted immediately and includes oxygen therapy and fluid resuscitation, with catheterization to monitor urine output and regular observation. Admission to a high-dependency unit should be considered if the patient is unstable or requires intensive input.

Further reading

Canale, S.T., 2006. Campbell's Operative Orthopaedics, eleventh ed, vols. 1–4. Mosby, St Louis.

Sweetland, H., Conway, K., 2004. Crash Course in Surgery. Mosby, Edinburgh.

After reading this chapter you should be able to:
- Describe a bone lesion on X-ray.
- Understand the difference between benign and malignant lesions on X-ray.
- Investigate a patient with an incidental bone lesion on X-ray.
- Classify bone tumours and know which types are most common.
- List which tumours most commonly metastasize to bone.
- Describe symptoms associated with bone metastasis.
- Describe typical X-ray features of primary and secondary bone tumours.
- Outline available treatments for primary and secondary bone tumours.
- Define different benign and malignant bone tumours, including chondromas and sarcomas.
- Give examples of haemopoietic disease which can present with bone destruction.
- Give a prognosis for individual malignant tumours.

This chapter concerns bone tumours (benign and malignant; primary and secondary) and other malignant conditions presenting as a musculoskeletal disorder. The patient may present with symptoms directly attributed to the tumour, and further investigation reveals the pathology. Conversely the tumour may be discovered incidentally as a lesion on X-ray, when the X-ray was taken for another reason such as minor trauma and an abnormality is found. Examples include a chest X-ray taken for respiratory disease showing a lesion in the clavicle or a pelvic X-ray taken for hip disease showing metastatic prostate carcinoma.

Benign lesions are quite common. Thankfully, primary bone malignancy is extremely rare. Secondary bone tumours are common in the elderly. It is important to remember that infection and metabolic bone disease can present as a bone lesion.

Benign tumours/disorders

- Osteochondroma.
- Osteoid osteoma.
- Enchondroma.
- Bone cysts.
- Fibrous dysplasia.

Malignant tumours

- Primary:
  - Osteosarcoma.
  - Ewing's sarcoma.
  - Chondrosarcoma.
- Secondary—metastatic deposit:
  - Breast.

- Lung.
- Prostate.
- Renal.
- Thyroid.
- Bowel.
- Haemopoietic diseases:
  - Myeloma.
  - Leukaemia.
  - Lymphoma.

Infection

- Osteomyelitis.

Metabolic bone disease

- Paget disease.

While the clinical features, treatment and prognosis will depend upon the specific pathology, the way in which a bone tumour is approached remains the same. We will address the general approach to the history, examination and investigation to bone tumours, and discuss the individual pathologies separately.

HISTORY

The following points must be elicited in the history, looking for clues as to the diagnosis.

Age of patient

Certain lesions such as bone cysts are more common in children, and other benign bone lesions such as enchondroma usually occur in young adults.

Overall, primary malignant tumours are very rare and metastatic bone disease is a disease of the elderly.

Pain

Although the patient may not have offered pain as a symptom initially, when a lesion is discovered the patient must be asked if the area is painful. The patient may have ignored any pain or just put it down to 'arthritis playing up'.

Pain that is severe and does not respond to simple analgesia, particularly if night pain is a feature, suggests a malignant process.

Swelling

Benign lesions are more likely to present with swelling, particularly osteochondroma, a lesion commonly found around the knee.

Malignant tumours may have pain and swelling but it is rare for a bone tumour to present with swelling only.

General health

General features of ill health such as tiredness, weight loss, poor appetite and fever suggest a systemic illness such as malignancy, haemopoietic disorders or infection.

Primary bone malignancy is unlikely to present with widespread features of malignancy as patients will usually present with pain and swelling before these general features have developed.

It is important to ask about any other areas of pain in the musculoskeletal system, particularly if considering widespread metastatic disease.

Past medical history

A previous history of carcinoma is extremely important when dealing with such a patient. The lesion should be treated as a metastatic lesion until proven otherwise.

Breast malignancy can be dormant for many years prior to representing with metastases.

EXAMINATION

Site

Different lesions are more common in certain locations, for example enchondromas are more common in the hand.

Secondary bone metastases tend to be found in the central skeleton.

Limb examination

Examination of the affected limb will usually be normal.

Tenderness, redness and swelling would be present in:

- Impending or actual fracture associated with a bone metastasis.
- Osteomyelitis.
- Osteoid osteoma.
- Malignant primary bone tumour.

Malignant secondaries or bone lesions from haemopoietic diseases rarely show any external features.

Generalized

In secondary malignancy with unknown primary, it is important to examine:

- Breast (for carcinoma).
- Chest (for lung tumours).
- Abdomen (for renal or bowel tumours and evidence of haemopoietic disease such as liver and spleen enlargement).
- Per rectum (PR) (prostate).
- Thyroid (for carcinoma).

INVESTIGATION

The X-ray

It is important to obtain two views taken at 90° (orthogonal) to one another and to obtain full-length views of the entire bone (to ensure there are no further lesions along the same bone).

Most benign lesions need no further investigation and repeat X-rays after 6 months are useful to ensure the bone lesion does not change in appearance and develop any sinister features.

Describing bone lesions on X-ray

> **COMMUNICATION**
>
> Practise describing bone defects and lesions whenever possible.

1. Name and age of patient.
2. Site – which bone and where in the bone:
   - The lesion can be in the diaphysis (shaft), metaphysis (cancellous bone between the growth plate and shaft) or epiphysis (between the growth plate and the joint).
   - The lesion can primarily affect either the cortex or medulla of the bone.

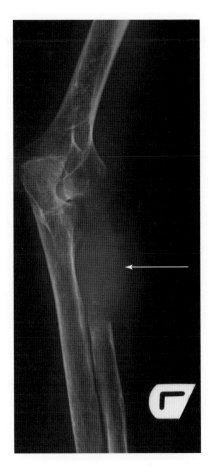

Fig. 22.1 Lytic lesion (proximal radius) is suggestive of malignancy.

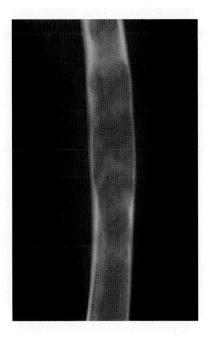

Fig. 22.2 Fibrous dysplasia. (Reproduced from Hochberg MC, Silman AJ, Smolen JS et al. (eds) (2011) Rheumatology, 5th edn. London: Mosby, with permission).

6. What is the lesion doing to the bone?
   - Cortical destruction is typical of a malignant process.
   - Cortical thinning does occur in benign disease due to expansion.

Further investigation

Further investigation is only necessary if there is doubt about the diagnosis or to confirm or exclude malignancy.

> **COMMUNICATION**
>
> It is not uncommon for patients to present with a lesion on X-ray to find they have metastatic disease from an unknown primary. Make sure this news is broken in the right way, preferably once all the information is available and with relatives and nursing staff present.

Blood tests

- A full blood count may show anaemia of chronic disease.
- Liver function tests could be deranged if liver metastases are present.
- The calcium profile is often raised in generalized malignancy, and alkaline phosphatase is raised in Paget disease.

3. Appearance:
   - The lesion can be lytic (e.g. breast metastasis) (Fig. 22.1), sclerotic (e.g. prostate metastasis), mixed or calcified (enchondroma).
   - Ground glass (fibrous dysplasia) (Fig. 22.2).
   - Abnormal bony architecture, e.g. post-osteomyelitis.
4. Zone of transition:
   - A well-defined border between the lesion and the normal bone suggests a benign slow-growing lesion (it is clearly demarcated).
   - A broad, irregular or indistinct zone of transition where the change from abnormal to normal is poorly defined suggests a malignant process (Fig. 22.3).
5. What is the bone doing in response?
   - A significant periosteal reaction, with Codman triangle (elevation of periosteum) (see Fig. 22.7B), onion skinning (Fig. 22.4A) and sunray spicules (Fig. 22.4B), is a feature of malignancy.
   - Infection can also cause a periosteal reaction.

Fig. 22.3 A poorly defined zone of transition (arrow) suggests malignancy.

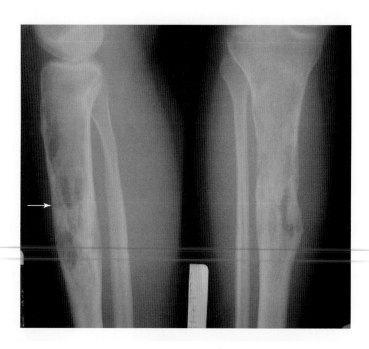

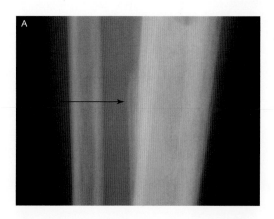

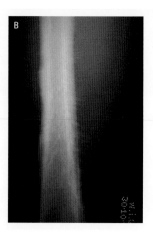

Fig. 22.4 Primary bone tumour showing: (A) onion skinning (arrow) and (B) sunray spicules.

- C-reactive protein (CRP) and erythrocyte sedimentation rate (ESR) are raised in infection or malignancy.
- A very high ESR suggests myeloma. It is confirmed with serum electrophoresis and urinary Bence Jones proteins.
- Prostate-specific antigen (PSA) is elevated in prostate malignancy.
- Carcinoembryonic antigen (CEA) is elevated in bowel carcinoma.

Isotope bone scan

This is a very useful tool to detect further lesions in malignancy or to see if a lesion is active (i.e. hot on bone scan). Infection will show up 'hot', as will malignant lesions.

Of the benign lesions, only osteoid osteoma will show increased uptake.

Computed tomography (CT)

CT is used to confirm osteoid osteoma.

Magnetic resonance imaging (MRI)

MRI can detect early metastatic lesions before X-ray features are apparent.

It is also used to define the extent of malignant bone tumours and can help to distinguish between benign and malignant lesions.

Biopsy

It can be very difficult to be certain of the diagnosis in some cases. A biopsy will prove whether the tumour is benign or malignant and exclude infection as the cause.

PRIMARY BONE TUMOURS

Primary tumours of bone can be benign or malignant.

Benign bone tumours

Enchondroma

An enchondroma is a benign bone lesion of cartilaginous origin.

Incidence

Enchondromas are quite common, occurring usually in adulthood.

Aetiology and pathology

Enchondromas develop from aberrant cartilage ('chondroma') left within bone ('en'). They are usually found in the metaphysis of long bones (femur or humerus) but are also common in the hand (Fig. 22.5).

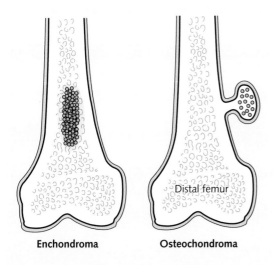

Enchondroma   Osteochondroma
Distal femur

Fig. 22.5   Benign cartilage tumours.

Clinical features

An enchondroma is usually asymptomatic and may be found incidentally. Large lesions causing cortical erosion can be painful and the patient may notice a swelling, particularly in the hand.

Diagnosis and investigation

Typical features on X-ray show a well-demarcated calcifying lesion in the metaphysis of the bone. Serial X-rays may be obtained to make sure the lesion is not growing rapidly.

Treatment

Usually no treatment is required, but if the lesion is significantly painful or associated with fracture, excision or curettage may be performed.

Osteochondroma

Incidence

This is the most common benign bone lesion, presenting from childhood through to adult life.

Aetiology and pathology

The lesion develops from aberrant cartilage remaining on the surface of the cortex. It is usually found around the knee, most commonly on the distal femur (see Fig. 22.5).

The pathological appearance is of a bone lesion continuous with the cortex of the bone, capped with hyaline cartilage. It can be sessile or pedunculated (see Fig. 22.5).

Clinical features

The majority are asymptomatic, presenting incidentally or as a swelling. Rarely, pain or pressure effects on nerves or vessels occur.

Diagnosis and investigation

The typical appearance of a pedunculated lesion in continuity with the cortex clinches the diagnosis. If there is doubt, CT or MRI may reassure.

Treatment

Usually no treatment is needed; rarely, excision is carried out, if symptomatic.

Prognosis

It is extremely rare for either osteochondroma or enchondroma to undergo malignant change.

Osteoid osteoma

Osteoid osteoma is a painful, self-limiting benign bone lesion.

Incidence

The lesion is uncommon, usually presenting between 5 and 30 years of age.

Aetiology and pathology

It is caused by a nidus of osteoblasts located in the cortex of bone, and is usually found in the tibia, spine or femur.

Clinical features

Patients have intense pain, particularly at night. Tenderness over the lesion is usual. In the spine a scoliosis may be present.

Diagnosis and investigation

X-ray features show a radiolucent nidus surrounded by a dense area of reactive bone (Fig 22.6A). CT scans confirm and accurately locate the lesion (Fig. 22.6B).

Treatment

Pain is typically relieved by non-steroidal anti-inflammatory drugs. CT-guided ablation is now preferred over surgical excision.

Fig. 22.6 (A) X-ray showing an osteoid osteoma. (B) Computed tomography scan will confirm.

Prognosis

The tumour is eventually self-limiting.

Fibrous dysplasia

This is not strictly a bone tumour.

Incidence

Fibrous dysplasia is relatively common, usually presenting in the first three decades.

Aetiology and pathology

It is most commonly found in the tibia, femur and ribs, and is caused by developmental abnormality of bone with numerous fibrous proliferations.

Clinical features

The condition is usually asymptomatic, discovered as an incidental finding, but can present with pain, swelling, deformity or fracture.

Diagnosis and investigation

A typical ground-glass appearance is diagnostic (Fig. 22.2).

Treatment

No treatment is usually required, but if significant, curettage and bone grafting can be performed.

Malignant primary bone tumours

Primary malignant bone tumours are very rare indeed. We will discuss two of those most likely to be encountered.

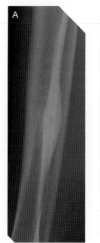
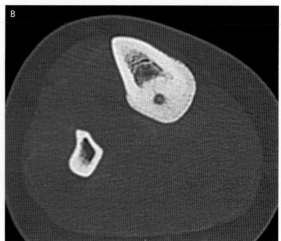

Osteosarcoma

Incidence

There are approximately 1–2 cases per million of population. Presentation is in adolescence and young adulthood or in the elderly where they develop in pagetic bones.

Aetiology and pathology

Paget disease or radiation can predispose, but most cases occur sporadically. The tumour is highly malignant and secretes osteoid. Local spread occurs quickly, destroying the cortex, but it may also metastasize.

The most common location is around the knee; other sites include the proximal humerus and femur.

Clinical features

The patient presents with pain and sometimes also swelling. Clinically there is usually warmth over the affected area and there may be a palpable mass.

Diagnosis and investigation

X-rays (Fig. 22.7) may show:

- An ill-defined lesion with an indistinct zone of transition (Fig. 22.7A).
- Sclerotic or lytic areas within the lesion.
- Cortical destruction.
- Codman triangle (elevation of periosteum) (Fig. 22.7B).
- Sunray spicules (calcification within the tumour but out of the bone).

Biopsy may be necessary to confirm the diagnosis. Further investigations such as CT and MRI are required to stage the lesion.

Treatment

A combined multidisciplinary team approach is adopted.

Preoperative chemotherapy followed by limb salvage surgery is performed if possible. Occasionally amputation is required.

Prognosis

Five-year survival is 60%.

Chondrosarcoma

Incidence

Chondrosarcoma are more prevalent with age, with most tumours arising after the age of 40. The peak incidence is approximately 8 cases per million at the age of 80. Men are more commonly affected than women.

Aetiology and pathology

A chondrosarcoma can either be a primary lesion or a secondary conversion of a benign cartilaginous tumour – such as osteochondroma or chondroma. A chondrosarcoma can be separated into low-grade and high-grade. Little difference can be seen histologically between a low-grade chondrosarcoma and a benign cartilaginous lesion. High-grade chondrosarcomas demonstrate a more abnormal cell structure, and consequently are more aggressive. The most common areas of growth are in the pelvis and around the hip.

Clinical features

Similarly to osteosarcoma, the main clinical features are that of pain and localized swelling. On examination there may be a bony mass palpable.

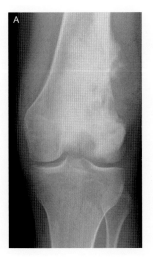
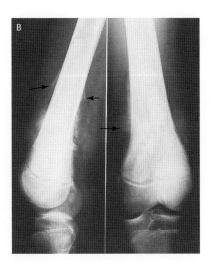

Fig. 22.7 X-rays of osteosarcoma. (A) Ill-defined lesion. (B) Codman triangles.

Diagnosis and investigation

X-rays usually show a lytic lesion with cortical destruction, with central calcification. Low-grade lesions may resemble benign cartilaginous lesion. CT or MRI may be required to investigate a lesion further.

Treatment

A multidisciplinary apporach is once again adopted. Chemotherapy and radiotherapy are less effective. Wide excision of the lesion is sometimes possible, as chondrosarcomas are slow-growing and metastasize late in the disease. However amputation may be the only viable option.

Prognosis

Prognosis is grade-dependent: 5-year survival for low-grade lesions is 90%, whereas for high-grade lesions it is 5%.

Ewing sarcoma

Incidence

Ewing sarcoma is extremely rare (less common than osteosarcoma), occurring between 5 and 25 years of age.

Aetiology and pathology

Histologically this is a small-cell sarcoma. It occurs as frequently in flat bones as in long bones, being most common in the femur or tibia (long bone), pelvis or vertebra (flat bones).

These tumours are highly malignant and often large at presentation.

Clinical features

Patients present with pain and may be unwell with a fever. Clinically the area is warm and swelling may be present.

Diagnosis and investigation

Diagnosis is usually made on X-ray appearance (Fig. 22.8), which is classically a lytic lesion with a laminated periosteal reaction (onion skinning). CT and MRI help to stage the lesion. Biopsy may be necessary.

Treatment

A combined multidisciplinary team approach is adopted.

Preoperative chemotherapy and radiotherapy followed by limb salvage surgery are performed if possible.

Prognosis

Five-year survival is 60%.

SECONDARY BONE TUMOURS

Incidence

Secondary bone tumours are the most common bone-destroying lesions in the older patient.

Aetiology and pathology

The tumours most likely to metastasize to bone are:

- Breast.
- Lung.
- Prostate.
- Renal.
- Thyroid.
- Bowel.

Metastatic lesions are most commonly found in the spine, pelvis, ribs and proximal long bones. The mechanism of metastasis is shown in Figure 22.9. Bone

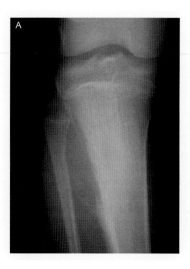
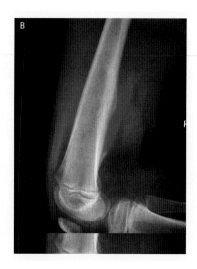

Fig. 22.8 X-rays of Ewing sarcoma.

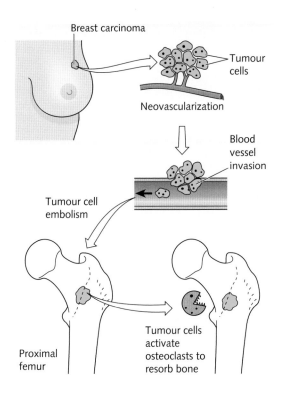

Breast carcinoma

Tumour cells

Neovascularization

Blood vessel invasion

Tumour cell embolism

Proximal femur

Tumour cells activate osteoclasts to resorb bone

Fig. 22.9 Mechanism of long-bone metastasis.

is destroyed by metastatic disease and weakened, predisposing to fracture. The majority of metastases appear osteolytic but those from prostate cancer appear sclerotic.

Clinical features

Patient with a known primary

The patient has a clear history of previous malignancy, which in the case of breast carcinoma may have been many years previously. Unrelenting bone pain in the axial skeleton then makes the patient seek medical help. Night pain is often a feature that does not respond to simple analgesia. There may be constitutional symptoms such as weight loss and malaise.

Patient with no known primary

The patient presents with bone pain as described above but with no history of previous malignancy. In this case it is important to ask about symptoms suggestive of malignancy such as cough and haemoptysis (lung), urinary symptoms (prostate) or change in bowel habit (bowel). Patients often do not have any symptoms of

the primary. Clinical examination should concentrate on likely sources of primary tumours; therefore examine:

- Breast.
- Chest.
- Prostate (per rectum).
- Thyroid.
- Abdomen (kidney and bowel).

Fracture

Usually the patient has a history of bone pain preceding the event (usually minor trauma) that caused the fracture. The patient is then either admitted or seen in a fracture clinic.

> **HINTS AND TIPS**
>
> Patients who present with significant fractures after a very minor injury (e.g. after lifting a suitcase) may have a malignancy.

Spinal cord compression

Patients with malignancy can present 'off their legs' with weakness and a demonstrable spinal level (change in sensation corresponding to the vertebral level affected). There may be a history of preceding spinal bony pain and then weakness, numbness and loss of bladder and bowel control – cauda equina syndrome. Urgent radiotherapy may shrink the tumour and preserve spinal cord function.

> **HINTS AND TIPS**
>
> It can be a very difficult decision whether or not to operate on a patient with spinal cord compression in the presence of malignancy. There are significant risks of surgery but most spinal surgeons will try to stabilize the spine if at all possible to preserve the patient's mobility and dignity. Patients will know they are terminally ill but will not want to spend the last few months of life immobile and incontinent.

> **HINTS AND TIPS**
>
> Spinal bony pain in patients with known metastatic disease needs investigation and treatment before spinal cord compression results.

Diagnosis and investigation

Any bone-destroying lesion could be due to infection or malignancy

- Check the white cell count and inflammatory markers – CRP and ESR. These are raised in infection but may also be raised in malignancy (myeloma).
- Further blood tests may identify the primary such as CEA or PSA.
- Plain X-rays will usually show an osteolytic lesion; however, significant bone loss (>50%) is needed before it is apparent on X-ray examination.

- If strong clinical suspicion exists then an MRI scan is more sensitive.
- Cortical thinning suggests impending fracture.
- A bone scan will be hot and is useful to exclude further distant lesions.
- In an unknown primary, further investigation to find the primary is warranted (Fig. 22.10).

Treatment

Treatment depends on the primary and on the life expectancy of the patient. A multidisciplinary approach is required involving oncologists.

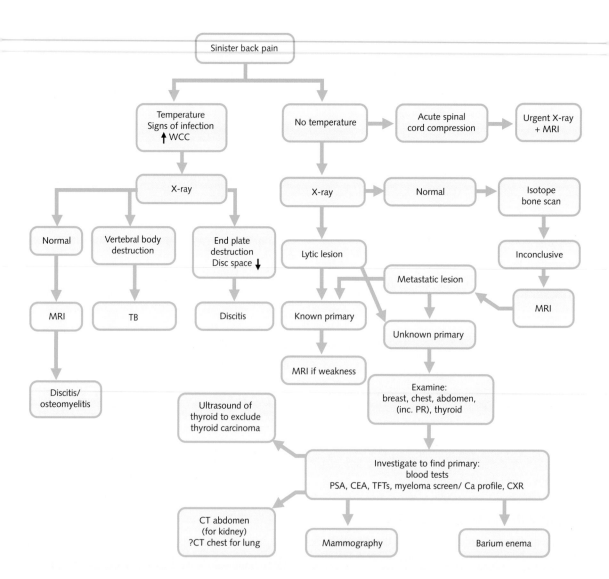

Fig. 22.10 Algorithm for the investigation of sinister back pain. Ca, calcium; CEA, carcinoembryonic antigen; CT, computed tomography; CXR, chest X-ray; MRI, magnetic resonance imaging; PR, per rectum; PSA, prostate-specific antigen; TB, tuberculosis; TFTs, thyroid function tests; WCC, white cell count.

Conservative

- Adequate analgesia and splintage.
- Radiotherapy is used frequently for bony metastatic pain.
- Chemotherapy may have a role in certain tumours.
- Hormonal therapy is useful in breast disease.
- Intravenous bisphosphonates are now being used to inhibit osteoclastic resorption of bone.

Surgical

- Intramedullary fixation of long bones is performed for fracture or impending fracture.
- Joint arthroplasty is sometimes used around the hip and shoulder.
- Spinal decompression and stabilization for acute cord compression.

Prognosis

The prognosis depends on the primary.

> **HINTS AND TIPS**
>
> Patients with renal tumours and a solitary metastasis may be cured by resection of both.

HAEMOPOIETIC DISEASES

Lymphoma and myeloma can present with bone destruction.

Lymphoma

Incidence

Lymphoma is rare but can occur at any age.

Aetiology and pathology

Lymphoma is a small-cell bone tumour arising from the marrow, which can occur in any bone, most commonly around the knee.

Diagnosis and investigation

- X-rays show a long lesion with mottled bony destruction.
- Isotope bone scanning excludes further lesions.
- Biopsy confirms the diagnosis.

Treatment

Chemotherapy and irradiation are commonly used in conjunction.

Myeloma

Incidence

This is a rare tumour, occurring between 50 and 80 years of age.

Aetiology and pathology

Lesions are due to a plasma cell malignancy, and are usually found in the spine, ribs or clavicle.

Clinical features

Bony pain is common and there may be a pathological fracture. Systemic symptoms of fatigue and fever are very common.

Diagnosis and investigation

Patients will have a high ESR and may have hypercalcaemia. Serum electrophoresis for immunoglobulins and urinary analysis for Bence Jones proteins confirm the diagnosis.

X-rays show classic punched-out lytic lesions. MRI and CT are of less use than X-rays.

Treatment

Chemotherapy is the mainstay with surgical stabilization or radiotherapy for impending fracture.

Prognosis

Overall prognosis is poor, with survival averaging 2 years.

LEUKAEMIA

The last malignancy to mention is leukaemia – a malignancy of white blood cells.

Leukaemia is the most common malignancy of childhood and about one-third of patients have bone pain. Leukaemia can also present with an acutely hot, swollen joint very similar to septic arthritis.

Further reading

Canale, S.T., 2006. Campbell's Operative Orthopaedics, eleventh ed, vols. 1–4. Mosby, St Louis.

Orthoteers website: http://www.orthoteers.co.uk.

Solomon, L., Warwick, D., Nayagan, D. (Eds.), 2001. Apley's System of Orthopaedics and Fractures, eighth ed. Hodder Arnold, London.

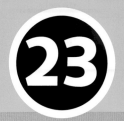
After reading this chapter you should be able to:
- Define what is meant by a 'locked knee' and give causes.
- Outline how to treat meniscal tears and describe which tears should be repaired.
- Describe the classical history of an anterior cruciate ligament (ACL) rupture and how this differs from a meniscal tear.
- Understand the mechanism of collateral ligament injuries and how these should be managed.
- Describe why the patella does not normally dislocate and describe which two groups of people suffer patellar dislocations.
- Describe shoulder anatomy and explain why this is the joint most prone to dislocation.
- Classify shoulder dislocations and know how to manage them.
- Outline the surgical indications for treatment of ACL and posterior cruciate ligament (PCL) ruptures and also shoulder and patellar dislocation.
- Diagnose and manage ankle sprains.

KNEE INJURIES

Introduction

The knee is commonly injured in sport – particularly football, rugby and skiing.

We will discuss injuries to the menisci, ligamentous injuries of the knee and patellar dislocation.

Meniscal injuries

The menisci are two semicircular fibrocartilage structures that lie between the femoral and tibial articular surfaces (Fig. 23.1). They act as 'shock absorbers' and are prone to injuries caused by the large forces crossing the knee.

Incidence

Meniscal injuries are common, usually occurring in young adult patients who participate in sports.

Pathology and aetiology

The medial meniscus is more commonly injured because it is fixed, in comparison to the more mobile lateral meniscus.

Meniscal tears can be traumatic or degenerative:

- Traumatic tears. The meniscus is normal and injury usually occurs after landing or twisting with the knee flexed. This can be associated with a ligamentous injury, such as an ACL tear. A chronically unstable knee is prone to further tears.
- Degenerative tears. These occur in an older population through abnormal cartilage. They may occur with little or no injury.

Types of meniscal tears (Fig. 23.2)

1. Bucket handle. The tear extends over a distance, remaining attached at the anterior and posterior horns. A locked knee results when a large bucket-handle tear flips over and becomes trapped in the joint, resulting in loss of complete extension.
2. Radial.
3. Horizontal cleavage.
4. Flap/parrot beak.

Of clinical importance is how peripheral the tear is. Very peripheral tears occur through vascular tissue and are amenable to repair, as these tears can heal. Meniscal tears further away from the blood supply (i.e. further into the knee) cannot heal.

Meniscal cysts result from synovial fluid being pumped into the meniscal tear. A valve effect means the fluid in the cyst cannot drain back into the knee (see Fig. 23.2).

Clinical features

Patients usually give a history of injury while playing sport, with the incident occurring during a tackle or when twisting or changing direction.

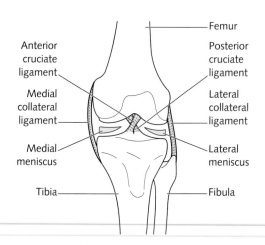

Fig. 23.1   Basic anatomy of the knee.

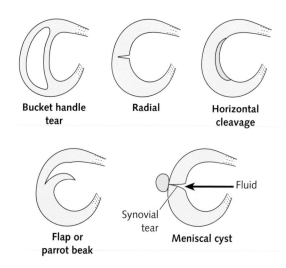

Fig. 23.2   Meniscal lesions.

A patient may present immediately after injury with a painful locked knee, or with a gradual chronic nagging pain with associated swelling over months or years following minor injury. In the chronic setting the symptoms are often intermittent in character.

Mechanical symptoms such as locking and catching suggest meniscal pathology. A 'clicking joint' does not necessarily mean there is pathology.

A more major injury with acute swelling and instability suggests associated ligamentous injury.

Examination may reveal:

- A locked knee.
- An effusion:
  - A large acute effusion suggests a very peripheral tear (which bleeds) or an associated injury.
  - A small chronic effusion is common.
- Joint line tenderness: this is an important part of the examination and is usually positive in a patient with a torn meniscus.
- A meniscal cyst, which may be palpable over the lateral joint line.

A variety of special tests are described for meniscal tears (such as McMurray's test), and none is very reliable.

Diagnosis and investigation

In most cases the diagnosis is made solely on the basis of history and examination.

X-rays are usually normal and are performed to exclude fracture or osteoarthritis or other rare causes of knee pain.

Magnetic resonance imaging (MRI) is very useful to confirm the presence of torn menisci, particularly in patients with a dubious history.

The most accurate way to confirm the diagnosis is with arthroscopy of the knee.

Management

Conservative

Initially RICE (rest, ice, compression, elevation) is used for an acutely swollen knee. Early physiotherapy is essential to encourage movement.

Surgical

Surgery is now performed using arthroscopic techniques. For peripheral bucket-handle tears, meniscal repair has the advantage of retaining the meniscus.

For tears not amenable to repair, meniscal resection is commonly performed. Partial meniscectomy removes the damaged portion only, leaving a stable rim and reducing the risk of osteoarthritis in the future.

Prognosis

Removal of a significant portion of a meniscus can lead to osteoarthritic changes developing in the knee because of increased load on the articular surface.

Ligamentous injuries of the knee

Anterior cruciate ligament

Incidence

One per 3000 of the population per year are affected.

Aetiology and pathology

The ACL is the primary restraint to anterior tibial translation, and a restraint to rotation. The mechanism of injury is usually a twisting or valgus strain pattern of injury commonly occurring in soccer or skiing (Fig. 23.3).

The knee is usually extended or slightly flexed with the foot fixed. Associated injuries to the medial collateral ligament (MCL) and either meniscus are common (the terrible triad). The patient often hears a 'pop' or feels 'something go' inside the knee.

ACL-deficient knees are liable to further meniscal tears.

Clinical features

With an acute ACL rupture, the patient will be unable to play on and may have to be carried from the field. Many patients present a long time after injury with symptoms of instability.

Swelling typically occurs within the timeframe of minutes to hours, unlike meniscal tears, which swell over 24 hours, because the ACL is more vascular than the menisci.

Once initial symptoms have settled, the patient may complain of giving way of the knee. This occurs when the patient tries to turn rapidly. Classically the patient will report being able to run in a straight line but not being able to 'twist and turn'. This giving way or instability is painfree.

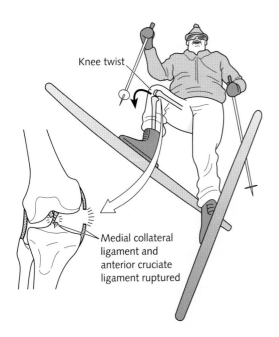

Knee twist

Medial collateral ligament and anterior cruciate ligament ruptured

Fig. 23.3 Mechanism of injury in anterior cruciate ligament rupture.

Clinically, patients have a tense effusion after an acute injury.

The anterior drawer, Lachman and pivot shift tests are positive (see Ch. 2).

Diagnosis and investigation

The majority can be diagnosed clinically.

In some patients it is difficult to elicit positive examination findings and in those patients an MRI scan is useful to confirm the diagnosis.

X-rays will usually be normal.

Management

Conservative

Initial treatment is with RICE and physiotherapy. In the absence of instability the majority of patients can modify their activities and manage with a hamstring rehabilitation programme only.

Surgical

ACL reconstruction is indicated for functional instability of the knee. This can be performed either through open or arthroscopic surgery using a hamstring tendon or patellar tendon graft. Meniscal tears can also be addressed at the time of surgery.

Posterior cruciate ligament

The PCL is the primary restraint to posterior movement of the tibia on the femur.

Incidence

PCL injuries are rare.

Aetiology and pathology

PCL injuries occur either in sporting activities or from road traffic accidents (dashboard injury) (Fig. 23.4).

Classically it is a goalkeeper's injury in football, the mechanism of injury being the knee combining with an onrushing attacking player forcing the tibia backwards. The PCL can also rupture when the knee is forcibly hyperextended.

The majority of PCL tears occur in combination with other ligamentous injuries and, rarely, injuries to the politeal artery. It is important to check the distal vasculature in suspect cases of PCL rupture.

Clinical features

The patient will have a substantial injury to the knee and will usually be unable to bear weight. Swelling is usually less obvious than with an ACL injury. Patients complain less of instability than with ACL injuries. Clinically, patients will have a posterior sag and positive posterior drawer test.

Careful assessment is needed to look for associated injuries such as lateral collateral ligament (LCL) injuries.

Fig. 23.4 Mechanism of injury in posterior cruciate ligament injuries.

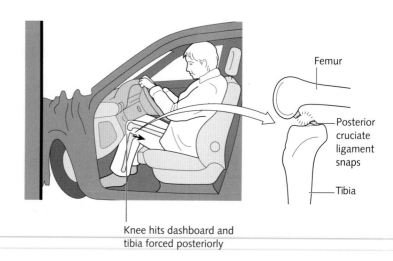

Femur

Posterior cruciate ligament snaps

Tibia

Knee hits dashboard and tibia forced posteriorly

Treatment

Conservative
Almost all isolated PCL injuries can be treated with rehabilitation alone.

Surgical
Patients with combined injuries or symptomatic instability require reconstruction.

Collateral ligament injuries

Incidence
MCL injuries are common injuries in isolation or combined with ACL injury, whilst LCL injuries are rare injuries.

Aetiology and pathology
In the case of MCL injuries there is a valgus strain pattern of injury. The injury can be complete or partial, and is frequently associated with ACL injury.

Isolated LCL injuries occur when a varus strain is placed on the knee (i.e. a hit from the medial side; Fig. 23.5).

Clinical features
Collateral ligament injuries are usually sporting injuries; the patient may feel 'something go' but an effusion is not a feature of an isolated collateral ligament tear (they are extra-articular structures). The patient will complain of pain and possibly instability.

When the MCL is injured there will be tenderness over the broad attachment of the MCL and opening up of the joint on valgus stress. In the normal knee the LCL is easily palpable as a cord-like structure. When the LCL is ruptured, the area is tender and indistinct. Opening up of the joint on the lateral side will be present on varus stress.

Management
Almost all isolated injuries heal well with conservative treatment. Treatment is with physiotherapy and bracing for 6 weeks. Minor tears heal well without bracing.

Surgical advancement is sometimes required for chronic unstable injuries.

Prognosis
The knee usually returns to normal after a period of rehabilitation.

Patellar dislocation

Introduction
The patella is prevented from dislocation by anatomical features such as a large lateral femoral condyle and the insertion of vastus medialis oblique and medial patellar femoral ligament (Fig. 23.6).

Incidence
Patellar dislocation is quite common.

Aetiology and pathology
Patellar dislocation can be habitual or traumatic.

Habitual dislocators are often young women with ligamentous laxity and a hypoplastic trochlea. This group gets recurrent dislocations after minor injuries, often without trauma, and are difficult to treat.

Traumatic dislocations occur during sports, usually with the knee slightly flexed with side impact. The dislocation occurs laterally and damage may occur to the joint surface as an osteochondral fracture. Structures along the medial border of the patella are torn.

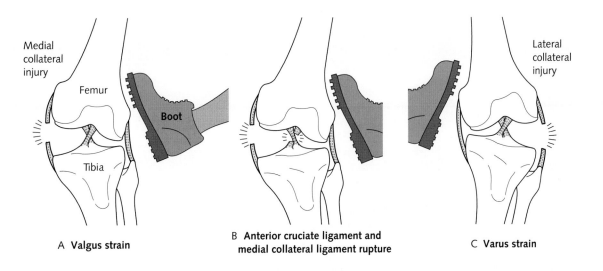

Fig. 23.5 Mechanism of injury in collateral ligament tears.

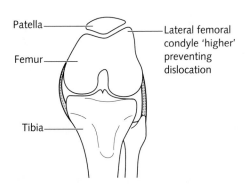

Fig. 23.6 Anatomical features that prevent lateral dislocation of the patella.

Clinical features

A first-time dislocation is extremely painful and the patient arrives in casualty with a history of 'dislocated knee'. The patella may have spontaneously reduced when the knee has been extended to allow transport. If not it will be laterally placed.

Often there is tenderness over the medial side of the knee and an effusion.

Later when the acute injury has settled the patient may have patellar apprehension and a J-sign. Habitual dislocators may show evidence of generalized laxity in other joints such as fingers, thumbs, elbows and knees (hypermobility syndrome). Both groups may have wasted or deficient vastus medialis.

Diagnosis and investigation

X-rays should be taken after reduction, including a tunnel and skyline view looking for any osteochondral defects.

Management

Conservative

Initial reduction is required, usually under sedation in the accident and emergency (A&E) department. A short period on crutches may be helpful. Immobilization is unhelpful.

Physiotherapy is required once pain and swelling allow improvement of range of movement and quadriceps strength.

Surgical

Osteochondral fractures should be repaired or removed arthroscopically.

Recurrent dislocations may require surgical realignment. Repair or reconstruction of the medial patellofemoral ligament is gaining in popularity.

SHOULDER DISLOCATION

Incidence

The shoulder is the most commonly dislocated large joint in the body.

Aetiology and pathology

The shoulder is at risk of dislocation because the joint has very little inherent bony stability, with reliance instead on capsule, labrum and rotator cuff muscles. The joint has 'sacrificed' stability for movement.

The dislocation can be anterior or posterior. Anterior dislocation (Fig. 23.7) accounts for 98% and usually occurs when the arm is forced back in a 'ball-throwing' position of external rotation and abduction. Posterior dislocations occur with epileptic seizures and electrocutions.

In anterior dislocation the labrum can be damaged anteroinferiorly, leaving a so-called Bankart lesion predisposing to further dislocations. Recurrent dislocations cause a Hill–Sachs lesion due to impaction of the glenoid on the posterior part of the humeral head.

In older patients the rotator cuff is torn rather than a Bankart lesion developing.

Clinical features

The patient is often a sports player – typically rugby – and has an acute injury to the shoulder, as described above. The injury is intensely painful and the shoulder is held supported by the other arm (Fig. 23.8).

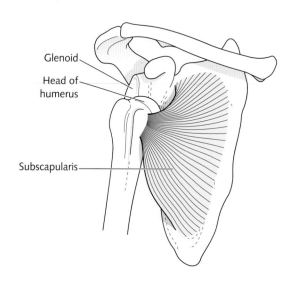

Glenoid

Head of humerus

Subscapularis

Fig. 23.7 Anterior dislocation of the humerus.

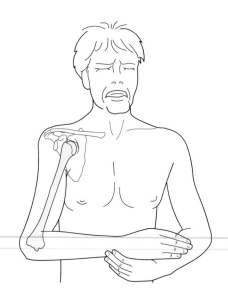

Fig. 23.8 Abnormal shoulder contour in anterior dislocation of the humerus.

Examination findings include:

- Loss of normal contour.
- Palpable glenoid.
- Complete loss of movement.

Check that the axillary nerve is functioning before and after any intervention.

Diagnosis and investigation

Anterior dislocation is usually obvious and confirmed with X-rays (always performed to exclude a fracture).

Posterior dislocation is often missed as the initial anteroposterior X-ray looks normal to the untrained eye. This should be suspected in any patient who has fixed internal rotation of the shoulder. The 'light bulb sign' (Fig. 23.9A) should raise suspicion but the diagnosis is made on axillary view (Fig. 23.9B) or computed tomography scan.

Treatment

Conservative

The dislocation needs to be promptly reduced in the A&E department under sedation.

Posterior dislocation often requires a general anaesthetic and may need open reduction.

Once the dislocation is reduced, the joint is rested in a collar and cuff and once the pain has settled, supervised early rehabilitation with the physiotherapist can commence.

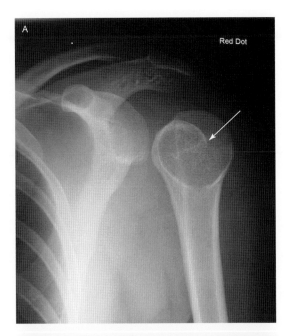

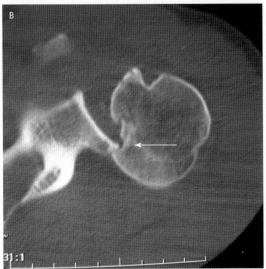

Fig. 23.9 Posterior dislocation of the shoulder: (A) Anteroposterior X-ray showing the 'light bulb' sign; (B) computed tomography scan showing axillary view. There is posterior subluxation of the head with impaction of the head from the glenoid rim (arrowed).

Surgical

Surgery is reserved for the recurrent dislocations to repair bone or labral defects.

Prognosis

A young male sportsman has an 80% chance of recurrent dislocation following anterior dislocation of the shoulder.

In the more elderly population shoulder stiffness is more of a problem than recurrence.

HINTS AND TIPS

Your current textbook may advise 6 weeks' immobilization for patellar and shoulder dislocations to allow the 'soft tissues to heal'. This is old-fashioned thinking and a short period of rest (3–5 days) is now followed by early rehabilitation.

ANKLE SPRAIN

Incidence

Ankle sprains are very common injuries, lateral more so than medial.

Aetiology and pathology

These injuries are commonly found on the sports field but anyone can have an ankle sprain. The mechanism of injury is inversion or eversion with damage to the lateral ligament and medial ligament complexes respectively.

In a lateral ligament sprain the talus tilts in varus in the ankle mortice, and the anterior talofibular and calcaneofibular ligaments are torn (Fig. 23.10). In a medial ligament sprain the talus tilts in valgus in the ankle mortice, and the deltoid ligament complex is torn.

Clinical features

The patient experiences pain and may feel 'something go'; swelling occurs rapidly.

Chronic ankle instability leads to giving way of the joint.

Clinically the patient has a variable amount of swelling and tenderness over either the lateral or medial ligament complex.

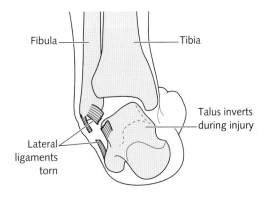

Fig. 23.10 Ankle ligament rupture.

Patients may have instability of the ankle joint with a positive anterior drawer test and opening of the lateral side.

Diagnosis and investigation

X-rays are performed only if there is bony tenderness or inability to weight bear (Ottawa ankle rules).

Management

Conservative

All sprains are treated conservatively initially with analgesia, RICE and physiotherapy.

Surgical

Arthroscopy of the ankle is sometimes performed for associated osteochondral injuries.

Rarely, ligament reconstruction is required for a chronically unstable ankle.

Further reading

Orthoteers website: http://www.orthoteers.co.uk.

Solomon, L., Warwick, D., Nayagan, D. (Eds.), 2001. Apley's System of Orthopaedics and Fractures. eighth ed. Hodder Arnold, London.

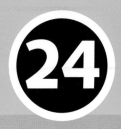
After reading this chapter you should be able to:
- Recognize problems affecting tendons (tendinopathy, tenosynovitis and tendon rupture).
- Know how to recognize, investigate and treat bursitis.
- Understand which factors predispose to Dupuytren contracture.

INTRODUCTION

Soft-tissue disorders are common. They are responsible for many days of absence from work and contribute significantly to the workload in primary care, accident and emergency departments, and rheumatology and orthopaedic clinics. This chapter will discuss the presentation, diagnosis and management of some common soft-tissue lesions.

TENDON LESIONS

The three main pathologies that affect tendons are:
1. Tendinopathy.
2. Tenosynovitis.
3. Rupture.

Tendinopathy

Definition

Pain arises from strain or injury to tendons and their insertions to bone. The term 'enthesopathy' is used to describe cases with a significant periosteal component, such as lateral or medial epicondylitis.

Aetiopathogenesis

The pathogenesis of tendinopathy is poorly understood. Some cases occur as part of a systemic inflammatory condition and others are related to injury from overuse. However, most cases of tendinopathy are idiopathic.

Clinical features

The most frequent sites of tendinopathy are the:
- Shoulder.
- Elbow.
- Achilles tendon.

Patients complain of pain that is worsened by active movement. Examination findings include:
- Tenderness of the tendon and its insertion.
- An increase in pain when active movement is performed against resistance.
- Soft-tissue swelling (not always present).

An example: tennis elbow and golfer's elbow

In these conditions, pain is centred around the lateral and medial epicondyles respectively, although it may radiate distally from the elbow. The examination findings are as follows.

Tennis elbow
The common extensor origin, at the lateral epicondyle, is tender and pain is exacerbated by resisted wrist extension (Fig. 24.1A).

Golfer's elbow
The common flexor origin, at the medial epicondyle, is tender and pain is exacerbated by resisted wrist flexion (Fig. 24.1B).

Investigation

Tendinopathy can be diagnosed clinically and investigations are often unremarkable. Radiographs may show abnormalities, such as calcification in chronic rotator cuff disease. Ultrasound may also detect changes in the tendon and surrounding tissue.

Management

The interventions shown below may lead to improvement of symptoms. The strategies at the top of the list should be employed early in the disease process, whilst those at the bottom should be reserved for resistant cases:

- Rest or avoidance of precipitating cause.
- Non-steroidal anti-inflammatory drug therapy.

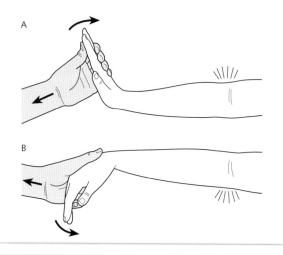

Fig. 24.1 The pain of tennis elbow is exacerbated by resisted wrist extension (A). The pain of golfer's elbow is exacerbated by resisted wrist flexion (B).

- Local corticosteroid injection.
- Physiotherapy/ultrasound therapy.
- Surgery.

Tenosynovitis

Definition

Tenosynovitis is inflammation of the synovial lining of a tendon sheath.

Aetiology

The two main causes are:

1. Inflammatory arthritis.
2. Trauma.

Trauma is usually repetitive or unaccustomed movement.

Clinical features

Patients present with pain in the region of the affected tendon. Common sites of tenosynovitis are the abductor pollicis longus and extensor pollicis brevis tendons (De Quervain tenosynovitis) and finger flexors. On examination, the tendon is swollen and tender, and crepitus may be felt on palpation.

A trigger finger or thumb results from tenosynovitis of the flexor tendons. A nodule can develop on the tendon in response to constriction of the tendon sheath. The nodule 'catches' as it enters or leaves the flexor tendon pulleys and a 'snapping' or 'flicking' movement of the digit occurs on flexion or extension. In severe cases the digit may be held in flexion, requiring the patient to release the 'triggered' digit with the other hand.

Management

Treatment includes rest, splinting and local corticosteroid injection. Surgical decompression of the tendon sheath may be required.

Tendon rupture

Aetiology

Tendon rupture may result from chronic inflammation and degeneration or trauma. For example, rupture of the extensor tendons of the fingers is often seen in rheumatoid arthritis.

Clinical features

The resulting clinical features are loss of movement at the joint to which the tendon provides power, deformity and sometimes swelling. After rupture of the long head of biceps tendon, a bulge formed by the lateral muscle belly is seen in the upper arm – 'Popeye's' sign. Extensor tendon rupture at the distal phalanx can occur after a direct blow to the fingertip, causing aggressive flexion of the distal interphalangeal joint. It results in an inability to extend the flexed distal interphalangeal joint ('mallet finger') (Fig. 24.2).

Management

Sometimes no intervention may be required, such as a long head of biceps tendon rupture, as function is preserved with other muscles – in that case, short head of biceps, brachialis and supinator. Sometimes splintage is all that is required – a mallet splint in the case of a mallet finger. However surgery is often required to restore function. This may require a direct repair of the tendon or a tendon transfer.

BURSITIS

Bursae are small sacs of fibrous tissue that are lined with synovial membrane which secrete synovial fluid. They

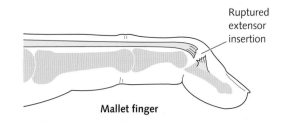

Ruptured extensor insertion

Mallet finger

Fig. 24.2 'Mallet finger'.

reduce friction where ligaments and tendons pass over bone. Inflammation of a bursa (bursitis) can be idiopathic, part of a systemic inflammatory disease or due to injury, infection or gout. Some types are notifiable industrial disorders (e.g. coal miner's 'beat' knee).

Olecranon bursitis, prepatellar bursitis and trochanteric bursitis are common and their clinical features and management are discussed below.

Olecranon bursitis

This can be precipitated by excessive friction at the elbow, for example by resting the elbow on a desk. Septic olecranon bursitis causes pain on elbow flexion. Idiopathic and traumatic cases are usually only painful when pressure is applied to the bursa; movement of the elbow is not usually uncomfortable or impaired. On examination the bursa is distended and tender.

Bursal fluid should be aspirated to exclude infection and improve symptoms. Local corticosteroid injection is effective in non-septic cases. Infection should be treated with appropriate antibiotics.

> **COMMUNICATION**
>
> Soft-tissue lesions are commonly precipitated by overuse injuries. It is therefore important to ask patients about their work and leisure activities.

Prepatellar or infrapatellar bursitis (housemaid's or carpetfitter's/ clergyman's knee)

This is common in people such as carpet fitters who spend a lot of time kneeling. A hot, red swelling develops over the front of the patella. Active knee extension is usually quite painful. Infection and gout should be excluded by aspirating fluid. Treatment involves rest. Recurrent episodes may require surgical excision of the bursa. Antibiotic therapy should be given for sepsis.

While aspiration of a prepatellar or olecranon bursitis may be useful in the diagnosis of infection or gout when there is doubt regarding diagnosis, serial aspiration should be avoided as this predisposes the patient to sinus formation and chronic infection. Infected bursitis that fails to settle with antibiotics requires formal incision and drainage.

Trochanteric bursitis

The trochanteric bursa is located lateral to the greater trochanter of the femurs and allows motion of the fasica lata over the trochanter. When this bursa becomes inflamed the patient will develop pain over the affected trochanter, exacerbated by movement. Patients will often complain of 'hip pain'; however careful questioning and examination will identify pain localized to the trochanter as opposed to the groin or adductor or buttock pain of hip joint pathology. Treatment consists of physiotherapy in the first instance, with steroid injections used in more severe cases. Persistent and debilitating trochanteric bursitis may require surgery.

DUPUYTREN CONTRACTURE

Definition

Dupuytren contracture is a common condition, characterized by fibromatosis of the palmar fascia, resulting in flexion contractures of the metacarpophalangeal and interphalangeal joints of one or more fingers.

Fibromatosis may affect other areas of the body – plantar fascia (Ledderhose disease), penis (Peyronie disease) or knuckle pads (Garrod disease). It is important to ask whether the patient has any symptoms or deformity elsewhere.

Incidence

Before the age of 55, the incidence of Dupuytren contracture is much higher in men than in women. After this time the incidence is equal.

Aetiology

Several factors predispose to Dupuytren contracture. These are shown in Figure 24.3. Historically Dupuytren contracture was felt to be a disease of northern Europeans, and whilst there is a preponderance, it is also common in those of Mediterranean or Japanese descent.

Clinical features

The ulnar side of the hand is most commonly affected. Patients complain of an inability to extend one or more fingers, usually the ring and little fingers. It is rarely (perhaps never) painful. The fibromatosis may remain stable or progress. Progressive cases can result in marked deformity and loss of function, with the fingers held in a fixed position curled into the palm.

Fig. 24.3 Factors associated with Dupuytren contracture
Family history of Dupuytren contracture
Hepatic cirrhosis
Diabetes mellitus
Anticonvulsant therapy

Fig. 24.4 Dupuytren contracture of the palmar fascia (arrow).

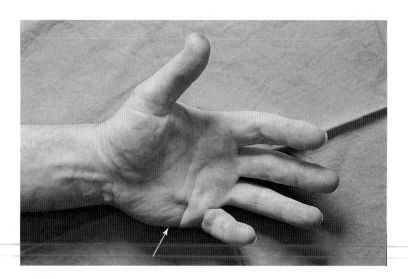

In early cases, nodules may be felt in the palm or on the palmar surface of the finger. In more advanced cases, flexion at the metacarpophalangeal joints is seen (Fig. 24.4) and the palm of the hand cannot be placed flat on a table (positive table-top test). In severe cases the proximal and distal interphalangeal joints are involved.

Management

The most effective treatment is surgery. The decision to progress to surgery can either be made when the patient has a positive table-top test, or when the deformity starts to affect the patient's quality of life. Palmar fasciectomy is the most commonly performed procedure. Complete correction of the deformity is more difficult the more advanced the disease. There is a risk of recurrence postoperatively.

Further reading

Hazleman, B., Riley, G., Speed, C. (Eds.), 2004. Soft Tissue Rheumatology. Oxford University Press, Oxford.

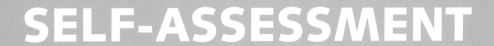

SELF-ASSESSMENT

Question 1

An 85-year-old man presents to his GP with low back pain for 2 days. Over the previous 3 years, he noticed that his shirts seemed to be getting longer but not looser. He had a previous rib fracture 1 year ago after falling off his seat. A blood test is performed and the results are as follows:

	Patient data	Normal range
Calcium	2.38 mmol/L	2.12–2.65 mmol/L
Phosphate	1.1 mmol/L	0.8–1.4 mmol/L
Alkaline phosphatase	98 iu/L	30–150 iu/L

Which is the most likely diagnosis?

A. Myeloma.
B. Osteomalacia.
C. Osteoporosis.
D. Paget disease.
E. Tuberculosis.

Question 2

A 58-year-old woman presents to her physician with hip pain for 3 weeks. On examination, she has bowing of her tibias. She seems to have difficulty hearing and the doctor has to keep repeating himself. Her father has similar bowing of tibias.

What is the most appropriate next step in diagnosis?

A. Bone biochemistry.
B. Coeliac serology.
C. Dual-energy X-ray absorptiometry (DEXA) bone scan.
D. Magnetic resonance imaging (MRI) tibia.
E. Test for rheumatoid factor.

Question 3

A 53-year-old man presents to his GP with a headache for 3 days. The pain is only on the left side of his head and radiates into his scalp. He has no vision problems or pain in his jaw when eating but he feels pain when he combs his hair. The pain is constantly there and is only relieved temporarily by paracetamol.

What investigation is most useful in confirming the diagnosis?

A. Antineutrophil cytoplasmic antibody (ANCA).
B. Erythrocyte sedimentation rate (ESR).
C. Lumbar puncture.
D. MRI of aortic arch.
E. Temporal artery biopsy.

Question 4

A 75-year-old man develops pain in his right wrist and right third metacarpophalangeal (MCP) joint. The joint is swollen, red, warm and tender. He is right-handed and cannot hold his pen properly because of the pain. Joint aspiration shows rhomboid calcium pyrophosphate crystals. On X-ray, chondrocalcinosis, subchondral sclerosis and osteophytes are seen of his wrist and MCP joint. The patient was given co-codamol for pain relief.

What is the most effective next step in management for his acute problem?

A. Antibiotics.
B. Disease-modifying antirheumatic drug (DMARD) therapy.
C. Joint replacement.
D. Physiotherapy.
E. Splinting.

Question 5

A 22-year-old man develops an acute swelling of his right knee and ankle with painful heels. There was no trauma. He had conjunctivitis and fever 1 week ago. His bloods and urine are taken for culture; results come back as 'nothing cultured'.

Which of the following is unlikely to be a pathogen?

A. *Chlamydia trachomatis.*
B. *Escherichia coli.*
C. *Haemophilus influenzae.*
D. *Neisseria gonorrhoeae.*
E. *Salmonella typhi.*

Question 6

A 65-year-old woman with stable rheumatoid arthritis of 8 years notices loss of sensation in her lateral 3½ fingers, palmar aspect.

What is the most appropriate therapy for her most recent condition?

A. Intramuscular gold injections.
B. Oral methotrexate tablets.
C. Oral steroid tablets.
D. Physiotherapy.
E. Splinting.

Single best answer questions (SBAs)

Question 7

A 33-year-old Asian woman comes to her physician complaining of fatigue, myalgia and weight loss. She finds it more painful to weight bear now as compared to 6 months ago. She is losing a lot of hair while brushing after a bath, and there is a non-itchy rash over her nose and cheeks.

What test is most likely to confirm the diagnosis?

A. Anti-double-stranded DNA antibodies.
B. ESR.
C. Lupus anticoagulant.
D. Skin biopsy of the rash.
E. Thyroid function test.

Question 8

A 58-year-old man presents to Accident and Emergency (A&E) with breathlessness. It is discovered that his breathlessness is caused by pulmonary hypertension. On further examination while in hospital, the man is found to have Raynaud phenomenon, calcinosis and sclerodactyly. He also complains of long-standing heartburn, for which he is taking omeprazole.

What is the most likely explanation for these findings?

A. Linear scleroderma.
B. Multiple sclerosis.
C. Paraneoplastic phenomena.
D. Systemic lupus erythematosus (SLE).
E. Systemic sclerosis.

Question 9

A 47-year-old business woman presents to her GP repeatedly with widespread joint pain. Her sleep is disrupted and she complains of fatigue and poor concentration; this makes her even more stressed at work. Having already undergone many different investigations, she finds it upsetting that doctors cannot find a diagnosis for her.

What is the best treatment strategy for this woman?

A. DMARD therapy.
B. Diet changes.
C. Exercise.
D. Joint injections.
E. Steroids.

Question 10

A 77-year-old man sees his physician for left knee pain, gradually getting worse over the past 1 month. He is finding it more difficult to weight bear on his left side and notices his knee joint is getting more swollen. Going for walks has become an arduous process, with his left knee becoming excruciatingly painful. Sometimes the pain wakes him up at night.

What would an X-ray of his knee show?

A. Hairline fracture.
B. Joint erosions.
C. Osteophytes.

D. Osteopenia.
E. Soft-tissue swelling.

Question 11

An 80-year-old man presents to his GP with pain in his finger joints for 6 months. He complains of not being able to button his shirts or hold his gardening tools properly. He has flattening of his knuckles, swan-neck deformities of his fingers and z-deformity of his thumbs. There is also a slight degree of ulnar deviation in his right hand. Both his parents had similar conditions.

What might you not see on X-ray of his hands?

A. Cyst formation.
B. Joint effusions.
C. Narrowed joint space.
D. Osteopenia.
E. Soft-tissue swelling.

Question 12

A 21-year-old man from Pakistan comes to his GP with progressive difficulty sitting forward in the mornings over a 3-month period and weight loss. Looking at him from the side, his GP observes a loss of lumbar lordosis.

What is the most likely diagnosis?

A. Ankylosing spondylitis.
B. Acute leukaemia.
C. Potts disease (tuberculosis of spine).
D. Prolapsed intervertebral disc.
E. Osteoporosis.

Question 13

A 45-year-old woman complains of dry eyes, dry mouth and a recent swelling at the side of her face. There is evidence of oral candidiasis and dental caries. She also mentions right shoulder and left knee tenderness, and sore joints in her feet. Her GP questions whether she has rheumatoid arthritis or SLE. Some tests are conducted.

Which is the most likely test to confirm the diagnosis?

A. Human immunodeficiency virus (HIV) test.
B. Schober test.
C. Schirmer test.
D. Transoesophageal echo.
E. Trendelenburg test.

Question 14

A 59-year-old obese man presented to his physician with acute onset of pain to his first metatarsophalangeal (MTP) joint. His first MTP joint was red, swollen, tender, warm and stiff. On further examination, the doctor found unusual white lumps at the end of two fingers. A joint aspiration was conducted.

What is the most likely finding from the joint aspiration?

A. Bacteria from joint infection.
B. Calcium pyrophosphate crystals.

C. Clear synovial fluid.
D. Pus.
E. Sodium urate crystals.

Question 15

A 53-year-old woman complains of bloody diarrhoea and abdominal pain. She also experiences fever, nausea and weight loss. A colonoscopy was conducted and ulcerative lesions on her rectum were seen. During this period of her bowel condition, she develops pain in her right knee and left shoulder. She felt that the intensity of her joint pains increased as her diarrhoea increased, and progressively got worse over the course of 2 weeks.

What is the most appropriate immediate management for this woman?

A. Biological therapies.
B. Non-steroidal anti-inflammatory drugs (NSAIDs).
C. Panproctocolectomy.
D. Prednisolone.
E. Sulfasalazine.

Question 16

A 60-year-old woman comes to her physician with pain and stiffness in both shoulders and in her hip for 3 weeks. There is worsening muscle weakness and she finds it difficult to move because of the pain. She also complains of a sudden-onset headache that came along with her joint pain 3 days ago. The headache is described as a 'left-sided headache going up into my scalp and jaw'. On palpation of the temporal region of her head, she said it is sore. There are no visual disturbances or seizures, but there is slight nausea.

What medication should be administered immediately?

A. Amitriptyline.
B. Carbamazepine.
C. Ibuprofen.
D. Morphine.
E. Prednisolone.

Question 17

An 80-year-old man who has known chronic renal failure starts developing bone tenderness and muscle weakness over the course of a month. He no longer goes around with his Zimmer frame because it is too painful. Blood tests are done for him and the results are as follows:

	Patient data	Normal range
Calcium	1.56 mmol/L	2.12–2.65 mmol/L
Phosphate	0.62 mmol/L	0.8–1.4 mmol/L
Alkaline phosphatase	198 iu/L	30–150 iu/L

What is not a possible consequence of his condition?

A. Skeletal deformity.
B. Tetany.
C. Polydipsia.
D. Convulsions.
E. Arrhythmias.

Question 18

A 67-year-old woman presents to her GP with difficulty rising from a chair. The doctor also notices erythematous plaques over her knuckles and also a lilac discoloration over her upper eyelids. He decides to conduct some investigations to confirm his diagnosis.

Which investigation would give the highest diagnostic yield?

A. Serum level of creatinine kinase.
B. ESR.
C. Antinuclear antibodies.
D. Chest X-ray.
E. X-ray of affected joints.

Question 19

A 45-year-old man presents to his GP with joint pain and stiffness in both wrists, knuckles and distal interphalangeal joints for 2 weeks. There is a slight degree of swelling in his right and left middle fingers, making them look like sausages. The GP notices that the man has dry skin along his hairline and at the back of his ears.

Which of the following nail changes is he most likely to have?

A. Keratoderma blenorrhagica.
B. Koilonychia.
C. Leuconychia.
D. Paronychia.
E. Subungual hyperkeratosis.

Question 20

A mother brings her 10-year-old son to see his physician because he complains of pain in both knees, and right hip. He has stopped wanting to play football for about 3 months, which she suspects was when the pain came on. His mother says that he did not want to come to see the doctor that day because he felt his joints 'were getting better'. Which of the following eye problems is the boy most at risk of developing?

A. Anterior uveitis.
B. Conjunctivitis.
C. Episcleritis.
D. Scleritis.
E. Scleromalacia.

Question 21

A 78-year-old man presents to his GP with thoracic back pain after a minor slip in his toilet. He feels he is 'shrinking' and attributes this to his becoming more 'hunchback from old age'.

What is the next most appropriate investigation to do for this man?

A. Calcium and vitamin D_3 levels.
B. DEXA bone scan.
C. HLA B27 testing.
D. MRI of whole spine.
E. Thoracic X-ray.

Question 22

A 56-year-old woman presents to her physician with pain shooting down her right leg from her back and also with sore knees. Both knees feel warm and walking causes pain. Bone biochemistry is done and the results are as follows:

	Normal range	Patient data
Calcium	2.12–2.65 mmol/L	2.38 mmol/L
Phosphate	0.8–1.4 mmol/L	1.1 mmol/L
Alkaline phosphatase	30–150 iu/L	220 iu/L

What is the most likely diagnosis in this woman?

A. Osteoarthritis.
B. Prolapsed intervertebral disc.
C. Paget disease.
D. Septic arthritis.
E. Stroke.

Question 23

A 60-year-old man, who used to work in the factory moving heavy machinery, presents to his physician with pain in his hips. He has great trouble sitting down and getting up because his hip joints are very stiff. There is also a Baker cyst at the back of his knees but he says that does not bother him too much. His main concern is the pain in his hips which has been ongoing for the past month; sometimes the pain creeps down to his knees. Resting makes it better and moving makes it worse.

What is the most appropriate next step in managing this man?

A. Glucosamine.
B. Hip X-ray.
C. Joint replacement.
D. Physiotherapy.
E. Trial of steroids.

Question 24

An 86-year-old woman comes to her GP with pain in her fingers and toes for 6 weeks. She explains that her knuckles feel tender, stiff and swollen; and so do her joints in her toes. Stiffness is maximum when she just wakes up but gets better as the day goes by. She also has a smooth firm subcutaneous lump on the extensor side of her elbow which is non-tender. Her past medical history states she has had a peptic ulcer with haemorrhage.

Which of the following would be best avoided in this woman?

A. Hydroxychloroquine.
B. Methotrexate.
C. Naproxen.
D. Prednisolone.
E. Sulfasalazine.

Question 25

A 55-year-old man comes to his doctor with an excruciating pain in his right first MTP joint since yesterday. The skin overlying the joint is very inflamed, swollen, red and warm and the joint is stiff and immobile. He walks with a limp. He had a similar episode before about a year ago which resolved and left him symptomless before this current episode broke out.

What is the most likely explanation for his condition?

A. There is degeneration of weight-bearing cartilage surfaces and subsequent eburnation of subchondral bone.
B. This is an autoimmune condition where T lymphocytes attack the synovial lining of joints, eventually causing erosion of cartilage and bone.
C. There is an ongoing secondary infection within the joint from an infection source at a distant site.
D. Hyperuricaemia leads to the formation of sodium urate crystals that get deposited in the synovium, causing inflammation.
E. Calcium pyrophosphate crystals have deposited in the joint.

Question 26

A 68-year-old woman comes to the clinic feeling tired, with myalgia and bone pain. The GP does a blood test and these are her results:

	Patient data	Normal range
Calcium	1.87 mmol/L	2.12–2.65 mmol/L
Phosphate	0.58 mmol/L	0.8–1.4 mmol/L
Alkaline phosphatase	202 iu/L	30–150 iu/L
Haemoglobin	10.3 g/dL	11.5–16.0 g/dL

	Patient data	Normal range
Mean call volume	101 fL	76–96 fL
Iron	9 µmol/L	11–30 µmol/L
Folate	1.9 µg/L	2.1 µg/L

Which investigation is the most useful in confirming her condition?

A. Anti-double-stranded DNA antibody.
B. Antiphospholipid antibody.
C. Anti-smooth-muscle antibody.
D. Anti-tissue transglutaminase antibody.
E. Anti-vitamin D_3 antibody.

Question 27

A 35-year-old woman presents to A&E with breathlessness, chest pain and haemoptysis. She receives thrombolysis and is relieved of her symptoms. She gives a past history of stillbirth and central retinal vein occlusion.

What is the most appropriate investigation for this woman?

A. Anti-double-stranded DNA antibody.
B. ANCA.
C. Antiphospholipid antibody.
D. Prothrombin time.
E. Venereal Disease Research Laboratory (VDRL) tests.

Question 28

A 58-year-old man presents to his GP with shortness of breath, bloody sputum, joint pain and a fever. His GP quickly admits him into hospital. Blood tests show that his urea and creatinine levels were abnormally high. Moreover, doctors noticed a 'saddle' look to his nose.

What is the most likely diagnosis for this man?

A. Pulmonary embolism.
B. SLE.
C. Churg–Strauss syndrome.
D. Essential cryoglobulinaemic vasculitis.
E. Wegener granulomatosis.

Question 29

A 72-year-old man presents with a 24-hour history of a painful swollen wrist, with no history of trauma. There is no significant past medical history. On examination he is apyrexial. The wrist is mildly erythematous and is tender on palpation with a decreased range of motion. X-rays of the wrist demonstrate chondrocalcinosis of the triangular fibrocartilage. CRP and ESR are mildly elevated and white blood cells are normal.

What is the most likely diagnosis?

A. Gout.
B. Septic arthritis.
C. Pseudogout.
D. Rheumatoid arthritis.
E. Haemarthrosis.

Question 30

A 24-year-old, normally fit and healthy woman presents with a 4-month history of gradually increasing pain in her left knee. There was no history of trauma. She is now having difficulty weight bearing, and is frequently woken at night with pain. She also notes weight loss in the same timeframe. X-rays of her knee demonstrate an expansile and lytic lesion in her distal femur, with cortical destruction and significant periosteal reaction.

What is the most likely diagnosis?

A. Tuberculosis.
B. Osteosarcoma.
C. Enchondroma.
D. Osteomyelitis.
E. Stress fracture.

Question 31

The majority of the blood supply to the femoral head in adults arises from:

A. Artery of ligamentum teres.
B. Lateral femoral circumflex artery.
C. Obturator artery.
D. Medial femoral circumflex artery.
E. Profunda femoris.

Question 32

The most common pathogen in septic arthritis in adults is:

A. *Streptococcus* sp.
B. *Mycobacterium tuberculosis*.
C. *Staphylococcus aureus*.
D. *Haemophilus influenzae*.
E. *Enterobacter* sp.

Question 33

A distal radius fracture with significant dorsal angulation is most likely to cause altered sensation in the distribution of which nerve:

A. Ulnar nerve.
B. Superficial radial nerve.
C. Medial cutaneous nerve of the forearm.
D. Median nerve.
E. Axillary nerve.

Question 34

A 30-year-old man presents with an intensely painful right proximal tibia with no history of trauma. He experiences the pain during the day and night. Of note, he states that aspirin relieves his pain significantly. On examination there is significant tenderness over the proximal tibial metaphysis. X-ray shows a small lucent area in the tibial metaphysis with dense sclerosis surrounding it.

What is the most likely diagnosis?

A. Enchondroma.
B. Osteoid osteoma.
C. Chondrosarcoma.
D. Osteochondroma.
E. Lymphoma.

Question 35

A 64-year-old man with a background of diabetes presents with a 24-hour history of progressive atraumatic left knee pain. He states he is unable to bend his knee and unable to weight bear. On examination he is pyrexial and he has a hot and erythematous left knee. He has a large effusion, virtually no range of movement and global tenderness around the knee.

What is the most important step in this man's management?

A. Anteroposterior (AP) and lateral X-rays of the knee.
B. Commence intravenous antibiotics.
C. Aspiration of the knee.
D. Bloods for inflammatory markers.
E. Ultrasound scan of the knee.

Question 36

Which of the following is not a risk factor in the development of Perthes disease?

A. Delayed bone age.
B. Hypothyroidism.
C. Low socioeconomic group.
D. Low-birthweight children.
E. Family history.

Question 37

A 13-year-old overweight boy presents with severe right hip pain, on a background of 2 weeks of groin pain. There is no history of trauma, and he is otherwise well. He is unable to weight bear, holds his hip in external rotation and flexion, and has a decreased range of motion in all axes because of pain. Inflammatory markers are normal. What is the likely diagnosis?

A. Perthes disease.
B. Septic arthritis.
C. Neck of femur fracture.
D. Osteoarthritis.
E. Slipped upper femoral epiphysis.

Question 38

A 15-year-old boy presents with bilateral knee pain, exacerbated by exercise. He cannot remember a specific episode of trauma. On examination he has prominent tibial tuberosities which are painful on palpation. He has a reduced range of flexion because of anterior knee pain, but has full extension. What is the diagnosis?

A. Osgood–Schlatters disease.
B. Osteochondritis dissecans.
C. Medial meniscal tear.
D. Osteoarthritis.
E. Bilateral tibial plateau fractures.

Question 39

In the case of a prolapsed vertebral disc, pain is caused when the nerve root is compressed by:

A. Annulus fibrosis.
B. Posterior longitudinal ligament.
C. Ligamentum flavum.
D. Nucleus pulposus.
E. Interspinous ligament.

Question 40

Which of the following is a sign of impending cauda equina syndrome?

A. Severe unilateral sciatic-type pain.
B. Bilateral sciatic-type pain.
C. Prolonged duration of symptoms.
D. Leg pain and altered sensation.
E. Muscle weakness.

Question 41

A 61-year-old retired brick layer presents with chronic back pain. He describes his pain as exacerbated by walking, particularly downhill, and radiating into his buttocks, thighs and calves bilaterally. Examination reveals a stooped gait and a reduced range of motion in the lumbar spine. His symptoms are exacerbated by extension of the spine.

What is the diagnosis?

A. Prolapsed intervertebral disc.
B. Mechanical back pain.
C. Spinal stenosis.
D. Spondylolisthesis.
E. Spinal malignancy.

Question 42

A locked knee is caused by:

A. Anterior cruciate ligament tear.
B. Radial meniscal tear.
C. Medial collateral ligament tear.
D. Bucket handle meniscal tear.
E. Tibial plateau fracture.

Question 43

A 18-year-old football player presents to A&E with a knee injury. He describes turning quickly and twisting his right knee, precipitating immediate pain. He states his knee was grossly swollen before he left the pitch. On examination there is a tense effusion, no joint line tenderness and a poor range of motion. Lachman test is positive, but otherwise the knee is stable.

What is the diagnosis?

A. Medial meniscal tear.
B. Posterior cruciate ligament tear.
C. Medial collateral ligament tear.
D. Patellar dislocation.
E. Anterior cruciate ligament tear.

Question 44

De Quervain tenosynovitis involves inflammation of which tendon sheath?

A. Extensor pollicis longus.
B. Abductor pollicis longus.
C. Extensor indicis.
D. Flexor pollicis longus.
E. Extensor carpi radialis longus.

Question 45

A 56-year-old woman with rheumatoid arthritis presents to her GP with a 6-month history of altered sensation and pain in both her hands, the right worse than the left. She describes pins and needle in her index, middle and ring fingers; and pain at night, which frequently wakens her from sleep. She also describes decreased grip strength. On examination there is wasting of the thenar eminences and percussion at the wrist crease exacerbates her symptoms.

What is the diagnosis?

A. Cervical radiculopathy.
B. Cubital tunnel syndrome.
C. Peripheral neuropathy.
D. Carpal tunnel syndrome.
E. Transient ischaemic attacks.

Question 46

A patient is admitted to an orthopaedic ward with a proximal tibia fracture whilst awaiting surgery. During the night the patient experiences a severe increase in pain. This is initially settled with opiate analgesia, but rapidly returns and eventually opiate analgesia is no longer effective.

What are you primarily concerned about?

A. Further displacement of the fracture.
B. Deep vein thrombosis.
C. Compartment syndrome.
D. Embolic arterial occlusion.
E. Nerve injury following the fracture.

Question 47

A man arrives in A&E following a car accident, with a suspected pelvic fracture. He is unresponsive, hypotensive and tachycardic. The first step in the management of this patient is:

A. Obtain intravenous access and commence fluid resuscitation.
B. Apply a pelvic binder.
C. Get an AP pelvis X-ray.
D. Cross-match the patient for type-matched blood.
E. Assess the airway whilst stabilizing the cervical spine.

Question 48

A 68-year-old women is seen 3 days following a total hip replacement. Initially progressing well, she suddenly develops sharp left-sided chest pain and shortness of breath. On examination she has a slight pyrexia (37.5 °C), is hypoxic on room air (Spo$_2$ 91%) and tachycardic (heart rate 110 bpm).

What is the cause of her symptoms?

A. Pulmonary thromboembolism.
B. Myocardial infarction.
C. Basal atelectasis.
D. Fat embolism.
E. Pneumothorax.

Question 49

A normally fit and well 45-year-old woman present to her GP with a lump on her wrist. She describes a 1-year history of a marble-sized lump on the volar aspect of her wrist. She states the lump comes and goes, and is not painful. On examination there is a 1×1 cm fluctuant lesion on the volar aspect of her left wrist. It is fixed to underlying tissues.

What is the most likely diagnosis?

A. Soft-tissue sarcoma.
B. Lipoma.
C. Ganglion.
D. Osteophyte.
E. Rheumatoid nodule.

Question 50

What is the tissue primarily involved in the development of Dupuytren contracture?

A. Flexor tendons.
B. Palmar fascia.
C. MCP joint capsule.
D. Flexor tendon sheaths.
E. Skin.

Question 51

A 38-year-old electrician presents with a painful swollen right knee. He states that over the past week his knee has become increasing more swollen and red and he now has a decreased range of motion. On examination there is a large erythematous swelling anterior to the patella, which is tender to palpate. There is thickened skin over the anterior of the knee. There is no effusion in the knee. He is able to flex his knee to 45° before he is limited by a combination of pain and tightness in the knee.
    What is the likely diagnosis?

A. Osteoarthritis.
B. Septic arthritis.
C. Baker cyst.
D. Patellar fracture.
E. Prepatellar bursitis.

Question 52

A 3-year-old girl is brought to A&E by her mother with a 24-hour history of a left leg limp. Her mother states there is no history of trauma. The child localizes the pain to her groin. The patient has an unremarkable past medical history, though her mother notes she had a cold last week. On examination the child is apyrexial and is systemically well. She is refusing to weight bear fully, and has a

decreased range of motion in all axes secondary to pain. X-ray shows no abnormality and her bloods are normal.
    What is the likely diagnosis?

A. Transient synovitis.
B. Septic arthritis.
C. Slipped upper femoral epiphysis.
D. Perthes disease.
E. Malignancy.

Question 53

What is the main principle when favouring internal fixation over casting of fractures?

A. Lower complication rate.
B. Cheaper.
C. Early mobilization.
D. Ensure union of fracture.
E. Less pain.

Question 54

In the case of septic arthritis in intravenous drug abusers, which of the following pathogens is most likely?

A. *Staphylococcus aureus*.
B. *Pseudomonas*.
C. Fungal infections.
D. *Streptococcus* sp.
E. All of the above.

Extended matching questions (EMQs)

Rheumatology

Question 1

A. Osteoarthritis.
B. Carpal tunnel syndrome.
C. Gout.
D. Trigger finger.
E. Dupuytren contracture.
F. Ulnar nerve palsy.
G. Pyrophosphate arthropathy.
H. Complex regional pain syndrome.
I. De Quervain's tenosynovitis.
J. Radial nerve palsy.
K. Psoriatic arthropathy.

You are examining the right hand of the patients below. Look at the description of the clinical findings and choose the most appropriate diagnosis from the list above.

1. The muscles of the hypothenar eminence are wasted. Abduction and adduction of the fingers are weak. Sensation over the little finger is reduced.
2. There is pitting of the fingernails. On palpation of the distal interphalangeal (DIP) joints of the middle and ring fingers, there is tender, boggy swelling. The whole length of the index finger is swollen and tender.
3. There is mild generalized swelling of the hand. The skin is pale, cool and extremely hypersensitive, to the extent that light touch produces severe pain. The radial and ulnar pulses are easily palpable.
4. When the patient opens his fist to extend his fingers, the middle finger responds more slowly than the others. In order to straighten the digit fully, the patient has to pull it with his other hand. The palm at the base of the finger feels lumpy.
5. There is bony swelling of all the DIP joints and the base of the thumb. Crepitus can be felt on movements of the thumb.

Question 2

A. Serum urate level.
B. Temporal artery biopsy.
C. Measurement of lupus anticoagulant and anticardiolipin antibodies.
D. Synovial fluid aspiration, Gram stain and culture.
E. Nerve conduction studies and electromyography.
F. Erythrocyte sedimentation rate (ESR).

G. Full blood count.
H. Plain X-ray of the hand and wrist.
I. Thyroid function test.
J. Plain X-ray of the knee.

What single investigation from the above list would be the most useful when trying to make a diagnosis in the following situations?.

1. A 63-year-old woman, who is taking low-dose oral corticosteroids and methotrexate for her rheumatoid arthritis, develops swelling and severe pain in her wrist. She is febrile with a temperature of 38.2°C and feels generally unwell.
2. A 28-year-old woman is admitted to hospital as an emergency with pleuritic chest pain. She is proven to have a pulmonary embolus and treated accordingly. She has no obvious risk factors for venous thromboembolism. Her past medical history includes recurrent migraines and three previous miscarriages.
3. A 72-year-old man presents with a headache and pain in his jaw when chewing food. He has noticed that the right side of his scalp is tender when he combs his hair.
4. A 36-year-old diabetic man complains of pain and tingling in his left thumb, index and middle fingers. This seems to be worse at night and stops him sleeping.
5. A 65-year-old man who has had one previous attack of gout develops severe pain in his knee. On examination, the joint is hot, swollen and tender. The patient is reluctant to weight bear.

Question 3

A. Rheumatoid arthritis.
B. Systemic sclerosis.
C. Systemic lupus erythematosus (SLE).
D. Polymyositis.
E. Polymyalgia rheumatica.
F. Kawasaki disease.
G. Primary Sjögren syndrome.
H. Takayasu arteritis.
I. Giant cell arteritis.
J. Wegener granulomatosis.

Read the clinical details of each patient below and decide which is the most appropriate diagnosis from the list above.

1. A 3-year-old boy develops an acute febrile illness. On examination, he is obviously unwell and has marked

cervical lymphadenopathy, an oligoarthritis and desquamation of the skin of his hands and feet.

2. A 44-year-old woman complains that her hands have become slightly swollen and feel tight and itchy. She also finds that her fingers become blue and painful in the cold weather. Apart from heartburn, for which she takes regular antacids, she was previously fit and well. The first thing that her family doctor notices when she walks into the consulting room is that she has a few telangiectasias on her face.

3. A 48-year-old man becomes acutely breathless and is admitted to hospital as an emergency. He deteriorates rapidly and is intubated and transferred to the intensive care unit for ventilation. A chest X-ray shows multiple shadows in both lung fields, consistent with severe infection or pulmonary haemorrhage. The patient's wife explains to the on-call doctor that he has been unwell for several months with symptoms of joint pain and intermittent skin rashes. He is under regular follow-up with an ear, nose and throat specialist because of recurrent epistaxis.

4. A 56-year-old woman consults her doctor with a 3-month history of weakness of her limbs. She is finding it increasingly difficult to climb the stairs and can no longer carry heavy bags of shopping. She has no pain, but feels very lethargic. Neurological examination of her limbs reveals normal tone and muscle bulk with no fasciculation. Proximal power is reduced at 3/5 in all four limbs. All reflexes are present and normal. Her plantar responses are flexor. Sensory examination is normal.

5. A 45-year-old woman is concerned because her eyes feel dry and gritty and are often red. Her mouth is also dry and she has to take frequent sips of water with her meals. Apart from occasional joint pain, she is otherwise well and has no significant past medical history. Her doctor organizes some blood tests, which reveal a mild normocytic anaemia with a slightly elevated ESR. An autoantibody profile shows the presence of anti-Ro and anti-La antibodies.

Question 4

A. Rotator cuff tendinitis.

B. Capsulitis.

C. Osteoarthritis.

D. Polymyalgia rheumatica.

E. Gout.

F. Ruptured long head of biceps.

G. Pancoast tumour.

H. Acute myocardial infarction.

I. Rheumatoid arthritis.

J. Bicipital tendinitis.

Read the clinical details of each patient below and decide which is the most appropriate diagnosis from the list above.

1. A 31-year-old woman presents with a 2-month history of left shoulder pain, which is gradually worsening. The pain is in the region of her deltoid muscle and is exacerbated by arm movements and lying on her left side. She is now struggling to reach behind her back to fasten her bra strap. On examination, the shoulder looks normal and has a full range of passive movement. However, active movements are painful, and the patient has a painful arc on abduction.

2. A 65-year-old diabetic man develops acute severe pain in his left shoulder whilst walking home from the pub. His wife is worried because he looks grey and sweaty and is slightly short of breath. He seems able to move his arm normally.

3. A doctor is called to a nursing home to visit an elderly woman with advanced dementia. The staff are concerned because they have noticed a swelling in her upper arm. On examination, the swelling is more obvious when the patient flexes her elbow. It feels soft on palpation and does not appear to be tender.

4. A 73-year-old woman presents with a 4-day history of pain in both shoulders. Her arms feel weak and extremely stiff. She has also had some pain in her thighs. The patient's doctor arranges some blood tests, which show that she has a normal full blood count and a very high ESR.

5. A 58-year-old man who suffers with chronic obstructive pulmonary disease is admitted to hospital for investigations. Over the past few weeks he has developed severe pain in his right shoulder and upper arm. The pain is continuous, day and night, and has not responded to any analgesia. The patient complains that he has been losing weight, is more breathless than usual and has coughed up a small amount of blood.

Question 5

A. Anti-dsDNA.

B. c-ANCA.

C. p-ANCA.

D. Anti-Sm.

E. Anticentromere.

F. Antigliadin.

G. Anticardiolipin.

H. Anti-Jo1.

I. Antihistone.

For each of the following patients, select the most characteristic autoantibody profile from the list above.

1. A 59-year-old woman presents with symptoms of Raynaud phenomenon and dysphagia. On examination, she has painful lesions on her fingers and facial telangiectasia.

2. A 23-year-old man consults his doctor complaining of joint pains, mouth ulcers, lethargy and a rash. His only past medical history is of severe acne, for which he takes minocycline.

3. A 60-year-old man develops acute renal failure. He has been unwell for some time with symptoms of joint

pain, skin rashes and several episodes of haemoptysis. On examination, he has a saddle-nose deformity.

4. A 45-year-old man presents with abdominal pain, weight loss and a skin rash. On examination, he has wasting of the small muscles of his hands and a purpuric rash on his legs.

5. A 30-year-old woman is admitted to hospital as an emergency with a left hemiparesis. She has a history of recurrent severe migraines, but does not have a headache at present. The doctor examining her notices the rash of livedo reticularis on her lower limbs.

Question 6

A. Gout.

B. Rheumatoid arthritis.

C. Pseudogout.

D. Haemophilia.

E. Septic arthritis.

F. Reactive arthritis.

G. Haemochromatosis.

H. Haemarthrosis.

Read the clinical details of each patient below and decide which is the most appropriate diagnosis from the list above.

1. A 68-year-old woman presents with a sore throat that she has had for a few days. She has been feeling generally unwell for the last 2 weeks. She has a swollen left wrist and swollen tender right knee and right ankle. She has a normal white cell count (WCC), high ESR and high C-reactive protein (CRP).

2. An 84-year-old woman with osteoarthritis develops a swollen warm right wrist. She has no other joint swelling and is otherwise well.

3. A 42-year-old man develops swelling of his second and third metacarpophalangeal (MCP) joints. He has no other swelling but has chondrocalcinosis on an X-ray.

4. A 65-year-old woman who has had a recent myocardial infarction develops an acutely swollen painful right knee.

5. A 70-year-old woman with inflammatory arthritis develops an acutely swollen painful left knee. She is systemically unwell.

Question 7

A. Osteoarthritis.

B. Rheumatoid arthritis.

C. Psoriatic arthritis.

D. Ankylosing spondylitis.

E. Diffuse idiopathic skeletal hyperostosis (DISH).

F. Gout.

G. Enteropathic arthritis.

H. Reactive arthritis.

The most likely diagnosis from the list above is:

1. A 30-year-old man presents with back pain and stiffness. It is worse in the morning and better by the end of the day.

2. An 80-year-old woman presents with swelling and pain of her proximal interphalangeal joints and DIPs of her hands. She has noticed that her joints are changing shape and that she is finding it more difficult to open bottles. Her mother also had similar-shaped hands.

3. A 64-year-old woman has abnormally shaped fingers and some fingers are shorter than others. She also has pitting of her nails.

4. A 40-year-old man has a painful swollen first metatarsophalangeal (MTP) joint. He has abnormal areas on his ears and a normal serum uric acid level.

5. A 42-year-old man has a swollen left knee and ulcerative colitis.

Question 8

A. Osteoporosis.

B. Paget disease.

C. Osteopenia.

D. Osteomalacia.

E. Rickets.

F. Hyperparathyroidism.

G. Lymphoma.

H. Myeloma.

The most likely diagnosis from the list above is:

1. A 7-year-old Asian boy presents with pain in his hips and knees. He has abnormally shaped legs, decreased serum calcium and raised alkaline phosphatase (ALP).

2. A 70-year-old man has hip pain and hearing problems. He has a raised ALP and high calcium.

3. A 60-year-old man presents with back pain, weight loss, raised calcium and high ESR.

4. An 80-year-old woman with rheumatoid arthritis presents with back pain and height loss.

5. A 60-year-old woman presents with renal failure, bone pain and low calcium.

Question 9

A. Churg–Strauss disease.

B. Polyarteritis nodosa.

C. Wegener granulomatosis.

D. Polymyositis.

E. Dermatomyositis.

F. Microscopic polyangiitis.

G. SLE.

H. Systemic sclerosis.

I. Behçet disease.

Extended matching questions (EMQs)

The most likely diagnosis from the list above is:

1. A 42-year-old man has asthma, proteinuria and a raised WCC.
2. A 40-year-old man presents with weakness of his hands, abdominal pain and blood in his urine. His antineutrophil cytoplasmic antibody (ANCA) is negative.
3. A 40-year-old Turkish man has mouth and scrotal ulcers. He has problems with his vision.
4. A 60-year-old man has a rash on his fingers and around his eyes. He is finding it difficult to stand from sitting and is losing weight.
5. A 60-year-old woman presents with chest pain, swollen painful joints and protein in her urine. Her ANCA is negative but she is antinunclear antibody-positive.

Question 10

A. Rheumatoid arthritis.
B. Osteoarthritis.
C. Fibromyalgia.
D. Psoriatic arthritis.
E. Gout.
F. Pseudogout.
G. Enteropathic arthritis.

The most likely diagnosis from the list above is:

1. A 60-year-old woman has painful joints, no swelling, normal ESR and normal CRP.
2. A 70-year-old woman who is overweight has painful knees. She is finding it difficult to climb stairs and finds that her knees lock and creak. Her ESR and CRP are normal.
3. A 60-year-old man has a swollen painful right knee. He has chondrocalcinosis on an X-ray.
4. A 68-year-old woman has swollen MCP joints bilaterally. She has stiffness in the morning for about an hour. She has raised ESR and CRP.
5. A 50-year-old man has a swollen left elbow and swollen right knee. He has stiffness for 2 hours in the morning. He has a raised ESR and CRP with a normal rheumatoid factor.

Question 11

A. Polymyositis.
B. Polymyalgia rheumatic.
C. Myasthenia gravis.
D. Muscular dystrophy.
E. Rheumatoid arthritis.
F. Cervical spondylosis.
G. Small cell lung cancer.

The most likely diagnosis from the list above is:

1. A 68-year-old woman has stiffness of both shoulders in the morning. She has difficulty brushing her hair. She

has a raised ESR. She has had no weight loss or weakness.
2. A 50-year-old woman has tenderness of her shoulders and thighs. She has weakness of her proximal muscles, raised inflammatory markers and no wasting.
3. A man has weakness of his arms and eyes. He gets weaker during the day. He has a normal ESR and CRP.
4. A 40-year-old man has weakness of his arms. He has proximal muscle wasting. His brother had similar symptoms.
5. A 40-year-old woman has pain and stiffness of both shoulders. She has swollen knees and hands. She has raised ESR and CRP.

Question 12

A. Wrist.
B. Knee.
C. MCPs.
D. MTPs.
E. DIPs.
F. Shoulder.
G. Elbow.

The most likely joint to be affected in the conditions below from the list above is:

1. Rheumatoid arthritis.
2. Gout.
3. Pseudogout.
4. Osteoarthritis.
5. Septic arthritis.

Question 13

A. Low C3, low C4.
B. Rheumatoid factor.
C. ANCA.
D. Anti-centromere.
E. Anti-RNP.
F. SS DNA.
G. Anti Jo-1.

The most appropriate antibody profile from the list above for the following conditions is:

1. Polymyositis.
2. SLE.
3. Sjögren syndrome.
4. Mixed connective tissue disease.
5. Wegener granulomatosis.

Question 14

A. Heberden nodes.
B. Photosensitive rash.
C. Telangiectasia.

D. Eosinophilia.

E. Back pain.

F. Onycholysis.

G. Nail pitting.

The most likely sign from the above list for the following conditions is:

1. Ankylosing spondylitis.
2. Osteoarthritis.
3. SLE.
4. CREST (calcinosis, Raynaud phenomenon, oesophageal dysmotility, sclerodactyly and telangiectasia).
5. Churg–Strauss disease.

Question 15

A. Methotrexate.

B. Sulfasalazine.

C. Azathioprine.

D. Infliximab.

E. Hydroxychloroquine.

F. Cyclophosphamide.

G. Rituximab.

Which drug from the above list is most likely to cause the following complications?

1. Haemorrhagic cystitis.
2. Bronchiolitis obliterans.
3. Hepatitis.
4. Optic neuritis.
5. Tuberculosis.

Orthopaedics

Question 1

A. Prostate metastasis.

B. Lung metastasis.

C. Myeloma.

D. Kidney metastasis.

E. Bowel metastasis.

F. Breast metastasis.

G. Osteosarcoma.

H. Thyroid metastasis.

I. Osteochondroma.

Read the clinical details of each patient below and decide which is the most appropriate diagnosis from the list above.

1. An 80-year-old man presents with pain in the hip. An X-ray shows a sclerotic lesion in the proximal femur with a poorly defined zone of transition. He has a history of hesitancy and poor stream.

2. A 10-year-old boy presents with a short history of severe pain around the knee. Examination reveals a tender mass just below the joint in the proximal tibia. An X-ray shows cortical destruction and periosteal elevation.

3. A 55-year-old man presents with a pathological fracture of his left clavicle after lifting a suitcase. On the X-ray there is a diffuse area of abnormal bone. The skull shows numerous lytic lesions and his ESR is 130 mm/h.

4. A 15-year-old girl presents with a gradual swelling around the knee. It occasionally gives a little discomfort. Examination reveals a hard mass over the distal femur. X-ray shows a pedunculated well-defined lesion in continuity with the cortex of the bone.

5. A 60-year-old woman presents with a complete flaccid paralysis of the legs. Prior to this she had 3 weeks of severe back pain. X-rays show complete collapse of T12 vertebra. Chest X-ray, abdominal and thyroid ultrasound scans are normal. The ESR is 30 mm/h and serum electrophoresis is normal.

6. A 66-year-old man who has been a lifelong smoker has pain in his right arm. A lesion is present in the proximal humerus on X-ray and his chest X-ray is abnormal.

Question 2

A. Anterior cruciate ligament rupture.

B. Medial meniscal tear.

C. Osteoarthritis.

D. Pseudogout.

E. Medial collateral ligament sprain.

F. Osteochondritis dissecans.

G. Patella dislocation.

H. Tibial fracture.

I. Posterior cruciate ligament injury.

J. Patellar tendon rupture.

Read the clinical details of each patient below and decide which is the most appropriate diagnosis from the list above.

1. A 30-year-old patient presents after a road traffic accident. The only injury is to the left knee which hit the dashboard of the car on impact. The knee is generally tender and has a large effusion and a posterior sag. X-ray shows no obvious fractures.

2. A 25-year-old woman is playing netball and twists her knee with the foot on the ground. The 'knee went in'. She hobbled off the court but was able to weight bear. Examination shows no effusion but tenderness medially above the joint line. Lachman test is negative.

3. A 55-year-old man presents with gradually increasing left knee pain over 6 months. He played football as a young man and has always had 'dodgy knees'. He remembers a few injuries but simply bandaged his knee and played again the week after. He stands with a varus deformity, and has a mild effusion with reduced range of movement and crepitus.

4. A 30-year-old woman has an accident on her first skiing holiday when her ski is caught in the snow at slow speed.

The boot stays in the ski and the right knee is twisted. She feels something go and the knee swells up immediately. Clinical examination is difficult due to pain but she does have an effusion.

5. A 35-year-old man presents with knee pain after a relatively minor injury at work several months ago. The knee was bent and twisted when carrying something down stairs. The knee was very sore initially but settled to some extent. He still has the feeling of something catching and doesn't fully trust the knee. Examination is normal apart from medial joint line tenderness and a small effusion.

6. A 36-year-old man suffers an injury playing rugby. He is not sure what happened exactly but was tackled and felt severe pain in his right knee. Examination shows swelling and tenderness below the patella. He is unable to straight-leg raise.

Question 3

A. Paget disease.

B. Osteomalacia.

C. Rickets.

D. Osteoporosis.

E. Myeloma.

F. Leukaemia.

G. Lymphoma.

H. Osteogenesis imperfecta.

I. Osteoid osteoma.

J. Hypercalcaemia.

Read the clinical details of each patient below and decide which is the most appropriate diagnosis from the list above.

1. A 70-year-old man presents with pain in both hips and thighs. The history is gradual but night pain is now a feature. Examination shows a normal gait but some restriction of hip movements, particularly hip internal rotation. His X-ray shows some early osteoarthritis of the hip but also areas of abnormal bone architecture in the pelvis and left femur. His ALP is 250 U/L.

2. A 12-year-old boy of Asian origin presents with joint aches and pains, particularly of the wrists. He a small and has some diffuse swelling over the wrists with tenderness. X-rays show widened epiphyses with cupping of the physis.

3. A 72-year-old woman presents with back pain and an obvious kyphosis. She had a fall several months ago, which made matters worse. She has no history of previous fractures. X-rays show loss of height in several thoracic vertebral bodies but the pedicles are intact. All blood tests are normal.

4. A 7-year-old boy presents with severe right hip pain. He has been unwell for several weeks with weight loss and various aches and pains but the hip pain has come on over the last 24 hours. Clinically the child looks unwell and any movement of the hip is extremely painful. He is apyrexial and his WCC is abnormal at 1.2×10^9/L. The

orthopaedic registrar is worried about septic arthritis and takes the patient to theatre for a washout of the right hip. The culture from theatre is negative.

5. A 10-month-old baby is brought to the casualty department for the fourth time unsettled and in pain. The child appears to localize pain to the right arm. The mother is sure she has not dropped the baby and has supervised the baby well. The Accident and Emergency (A&E) senior house officer thinks she might have a case of non-accidental injury and refers the baby to the paediatric doctors who admit the child. A full skeletal X-ray shows several rib fractures and a humeral fracture with a thin cortex and osteopenia.

6. A 14-year-old boy presents with severe right lower-leg pain which has been getting worse over 2 months. The pain is present at rest, and night pain is a feature. The pain is relieved by ibuprofen, prescribed by the GP. X-rays show a thickened cortex of the distal shaft of the tibia. A computed tomography (CT) scan shows a nidus within a cortical lesion.

Question 4

A. Osteoarthritis.

B. Rheumatoid arthritis.

C. Reiter syndrome.

D. Septic arthritis.

E. Gout.

F. Avascular necrosis.

G. Ankylosing spondylitis.

H. Enteropathic arthritis.

I. Psoriatic arthropathy.

Read the clinical details of each patient below and decide which is the most appropriate diagnosis from the list above.

1. A 65-year-old woman presents with a gradual history of pain in the first MTP joint. The pain is worse on walking, particularly when she pushes off from that foot. She is only able to wear certain shoes and finds her walking boots surprisingly comfortable. Examination shoes a bony lump over the dorsum of the metatarsal and diminished movements of the joint with crepitus. She has no other joint problems.

2. A 25-year-old soldier comes home on leave after being on duty for 3 months. She has been complaining of knee pain and swelling for several weeks. She has also recently been diagnosed by her GP as having conjunctivitis. Examination reveals a diffusely swollen knee with a large effusion and bilateral eye redness. She has recently also had dysuria.

3. A 40-year-old man presents with pain and swelling of his right hand with multiple swollen joints, particularly the MCP joints. He has had a rash over the extensor part of the arm, which has itched a bit but has never really troubled him.

4. An 80-year-old woman, a resident of a nursing home, is normally pleasantly confused and mobile around the

home. Over the last few days she has been unwell and has not used her right arm. She has become drowsy and listless and it is very difficult to obtain a history from her. There is swelling of her right shoulder, which she holds close to her body. Her temperature is 38.6°C and her WCC is 19 × 10⁹/L.

5. A 40-year-old man presents with an acutely inflamed left first MTP joint. He is a heavy drinker and works as a sales representative, entertaining clients a lot in the evenings. He is apyrexial and an X-ray is normal. His serum uric acid is normal.

6. A 28-year-old man presents with back pain over several months. He was a keen cricketer but is now unable to do the sports he enjoys because of pain and stiffness. The stiffness is worse in the morning. Clinically he has diminished movement of the lumbar spine, as demonstrated by Schober test. The sacroiliac joints are also tender. X-rays show calcification between vertebral bodies.

Question 5

A. Spondylolisthesis.

B. Spinal stenosis.

C. Prolapsed intervertebral disc.

D. Discitis.

E. Chronic musculoskeletal back pain.

F. Spinal metastases.

G. Acute low back pain.

H. Ankylosing spondylitis.

I. Abdominal aortic aneurysm.

J. Cauda equina syndrome.

Read the clinical details of each patient below and decide which is the most appropriate diagnosis from the list above.

1. A 60-year-old man presents with low back pain and aching in both legs. The pain is worse on walking and relieved by rest. The leg pain radiates down the leg and into both calves. Examination shows reduced movements of the spine and pain on extension. Sciatic stretch testing is normal. X-rays show osteoarthritis of the spine.

2. A 60-year-old woman has unrelenting low back pain which is not mechanical in nature. Night pain is severe and not relieved by simple analgesia. On examination she is pale and thin. Her abdominal system reveals a palpable liver edge. X-rays of her lumbar spine show loss of a pedicle (winking-owl sign).

3. A 56-year-old diabetic patient with chronic renal failure is admitted for dialysis. He also complains of new back pain. The patient becomes unwell with a raised temperature, a WCC of 22.5 × 10⁹/L, CRP 125 mg/L, and ESR 79 mm/h. The renal physicians treat him for line sepsis but he fails to respond. An X-ray of the lumbar spine 1 week later shows loss of disc space between L3–L4 with bony destruction of the end plates.

4. A 32-year-old GP presents with a short history of back pain after straining in the garden. He has bilateral leg

symptoms with pain radiating down both legs into the feet. He says the saddle area of his bottom feels odd when sitting down and he has difficulty passing urine. When he arrives in A&E he is in acute urinary retention and the crossover sign is positive.

5. A 30-year-old man complains of low back pain after digging at work. The pain does not radiate and is worse on movement. He feels well and examination shows muscle spasm, reduced movements and some tenderness across the lower lumbar spine.

6. A 15-year-old boy presents with increasing low back pain for 1 year. He is a county-level fast bowler and big things are expected of him. The pain does not radiate and is worse after prolonged activity. Examination shows a well boy with well-maintained spinal movements and normal neurology. Pain is significant on extension. Oblique X-rays of the lumbar spine show a typical Scottie dog appearance with a pars defect at L5–S1.

Question 6

A. Perthes disease.

B. Juvenile idiopathic arthritis.

C. Developmental dysplasia of the hip.

D. Congenital talipes equinovarus.

E. Slipped upper femoral epiphysis.

F. Septic arthritis.

G. Osteomyelitis.

H. Reactive arthritis.

I. Ewing tumour.

J. Osgood–Schlatter disease.

Read the clinical details of each patient below and decide which is the most appropriate diagnosis from the list above.

1. A 13-month-old baby presents with a limp as the child begins to walk. The left leg looks short when compared with the right. The child has a waddling gait but is not in obvious discomfort.

2. A 13-year-old boy presents with a 1-week history of left leg pain radiating from the groin down the thigh and into the knee. The pain is worse on activity and partially relieved by rest. Clinically he has an externally rotated left leg with pain on all movements. The anteroposterior X-ray of the hip shows a smaller epiphysis than on the right. The frog lateral view clinches the diagnosis.

3. A 12-year-old boy has been unwell for a few months with pain and swelling in his right knee. He has also been more tired than usual and not himself. On further questioning it becomes clear that other joints are involved. The right knee is swollen with a small effusion. At presentation he is noted to have decreased visual acuity in his right eye.

4. A 14-year-old boy is a keen footballer and presents with bilateral knee pain that is worse on movement and very tender if touched. On examination he is well and has tenderness over the tibial tubercle just beneath the patellar ligament.

5. A 7-year-old boy presents with a 1-year history of right knee pain, gradually increasing. He has a pronounced limp and has been off school for 1 month. On examination the right knee is normal but the hip is irritable and abduction is markedly decreased. X-rays show sclerosis of the femoral head.

6. An 8-week-old baby girl is very ill on the paediatric intensive care unit. She has features of sepsis, including a raised temperature and WCC, and blood cultures have grown *Staphylococcus aureus*. There is no obvious focus of infection. An ultrasound scan of both hips is normal.

Question 7

A. Tension pneumothorax.

B. Pelvic fracture.

C. Lumbar spine fracture/dislocation.

D. Wedge fracture lumbar spine.

E. Haemothorax.

F. Fracture of the seventh cervical vertebra.

G. Neck sprain.

H. Hip dislocation.

I. Osteomyelitis.

Read the clinical details of each patient below and decide which is the most appropriate diagnosis from the list above.

1. A 30-year-old man falls 6 metres from some scaffolding. On admission to the Emergency Room he complains of shortness of breath and chest pain. On examination he is cyanosed and unable to complete sentences. His trachea is deviated to the right, and he has absent breath sounds on the left side. Blood pressure is low, pulse rate is 120 bpm and oxygen sats are only 80% on high-flow oxygen.

2. A heavy steel girder falls directly on to a 45-year-old man on a construction site, crushing his lower abdomen. He is rushed to the Emergency Room and is noted to have bruising around his lower abdomen and groin. His airway and breathing are stable, but his blood pressure is low and he has tachycardia. Intravenous fluids are started, which correct the hypotension. On secondary survey, a doctor finds blood at the urethral meatus, and notes that the man has not passed urine.

3. A 23-year old woman loses control of her car at high speed and crashes. Unfortunately she is not wearing her seat belt and is ejected from the vehicle. When the paramedic arrives she complains of severe lower back pain, and says that she cannot feel her legs. When the paramedic examines her lower back he can feel a step in her lumbar spine. Later in hospital she is unable to pass urine, so a catheter is passed which drains 1000 mL of clear urine.

4. An 80-year-old man loses balance and falls on to his bottom on the pavement. He complains of lower back pain but is just about able to walk. His legs feel normal and he has normal bladder and bowel function. After 1 week the pain has not gone so he attends his general practice, and is sent for an X-ray.

5. A 32-year-old mountain biker goes over his handlebars and lands head first on the ground. He feels immediate neck pain but is otherwise normal. He rides home, but the pain is severe so his wife brings him to casualty. He tells the doctor that he remembers hitting his chin against his chest quite hard. Examination reveals tenderness at the level of C7. Neurological examination is normal. A lateral X-ray of the man's neck shows from C1 to C6 and is normal. The doctor therefore reassures the man and discharges him. On the way home the man develops tingling in his right little finger.

6. A 40-year-old lawyer is stationary in his car at the traffic lights. He is wearing his seatbelt. Suddenly he feels a shunt from behind as a van crashes into him at moderate speed. He gets out of his car. The back bumper has been damaged but otherwise the car is untouched. After 10 minutes the man notices that his neck feels stiff. He goes home, but during the night his neck becomes very painful, and he develops a headache.

Question 8

A. Physiotherapy.

B. Anti-inflammatory tablets.

C. Unicompartmental knee replacement.

D. Total knee replacement.

E. X-ray of the hip.

F. X-ray of the spine.

G. Realignment surgery.

H. Arthroscopy.

Read the clinical details of each patient below and decide which is the most appropriate action from the list above.

1. A 40-year-old heavy manual worker presents with a 2-year history of painful right knee. He says the pain is always on the inside of his knee and is worse after activity. He also gets stiffness and finds that the pain is starting to affect his ability to work. Examination reveals severe varus deformity of the knee. X-rays show arthritis in the medial compartment with a normal lateral compartment.

2. A 35-year-old plumber presents to clinic with pain in his right knee. This occurred after he stood up from a squatting position. His knee swelled over 24 hours. The pain is on the medial aspect of his knee and he cannot fully straighten his knee. On examination he has a moderate effusion and has lost 20° of extension.

3. A 67-year-old farmer presents with constant pain on the inside of his left knee. He still works as a farmer, but his pain is making it difficult. The pain is worse after walking, and despite painkillers he gets night pain which affects his sleep. On examination he has a swollen left knee, tenderness over the medial joint line and mild varus deformity with a good range of movement. Radiographs show osteoarthritis confined to the medial compartment.

4. A 55-year-old patient has been referred by her GP for a total hip replacement. She complains of left hip pain but

also complains of numbness in her buttock that radiates down into her foot. Pain is relatively constant but she does not find that hip movements worsen her symptoms. She has a good range of hip movement on examination. X-rays of her hip show mild osteoarthritis.

5. A 78-year-old retired miner presents with right knee pain. This is all over his knee and is associated with swelling and clicking. He has not slept properly because of the pain for the last 6 months and he can no longer cope with his symptoms. He has mild chronic obstructive airways disease, but is relatively fit otherwise. He lives alone, has stairs and normally walks with a stick. Examination reveals a fixed flexion deformity of 10° and a Baker cyst in the popliteal fossa. X-rays reveal loss of joint space, subchondral sclerosis and cyst, with large osteophytes. He would like an operation to help his pain.

Question 9

A. Hypovolaemia.
B. Sepsis.
C. Anaphylaxis.
D. Neurogenic shock.
E. Cardiogenic shock.
F. Drugs.
G. Epidural anaesthesia.

Read the clinical details of each patient below and decide which is the most appropriate diagnosis from the list above.

1. A fit 65-year-old woman returns to the ward 2 hours after a total hip replacement. The nurse is worried because her blood pressure is only 90/60 mmHg. Her pulse rate is 74 bpm and she has a good urine output. She feels well and capillary refill is 2 seconds. Her legs feel numb but sensation is slowly returning.

2. A 60-year-old man presents with a very painful right hip and feeling unwell. He has a history of type 2 diabetes mellitus and chronic obstructive airways disease for which he takes oral steroids. Recently he has had a 'bad chest', for which the GP gave antibiotics. On examination his hip is held in fixed flexion and he will not move it. His temperature is 38°C. Pulse is 120 bpm and blood pressure records 80/40 mmHg. His veins are distended and he has warm peripheries.

3. A 25-year-old kitchen fitter is ejected from his van at high speed when he crashes on a motorway. He has lower back pain but is alarmed because he can no longer feel his legs. When he arrives in the emergency department he is fully examined by the doctor, including a log roll and per rectum examination. This is normal apart from a boggy swelling at the level of L1 and loss of sensation and power in his legs. Pulse rate is 60 bpm and blood pressure is 100/50 mmHg.

4. The night doctor is called urgently to review an 80-year-old woman on the ward 4 days after a hemiarthroplasty for a fractured neck of femur. She looks very unwell. On examination she has a pulse of 110 bpm, shallow and rapid breathing with crepitations at the bases, a raised jugular venous pulse and is sweaty and clammy. Blood pressure is only 84/40 mmHg. The electrocardiograph (ECG) shows ST elevation in the lateral leads which is new compared with the preoperative ECG.

5. A 40-year-old man is being nursed in the recovery room in theatre after having a complex total hip replacement. His blood pressure is 90/50 mmHg despite 2 litres of intravenous fluids. His pulse rate is 120 bpm. His urine output is poor and he looks pale, sweaty and anxious. Capillary refill time is 5 seconds and his peripheries are cool.

Question 10

A. Anterior dislocation.
B. Posterior dislocation.
C. Bankart lesion.
D. Fracture of proximal humerus.
E. Rotator cuff tear.
F. Axillary nerve palsy.

Read the clinical details of each patient below and decide which is the most appropriate diagnosis from the list above.

1. A 25-year-old woman attends casualty holding her right arm. She landed awkwardly on her shoulder, which at the time was abducted. It is now very painful and she can barely move it. On examination there is loss of the normal shoulder contour and X-ray of the shoulder confirms the diagnosis.

2. A 20-year-old man is admitted to a medical ward following a prolonged epileptic seizure. As he regains consciousness he complains that his left shoulder is very painful.

3. A 45-year-old man attends clinic complaining that his shoulder 'clunks' when he moves it in certain positions. He has a history of an anterior shoulder dislocation 6 months ago.

4. A 65-year-old woman attends A&E; she fell on to her outstretched right arm after tripping on a kerb. Her shoulder is very painful and she has not been able to move it since. Examination reveals swelling and bruising over the shoulder. No movements are possible.

5. A 45-year-old man injures his right arm after falling off his mountain bike. Initially it was stiff and painful but improved with physiotherapy after a few weeks. He now has difficulty lifting anything heavy and his arm is weak when testing initial abduction.

Question 11

A. *Staphylococcus aureus*.
B. Anaerobic bacteria.
C. *Mycobacterium tuberculosis*.
D. Meticillin-resistant *Staphylococcus aureus* (MRSA).
E. *Haemophilus influenzae*.
F. *Neisseria gonorrhoeae*.
G. *Escherichia coli*.

Extended matching questions (EMQs)

Read the clinical details of each patient below and decide which is the most appropriate diagnosis from the list above.

1. A 2-year-old child is admitted with a hot, painful swollen left knee associated with a high fever. She will not move the knee because of pain. On further questioning it turns out that the child has never had any vaccinations because her mother has read in the newspapers that vaccinations are dangerous.
2. A 60-year-old woman with known osteoarthritis of her left hip is admitted feeling unwell with a high temperature. Her hip is now very painful and she will not allow the doctor to move it. She says she has been unwell recently with a 'water infection'.
3. A 51-year-old Caucasian woman presents with back pain. She has not been well for the last 3 months. Recently she has lost weight and had night sweats. She mentions that she lived in India for 10 years when she was 20. On examination she has a gibbus in the mid part of the thoracic spine and has tenderness on palpation.
4. A 10-year-old girl is admitted with pain in her left tibia and a fever. There is no history of recent illness. X-rays show osteomyelitis in the proximal tibia.
5. A farmer falls 3 metres from a ladder in his cattle yard. He sustains an open fracture of his tibia which is heavily contaminated.

Question 12

A. Salter–Harris fracture.
B. Simple fracture.
C. Pathological fracture.
D. Open fracture.
E. Complex regional pain syndrome (CRPS).
F. Compartment syndrome.
G. Non-accidental injury.

Read the clinical details of each patient below and decide which is the most appropriate diagnosis from the list above.

1. A 10-year-old boy falls out of a tree and lands on his left wrist. He cries immediately and his mother brings him to A&E because his wrist is deformed. When the doctor takes an X-ray he explains that the child has a fracture.
2. A 50-year-old man suddenly feels pain in his right thigh and falls to the ground. He is alarmed to find that his leg is badly angulated and X-ray in casualty confirms a fracture. He explains that he has had pain in this leg for some time, and over the last few months has had weight loss. He also mentions that he has been coughing up blood and worries that his lifelong smoking habit is the cause.
3. A 30-year-old footballer is kicked hard in his shin during a game. He doesn't feel too uncomfortable initially and can weight bear, but over the next 3 hours his pain becomes severe. The team doctor examines his leg and finds that his leg is swollen and tense. He has altered sensation over the dorsum of his foot and passive movement of his toes is extremely painful. Foot pulses are normal.

4. An 18-month-old girl is brought to A&E by her mother following a fall off the settee at home. She has a painful swollen forearm. Radiographs show a transverse fracture of the forearm with callus formation. The grandmother says that the arm hurt a few days ago.
5. A 46-year-old secretary falls from a ladder on to her forearm. Her arm is badly angulated and there is a tiny wound over the mid part of the forearm. The junior doctor straightens her arm and places it in a cast and brings her back to clinic 2 days later. His consultant reviews the case and is very angry.

Question 13

A. CT.
B. Magnetic resonance imaging (MRI).
C. Plain X-ray.
D. Bone scan.
E. Nerve conduction study.
F. Ultrasound scan.
G. Venous Doppler scan.

Read the clinical details of each patient below and decide which is the most appropriate investigation according to what you think the most likely diagnosis is.

1. A 56-year-old housewife says she gets pins and needles and pain, especially at night in her index, middle and half her ring fingers. This is relieved by hanging her hand over the end of the bed. She has a history of type 2 diabetes.
2. A 40-year-old woman reports a 6-month history of shooting pains from her left buttock, radiating down the back of her leg into her foot. She has altered sensation over the lateral aspect of her lower leg and the sole of her foot.
3. A 68-year-old man attends casualty with a swollen, tender left leg. He had a left total knee replacement 6 weeks ago. Movements of his ankle are quite painful.
4. A 30-year-old man presents with a lump on the palmar aspect of his left wrist. He has had this for many years but recently it has slightly increased in size and can be painful as it catches on his watch. On examination it is mobile to the skin and underlying muscle and soft and has smooth round borders. It is not pulsatile.
5. A 56-year-old man has renal cell carcinoma. He complains of pain in his right forearm.

Question 14

A. Ulnar nerve compression.
B. Cervical rib.
C. Pancoast tumour.
D. Carpal tunnel syndrome.
E. Axillary nerve palsy.
F. Radial nerve palsy.
G. C6/C7 cervical disc prolapse.
H. Peripheral neuropathy

Read the clinical details of each patient below and decide which is the most likely diagnosis from the list above.

1. A 21-year-old man complains of numbness in his little and ring fingers and over the medial aspect of his forearm with weakness of his hand. This only seems to occur in certain positions, especially when his arm is raised above his head. His hand also turns white on occasions. There is wasting of the small muscles of the hand.
2. A 65-year-old heavy smoker complains of weakness in his left hand. He has had a persistent cough for the last 3 months and has lost 13 kg in weight. On examination he has wasting of the small muscles of the hand. The doctor also notes that he has a constricted pupil on the left side with drooping of the eyelid and dry skin over the left side of his forehead.
3. A 26-year-old man crashes his motorbike at 40 mph. He sustains a spiral fracture to the mid shaft of his right humerus. He has altered sensation over the first dorsal web space of his right hand and has weakness of extension of his wrist, fingers and thumb.
4. A 40-year-old woman develops a sudden onset of severe neck pain after turning suddenly. This is associated with pain in her middle finger and weakness straightening her arm. She has no significant past medical history.
5. A 40-year-old man is tackled heavily during a rugby game and lands awkwardly on his left shoulder. His shoulder has lost its normal contour and he finds all movements painful. He notices some tingling over the outer aspect of his upper arm.

Question 15

A. Ataxic.

B. Trendelenburg.

C. Waddling.

D. Antalgic.

E. Foot drop.

F. High-stepping.

G. Shuffling.

H. Spastic.

Read the clinical details of each patient below and decide which is the most likely gait pattern from the list above.

1. A 62-year-old man presents with pain in his left hip which he has suffered with for many years. X-rays show osteoarthritis. When asked to stand on his left leg his pelvis drops. When standing on his right leg his pelvis tilts up.
2. A 35-year-old football hooligan is seen in clinic saying that he can't walk properly. He was involved in a fight 6 weeks ago and says the policeman hit him very hard just below his right knee with a truncheon. He has some numbness over the dorsum of his foot but has no pain. When he walks he brings his right knee much higher than the left.
3. A 10-year-old boy is seen in the orthopaedic clinic for review. When walking he displays muscular incoordination and has his feet quite wide apart. His old notes state that he had meningitis as an infant.
4. A 30-year-old woman is seen in clinic with a painful ankle after she twisted it falling down a kerb. When walking she hobbles and has a reduced-stance phase on the affected side.
5. An 8-year-old boy is seen in clinic with his mother. His lower-limb function has worsened over the last few years. He has flexed and adducted hips and walks with a stiff gait. His feet are in equinus.

SBA answers

1. C. Osteoporosis. Vertebral height loss, back pain from vertebral fracture and previous history of fracture are all suggestive. Myeloma would cause back pain for weeks or months, hypercalcaemia and often raised alkaline phosphatase (ALP). Osteomalacia is a problem of vitamin D deficiency leading to inadequate mineralization – a low calcium level is likely. Paget disease would result in a raised ALP and is not associated with vertebral height loss. Systemic features such as sweats and weight loss would be expected in tuberculosis.

2. A. Bone biochemistry. The diagnosis is Paget disease, and bone biochemistry would detect raised ALP. Coeliac serology is appropriate when vitamin D deficiency is thought to be of dietary origin. DEXA confirms osteoporosis, MRI tibia may give images suggestive of Paget disease but an isotope bone scan is more likely to produce a characteristic picture, and MRI is an expensive test. Rheumatoid factor is not indicated unless rheumatoid arthritis is suspected.

3. E. Temporal artery biopsy. This has characteristic giant cells and is diagnostic. Skip lesions can occur. ANCA tends to be negative in giant cell arteritis. ESR would be raised in the vast majority of cases but is not specific or diagnostic. Lumbar puncture would be to exclude cerebrospinal fluid infection or subarachnoid haemorrhage. MRI of aortic arch may show arteritis but could be normal, too proximal or have atherosclerotic changes.

4. E. Splinting. This will allow the joint to rest and give pain relief. Aspiration has not grown organisms so antibiotics are not required. DMARDs are not indicated for pseudogout. Joint replacement would only occur for chronic pain or to improve function, not in an acute setting. Physiotherapy will be needed later once the inflammation has settled.

5. C. *Haemophilus influenzae,* which is a respiratory pathogen. Reiter syndrome is associated with gastrointestinal pathogens such as *Escherichia coli* and salmonella, and sexually transmitted infections such as gonorrhoea and chlamydia.

6. E. Splinting. This is useful at night to maintain the architecture of the carpal tunnel. Gold has no role in carpal tunnel syndrome – it is a DMARD. The same applies to methotrexate and steroids which are targeting joint inflammation. Physiotherapy tends not to be helpful. Injections of steroid, splints and surgical decompression are the mainstay of treatment.

7. A. Anti-double-stranded DNA antibodies would confirm SLE. ESR would be raised but is not diagnostic. Lupus anticoagulant is indicated if thrombosis or fetal loss has occurred, skin biopsy may help if it is subcutaneous lupus but in photosensitivity rash would not help reach a diagnosis. Thyroid disease is an important condition to exclude but would not confirm SLE.

8. E. Systemic sclerosis. He has features of CREST syndrome (calcinosis, Raynaud phenomenon, oesophageal dysmotility, sclerodactyly and telangiectasia). Linear scleroderma does not produce extracutaneous problems; multiple sclerosis is a chronic neurological condition; paraneoplastic phenomena generally are associated with few signs and not pulmonary hypertension; and SLE would not give calcinosis.

9. C. Exercise. Fybromyalgia is a condition of unclear cause but associated with chronic pain. Exercise regimens are most effective and assist pain control, combined with some antidepressants and on occasions psychological support. As there is no inflammation, DMARD, joint injections and steroids are not indicated. Dietary changes have no significant evidence of benefit.

10. C. Osteoarthritic changes include osteophytes, subchondral sclerosis, subchondral cysts and joint space narrowing. Fragility fracture would have a quicker timescale of deterioration, erosions are seen in inflammatory arthritis, osteopenia might be present as a consequence of disuse but is non-pathological and incidental, and although soft-tissue swelling might be seen on X-ray, it is an imaging modality for bone – clinical assessment can determine soft-tissue swelling!

11. B. Joint effusion is not easily determined by X-ray of small joints. Cyst and narrowed joint space might be seen in osteoarthritis, and while the history is of rheumatoid arthritis, it is likely that, in an 80-year-old, osteoarthritis changes will be concurrently present with rheumatoid arthritis change. Osteopenia occurs in rheumatoid arthritis due to disuse and soft-tissue swelling might be seen on X-ray (but note the answer to question 10, above).

12. A. Ankylosing spondylitis. He has an inflammatory history and loss of movement, is male and young. The weight loss might be due to concurrent inflammatory bowel disease. The main differential of tuberculosis should be considered carefully but, although this might cause weight loss, sweats and

lymphadenopathy would also be expected. A prolapsed disc would have a sudden onset, and osteoporosis should not cause weight loss in a young person.

13. C. A Schirmer test confirms dry eyes by tracking tear production on litmus paper. Parotitis and evidence of oral dryness, with subsequent caries, are suggestive. HIV should be excluded but no high-risk activity is mentioned. Schober test is for lumber spine movement. Transoesopageal echo looks for vegetations on heart valves in subacute bacterial endocarditis, but she has no signs of sepsis. Trendelenburg test assesses hip muscle weakness due to hip arthritis.

14. E. Sodium urate crystals are found in gout. The white lumps are tophi. Bacteria do need to be excluded in a hot joint but, given the concurrent tophi, gout is more likely. Calcium pyrophosphate (pseudogout) crystals tend to occur in the elderly, and in knees and wrists. Clear synovial fluid would be unlikely – inflammatory fluid tends to be slightly cloudy due to the white cell response. Pus is possible but white tophus more likely given the finger deposits.

15. D. Prednisolone will act fast to help settle the bowel and would address the joint pains too. Sulfasalazine may well be a good choice of drug once the bowel is settled. Other drugs for inflammatory bowel disease, such as azathioprine or cyclosporine, are not efficacious regarding the joint disease. Biological therapies might be required following failure of conventional drug approaches. NSAIDs may worsen the bowel symptoms and should be avoided. Panproctocolectomy is reserved for those who have failed medical therapy.

16. E. Prednisolone should be given if temporal arteritis is suspected in high doses of 1 mg/kg. Carbamazepine and amitriptyline have a role in trigeminal neuralgia. Ibuprofen and morphine will help pain but not treat the cause, and pain will return.

17. C. Polydipsia. Renal disease can cause failure of vitamin D metabolism, and osteodystrophy. Polydipsia is not a feature of osteomalacia. The hypocalcaemia can cause deformity, tetany, convulsions and arrhythmias.

18. A. Serum level of creatinine kinase. Dermatomyositis will produce inflamed muscles, which leak enzymes due to oedema in the cell. Creatinine kinase can then be detected and is often several orders of magnitude compared to normal. ESR is usually raised but non-specific, antinuclear antibodies may be positive for Jo-1 antibodies in polymyositis, chest X-ray should be done to exclude malignancy and X-ray of affected joints does not usually show erosions.

19. E. Hyperkeratosis occurs in psoriatic nails. Keratoderma is associated with reactive arthritis; koilonychia (spoon-shaped) is associated with iron deficiency. Leuconychia is a generally benign condition of white marks on the nail due to trauma or injury to the nail as it grows. Paronychia is an infection of the skin adjacent to the nail.

20. A. Anterior uveitis is associated with juvenile idiopathic arthritis and patients should be regularly reviewed by ophthalmology, as blindness can occur. Conjunctivitis is usually bacterial and may associate with reactive arthritis; episcleritis and scleritis can occur in rheumatoid arthritis as an extra-articular manifestation. Scleromalacia is the name given to blue-tinged sclera in rheumatoid arthritis or collagen disorders, and occurs as the sclera thins due to chronic scleritis.

21. E. Thoracic X-ray is needed to exclude vertebral wedge fracture. If present this virtually confirms osteoporosis and the requirement for prophylaxis in the form of bisphosphonates and vitamin D/calcium. DEXA would help confirm the diagnosis; HLA B27 testing is only useful for seronegative spondyloarthropathy where the diagnosis is in doubt. MRI of the whole spine might be considered if he had a new vertebral fracture and was contemplating vertebroplasty.

22. C. Back pain, knee pain with increased blood flow suggesting high bone turnover, associated with a raised ALP, suggest Paget disease. Prolapsed disc is possible but does not explain the knee warmth. Osteoarthritis should not cause a rise in ALP. Bilateral septic arthritis would be unusual and there are no signs of toxicity. Stroke tends not to cause pain.

23. B. X-ray will confirm osteoarthritis. Glucosamine may help, but evidence is scanty. Joint replacement equally, but the diagnosis needs to be confirmed first. Physiotherapy is of help with symptoms and function; steroids are not warranted as osteoarthritis is degenerative and usually not inflammatory.

24. C. Naproxen is an NSAID and the elderly are particularly at risk from NSAID gastrointestinal side-effects. Methotrexate should be used with care due to increased risk of marrow toxicity in this age group; prednisolone would give symptom relief quickly and sulfasalazine and hydroxychloroquine could be considered as DMARDS.

25. E. Response A refers to osteoarthritis, B to rheumatoid arthritis, C to septic arthritis and E to pseudogout.

26. D. Coeliac disease causes malabsorption of vitamin D and iron deficiency, folate deficiency and osteomalacia. Anti-DNA would be found in SLE but usually calcium metabolism is unaffected. Antiphospholipid syndrome is associated with thrombus, and low platelets, anti-smooth muscle can again be found in SLE or autoimmune liver disease; anti-vitamin D_3 antibody is not detectable by commercial assays.

27. C. Stillbirth and two vascular events suggest the antiphospholipid syndrome which is also associated with migraine, livedo, low platelets and SLE. Other autoantibodies should be checked given the association with SLE and the history of haemoptysis should exclude vasculitis (ANCA). A prothrombin time might be checked as part of a coagulopathy screen, and VDRL tests are rarely done now in the context of thrombosis, but can show false positives.

28. E. Wegener granulomatosis is a systemic, ANCA-positive vasculitis which can produce multisystem failure. Pulmonary embolism does not explain the renal failure, SLE is rare in men but might cause many of these symptoms, with the exception of the nasal deformity and bloody sputum. Churg–Strauss is a form of vasculitis associated with a high eosinophil count, and cryoglobulinaemic vasculitis produces ulceration and low complement levels and is usually insidious. It has an association with hepatitis C.

29. C. Pseudogout. Both gout and pseudogout would present insidiously without trauma, giving rise to elevated ESR and CRP. However the chondrocalcinosis of the triangular firbrocartilage on X-ray is highly indicative of pseudogout. The lack of temperature and normal white blood cell count mean that septic arthritis is unlikely, but this need to be definitively excluded via joint aspiration.

30. B. Osteosarcoma. Osteosarcoma is most common in the second and third decades of life, and frequently occurs around the knee. The symptoms of night pain and weight loss are suspicious of malignancy. The X-ray findings are typical of osteosarcoma.

31. D. Medial femoral circumflex artery. The majority of the blood supply to the femoral head in adults arises from the medial femoral circumflex artery; there is a lesser contribution from the lateral femoral circumflex artery. The artery of the ligamentum teres supplies a negligible blood supply in adults.

32. C. *Staphylococcus aureus*. *S. aureus* is the most common pathogen in septic arthritis in adults, followed by *Streptococcus* and *Enterobacter*. *S. aureus* is the most common pathogen in all ages.

33. D. Median nerve. A dorsally angulated distal radius fracture can cause compression of the median nerve, giving symptoms of carpal tunnel syndrome.

34. B. Osteoid osteoma. Osteoid osteoma presents insidiously, giving rise to intense pain and tenderness over the affected area, sometimes with a history of night pain. X-ray findings are of a central lucent nidus surrounded by a dense area of reactive bone. Salicylates greatly reduce the pain.

35. C. Aspiration of the knee. This man has a septic arthritis until proven otherwise. It is important that this is confirmed via joint aspiration as soon as possible. X-rays and blood test can be performed first but joint aspiration is the most important investigation. When possible, antibiotics should be withheld until after the joint aspiration has been performed.

36. B. Hypothyroidism. Hypothyroidism conveys no risk to developing Perthes disease. Hypothyroidism and other hormonal conditions are risk factors in slipped upper femoral epiphysis. Delayed bone age, low socioeconomic group, low birthweight and a family history are all risk factors of developing Perthes disease.

37. E. Slipped upper femoral epiphysis. This condition occurs in adolescents aged 11–14, and is more common in boys than girls. A background of chronic pain prior to the slip of the epiphysis is common. Patients hold their leg flexed and externally rotated for comfort.

38. A. Osgood–Schlatters disease. Osgood–Schlatters disease or traction apophysitis is common in adolescents, particularly boys, and after periods of rapid growth.

39. D. Nucleus pulposus. A disc prolapse occurs when part of the nucleus pulposus herniates through the annulus fibrosus and presses on a spinal nerve root.

40. B. Bilateral sciatic-type pain. Bilateral leg symptoms are suggestive of impending cauda equina syndrome.

41. C. Spinal stenosis. This man has spinal stenosis. The pain in his buttocks, thighs and calves is spinal claudication. Patients walk with a stooped gait so as to flex the lumbar spine and decrease their symptoms.

42. D. Bucket handle meniscal tear. The 'handle' part of a bucket handle tear flips over, becoming trapped in the joint and preventing full extension.

43. E. Anterior cruciate ligament tear. An anterior cruciate ligament tear is normally caused by a twisting injury to the knee. Patients will describe immediate pain and rapid swelling. Examination with reveal a large effusion, due to the haemarthrosis, and laxity in the AP axis. Lachman test and anterior drawer test are diagnostic.

44. B. Abductor pollicis longus. De Quervain tenosynovitis is inflammation of the tendon sheaths of abductor pollicis longus and extensor pollicis brevis.

45. D. Carpal tunnel syndrome. This woman has carpal tunnel syndrome. Her symptoms and their distribution are classical of carpal tunnel syndrome. Percussion at the wrist crease is Tinel test.

46. C. Compartment syndrome. The principal symptom of compartment syndrome is pain. Any patient who has a severe increase in pain following a fracture should be assessed for compartment syndrome. Proximal tibial fractures are at increased risk of developing compartment syndrome.

47. E. Assess the airway whilst stabilizing the cervical spine. In the assessment of any trauma patients, follow the ABCDE pathway and assess systems in order of

importance. Don't become distracted by the perceived main issue. All patients should be assumed to have a cervical spine injury until proven otherwise.

48. A. Pulmonary thromboembolism. Although rare, pulmonary thromboembolism is a recognized complication of arthroplasty surgery. The onset and nature of her symptoms are highly suggestive of this condition.

49. C. Ganglion. The history of a small fluctuant lesion surrounding a joint with an intermittent history is that of a ganglion.

50. B. Palmar fascia. Dupuytren contracture is a disease in which palmar fascia undergoes fibrosis and contracture

51. E. Prepatellar bursitis. Prepatellar bursitis is common in patients who work on their knees (e.g.

electricians, plumbers). His signs and symptoms suggest an obvious bursitis and do not highlight an intra-articular pathology.

52. A. Transient synovitis. With the history of a recent viral illness, and normal radiology and inflammatory markers, transient synovitis is most likely.

53. C. Early mobilization. The main principle of internal fixation is to allow early mobilization.

54. E. All of the above. Intravenous drug abusers inject themselves with potentially contaminated drugs, through a dirty needle. They are also frequently immunosuppressed and undernourished; consequently they are at risk of a wide range of infections. As a result they will require a broad range of antibiotics to cover potential pathogens.

Rheumatology

Question 1

1. F. Ulnar nerve palsy. The ulnar nerve supplies the muscles of the hypothenar eminence, including the interossei, which are responsible for finger abduction and adduction. See Figure 10.2 for the sensory distribution of the ulnar nerve in the hand.
2. K. Psoriatic arthropathy. The patient has inflammatory arthritis affecting the DIP joints and causing a dactylitis of the index finger. This is typical of a spondyloarthropathy. The nail changes are suggestive of psoriasis.
3. H. Complex regional pain syndrome. These are classical signs of complex regional pain syndrome. The skin may undergo dramatic colour changes from white to purple, and growth of hair and nails may be affected.
4. D. Trigger finger. This results from tenosynovitis of the flexor tendon.
5. A. Osteoarthritis. The first carpometacarpal joint and DIP joints are classical sites for osteoarthritis. The bony swellings of the DIP joints are called Heberden nodes.

Question 2

1. D. Synovial fluid aspiration, Gram stain and culture. This woman has septic arthritis until proven otherwise. Her risk factors for this include rheumatoid arthritis and corticosteroid therapy.
2. C. Measurement of lupus anticoagulant and anticardiolipin antibodies. The patient's venous thromboembolism, recurrent miscarriages and migraine may well be manifestations of the antiphospholipid antibody syndrome.
3. B. Temporal artery biopsy. The symptoms are suggestive of giant cell arteritis, and a temporal artery biopsy is the investigation of choice. The patient's ESR is likely to be high, but this is a non-specific rather than a diagnostic finding.
4. E. Nerve conduction studies and electromyography. These are classical symptoms of carpal tunnel syndrome.
5. D. Synovial fluid aspiration, Gram stain and culture. The first and most important step is to exclude septic arthritis in this man. It would be dangerous to assume that this is just another attack of gout.

Question 3

1. F. Kawasaki disease. This is a rare form of vasculitis that predominantly affects young children. Other clinical features include conjunctival congestion and coronary arteritis, which can lead to acute myocardial infarction.
2. B. Systemic sclerosis. This woman describes the early changes of scleroderma in her hands. She also has Raynaud phenomenon, symptoms of oesophageal involvement and telangiectasia, which are all features of limited systemic sclerosis.
3. J. Wegener granulomatosis. This is a small-vessel vasculitis that had a very high mortality rate before the introduction of cyclophosphamide. This patient has had a life-threatening pulmonary haemorrhage. Renal complications can also be very serious. See Figure 14.19 for details of other clinical features of Wegener granulomatosis.
4. D. Polymyositis. This painless, symmetrical proximal myopathy is consistent with polymyositis. Polymyalgia rheumatica causes proximal pain and stiffness, so is less likely.
5. G. Primary Sjögren syndrome. Dryness of the eyes and mouth, arthralgia and positive anti-Ro and anti-La antibodies are all features of Sjögren syndrome.

Question 4

1. A. Rotator cuff tendinitis. The site of the pain is typical of a rotator cuff problem. Passive movements of the joint are full, making glenohumeral arthritis or capsulitis unlikely. A painful arc is often seen with supraspinatus tendinitis.
2. H. Acute myocardial infarction. Cardiac pain is often referred to the shoulder and is not always felt in the anterior chest. This man's pain is unaffected by movements of the joint, making a musculoskeletal cause less likely. He is diabetic, so has at least one risk factor for ischaemic heart disease. The sweating and shortness of breath are common symptoms of cardiac ischaemia.
3. F. Ruptured long head of biceps. This is more common in the elderly and may follow only minimal trauma. It is painless and produces a bulge anteriorly in the upper arm.
4. D. Polymyalgia rheumatica. This patient is elderly and has proximal pain in both her shoulder and pelvic girdles, associated with stiffness and weakness.

These symptoms are consistent with polymyalgia rheumatica, a diagnosis which is supported by the raised ESR.

5. G. Pancoast tumour. A Pancoast tumour is a carcinoma of the lung that invades the brachial plexus, causing pain in the upper limb. This man has chronic lung disease and is likely to be a smoker. The fact that his pain continues through the night and is unresponsive to analgesia raises the suspicion of malignancy. Weight loss and haemoptysis are both symptoms seen with lung carcinoma.

Question 5

1. E. Anticentromere. This patient has limited systemic sclerosis, which is strongly associated with anticentromere antibodies.
2. I. Antihistone. This man has drug-induced SLE, as a consequence of his minocycline therapy. Antihistone antibodies are commonly found in this condition.
3. B. c-ANCA. This man has Wegener granulomatosis. Eighty per cent of patients are c-ANCA-positive.
4. C. p-ANCA. This patient has polyarteritis nodosa, which is associated with p-ANCA.
5. G. Anticardiolipin. This patient has antiphospholipid antibody syndrome.

Question 6

1. F. Reactive arthritis. This patient has had a preceding infection and there is a short history of swollen joints.
2. C. Pseudogout. Wrist is a common presentation and this is the right age group.
3. G. Haemachromatosis. This typically affects these joints. Check ferritin.
4. H. Haemarthrosis. The patient recently had a myocardial infarction and therefore is taking several antiplatelet drugs.
5. E. Septic arthritis. Patients with rheumatoid arthritis can have septic joints.

Question 7

1. D. Ankylosing spondylitis.
2. A. Osteoarthritis. Classical nodal osteoarthritis.
3. C. Psoriatic arthritis. This woman has a severe form of psoriatic arthritis called arthritis mutilans.
4. F. Gout. Uric acid can often be normal.
5. G. Enteropathic arthritis.

Question 8

1. E. Rickets. This is due to low vitamin D.
2. B. Paget disease.

3. H. Myeloma, which often presents with bone pain. Check protein electrophoresis.
4. A. Osteoporosis. Patients with rheumatoid arthritis often have steroids, which are a risk factor for osteoporosis.
5. D. Osteomalacia. This is like rickets but in adults.

Question 9

1. A. Churg–Strauss disease, which classically presents with eosinophilia.
2. B. Polyarteritis nodosa, due to microaneurysms.
3. I. Behçet disease, which is more common in the Mediterranean.
4. E. Dermatomyositis. Classical heliotopic rash and goitrous papules, proximal weakness. Related to malignancy.
5. G. SLE.

Question 10

1. C. Fibromyalgia. Diagnosis of exclusion. No joint swelling and normal inflammatory markers.
2. B. Osteoarthritis.
3. F. Pseudogout.
4. A. Rheumatoid arthritis. Symmetrical distribution and most commonly affects MCP joints.
5. D. Psoriatic arthritis. Inflammatory history with asymmetrical distribution.

Question 11

1. B. Polymyalgia rheumatica.
2. A. Polymyositis.
3. C. Myasthenia gravis. Weakness worse with exercise and affects all muscles.
4. D. Muscular dystrophy. Genetic.
5. E. Rheumatoid arthritis.

Question 12

1. C. MCPs.
2. D. MTPs.
3. B. Knee.
4. B. Knee. Weight-bearing joint.
5. B. Knee.

Question 13

1. G. Anti Jo-1.
2. A. Low C3, low C4.
3. B. Rheumatoid factor. 100% of patients are positive for rheumatoid factor.
4. E. Anti-RNP.
5. C. ANCA. Classically c-ANCA.

Question 14

1. E. Back pain.
2. A. Heberden nodes. Bony swelling of DIPs.
3. B. Photosensitive rash.
4. C. Telangiectasia.
5. D. Eosinophilia.

Question 15

1. F. Cyclophosphamide. Therefore given with mesna.
2. A. Methotrexate. Therefore baseline chest X-ray required.
3. A. Methotrexate. Therefore regular monitoring of liver function tests.
4. E. Hydroxychloroquine.
5. D. Infliximab.

Orthopaedics

Question 1

1. A. Prostate metastasis. The history of urinary dysfunction suggests prostate. Metastases from prostate cancer are sclerotic (the others being lytic).
2. G. Osteosarcoma. Although rare, primary malignant tumours do occur in children and metastases are unheard of in this age group. The level of pain is suspicious but it is the X-ray features that give away the diagnosis.
3. C. Myeloma. The fracture under normal loads should raise suspicion. The X-ray features are typical of myeloma, as are the high ESR and skull lesions.
4. I. Osteochondroma. The history is benign, of mild discomfort over long periods, and the X-ray appearance is typical of a benign lesion, in this case an osteochondroma.
5. F. Breast metastasis. You were not told that she had a breast lump. She has a malignant spinal lesion causing spinal cord compression. The normal investigations exclude all the other potential sources of primary malignancy (except bowel carcinoma, but this rarely metastasizes to the spine), leaving breast carcinoma as the most likely.
6. B. Lung metastasis. The history of smoking and an abnormal chest X-ray give away the diagnosis.

Question 2

1. I. Posterior cruciate ligament rupture. The history is typical, with a backwardly directed force on the tibia. The posterior sag is pathognomonic for posterior cruciate ligament rupture.
2. E. Medial collateral ligament sprain. The history suggests medial ligament sprain and the fact that she could bear weight afterwards suggests a less serious injury. Tenderness at the joint line would be the meniscus but above is more likely to be medial collateral. The absence of an effusion excludes an anterior cruciate ligament rupture.
3. C. Osteoarthritis. The history is typical for osteoarthritis with gradually increasing pain, a varus deformity and crepitus.
4. A. Anterior cruciate ligament rupture. The history of a skiing injury and the patient hearing a pop or feeling something go are typical. The presence of an effusion makes it more likely. Often knees such as these are difficult to examine initially but later will have positive Lachman and pivot shift tests.
5. B. Medial meniscal tear. The history of twisting injury, things settling but persistent niggling symptoms is typical. Joint line tenderness and an effusion also suggest meniscal injury.
6. J. Patellar tendon rupture. In this case the history is not helpful but examination findings of loss of straight-leg raise with swelling and tenderness below the patella give the diagnosis.

Question 3

1. A. Paget disease. The abnormal bony architecture and high alkaline phosphatase give the diagnosis.
2. C. Rickets. The history is typical for rickets, as are the clinical and X-ray features.
3. D. Osteoporosis, presenting with vertebral fractures. The history with deformity and X-ray features all point to osteoporotic vertebral fractures. The normal blood tests exclude pathological causes of fractures.
4. F. Leukaemia. The history of prolonged illness with aches and pains suggests a generalized disorder. The low WCC is also suggestive of a haematological disorder and a sterile hip washout makes septic arthritis very unlikely. Leukaemia does occasionally present with musculoskeletal symptoms.
5. H. Osteogenesis imperfecta. The history of 'spontaneous' or low-violence fractures is typical. These cases are often initially diagnosed as non-accidental injury but here the X-ray shows abnormal bone.
6. I. Osteoid osteoma. The history is typical, with intense pain relieved by non-steroidal anti-inflammatory drugs. The X-ray and CT finding are typical.

Question 4

1. A. Osteoarthritis of the first MTP joint (hallux rigidus). The pain in the toe-off stage is typical as the patient has lost extension. Walking boots can relieve the pain by minimizing this movement. Clinical features are typical of osteoarthritis anywhere, with osteophytes (dorsal bump) and crepitus.

2. C. Reiter syndrome. A syndrome of arthritis, conjunctivitis and urethritis. It is more common in men but does occur in women.

3. I. Psoriatic arthropathy. Commonly affects the hands, which can be significantly deformed.

4. D. Septic arthritis. Can be a difficult diagnosis to make in the elderly. Her raised WCC and temperature point to an infective cause.

5. E. Gout. Typical history and the usual joint. The serum uric acid is often normal during an acute episode.

6. G. Ankylosing spondylitis. The condition tends to present in early adult life and the spine is commonly affected and stiffens, eventually ankylosing. The sacroiliac joints are commonly involved.

Question 5

1. B. Spinal stenosis. The history is typical and pain is often worse on extension. The X-ray often only shows osteoarthritis and a CT or MRI scan will confirm the presence of spinal stenosis.

2. F. Spinal metastases. The history sounds sinister, with unrelenting pain. The X-ray showing loss of the pedicle (winking-owl sign) means bony destruction by tumour.

3. D. Discitis. Often this condition presents late after the patient has had a number of normal investigations. This patient is at risk of sepsis, having diabetes and chronic renal failure. The X-ray shows the typical features of long-standing discitis.

4. J. Cauda equina syndrome. This is a typical history. Bilateral symptoms are suspicious. Any patient with sciatica and new urinary or bowel disturbance should be investigated urgently.

5. G. Acute low back pain. Very common and usually resolves. Note the absence of leg pain.

6. A. Spondylolisthesis. Fast bowlers in cricket are at increased risk. The X-ray features in this case are diagnostic.

Question 6

1. C. Developmental dysplasia of the hip. Late-presenting developmental dysplasia of the hip presents with a painless limp and leg-length discrepancy. All the other conditions on the list will present with pain.

2. E. Slipped upper femoral epiphysis. The patient is the correct age and the history of pain is typical. The femoral head in slipped upper femoral epiphysis rotates posteriorly and leaves an externally rotated leg. The frog lateral X-ray shows the slip more obviously than the AP X-ray.

3. B. Juvenile idiopathic arthritis. Presentation with a monoarthritis is common, with other joints involved later. Generalized symptoms suggest a systemic disorder. The presence of eye symptoms is worrying as blindness can result.

4. J. Osgood–Schlatter disease. The disease is often bilateral and occurs during the adolescent years. Tender swollen tibial tuberosities are present bilaterally.

5. A. Perthes disease. The boy is the right age to have Perthes and the history of knee pain is typical. The loss of abduction is worrying as it could mean impending joint subluxation. The sclerosis of the femoral head is due to avascular necrosis.

6. G. Osteomyelitis. Diagnosis is difficult in the very young child. In this case the child clearly has an infection. In the absence of an obviously swollen joint and with a normal hip ultrasound scan, the most likely cause is osteomyelitis.

Question 7

1. A. Tension pneumothorax. This occurs after trauma creates a one-way valve in the lung or chest wall. This means that air flows into the chest cavity, but not out again, which collapses the lung, causing hypoxia. The mediastinum is displaced to one side, which reduces venous return to the heart and therefore cardiac output. This causes hypotension. This is life-threatening and requires immediate decompression with a large-bore needle (before a chest X-ray is sought!), followed by insertion of a chest drain.

2. B. Pelvic fracture. The mechanism here suggests that this poor man has had a heavy crush injury to his pelvis. Venous bleeding can be massive with pelvic fractures, and can even be fatal. The man's hypotension and tachycardia are signs of hypovolaemic shock. Associated bladder and urethral injuries are not uncommon, and this man may have either a ruptured bladder or a urethral tear, which would explain the blood at his urethral meatus and inability to pass urine. He should have a retrograde urethrogram before attempted catheterization.

3. C. Lumbar spine fracture/dislocation. This is a high-energy injury, and the lumbar spine fracture dislocation is associated in this case with transection of the spinal cord. Therefore there is no function below the level of the injury, including nerves to the legs and sacral nerves to the bladder and bowel. The prognosis in this case is very poor.

4. D. Wedge fracture lumbar spine. This is likely to be an osteoporotic wedge fracture. This is a low-energy fracture. It is also important to consider other pathological causes such as myeloma or bone metastasis from a primary malignancy.

5. F. Fracture of the seventh cervical vertebra. Unfortunately the doctor has missed the diagnosis of a C7 fracture. This is because the X-rays did not show the whole of the cervical spine. Adequate trauma X-rays for neck injuries are an AP and lateral showing C1 to the top of the first thoracic vertebrae and an odontoid peg view. This patient has a potentially unstable fracture from a significant hyperflexion injury, and there is now compression of the right eighth cervical nerve root (learn dermatomes!).

6. G. Neck sprain. This is a classic case of a neck sprain. The damage to the car suggests that this is a low-speed crash, and the delayed onset of pain is crucial in making the diagnosis. Patients with significant neck injuries (fractures or ligament tears) develop immediate pain. A neck sprain requires simple analgesia and neck exercises to prevent more stiffness from developing.

Question 8

1. G. Realignment surgery. This man is developing medial compartment osteoarthritis in his knee because of his varus deformity. This results in increased load through the medial part of the knee joint and therefore earlier wear. He is too young for a joint replacement but realignment surgery will correct his deformity so that there is less wear on the medial side. This will hopefully slow down the progression of his osteoarthritis, but he may require a joint replacement when he is at a suitable age.

2. H. Arthroscopy. This man has a locked knee secondary to a medial meniscal tear. The meniscus can get trapped in the joint and tears as the knee extends. The meniscus is not very vascular and therefore the bleeding is slow and swelling occurs over 24 hours. An arthroscopy will identify the tear and it can then either be repaired or excised.

3. C. Unicompartmental knee replacement. This man has developed medial joint line osteoarthritis but his knee is otherwise well preserved. A unicompartmental knee replacement is designed to treat just the affected area of the knee. Its advantage over a total knee replacement is that it is a smaller operation and has a shorter recovery time.

4. F. X-ray of the spine. The doctor has not properly examined this woman. The X-ray changes of the hip are very mild and would not explain the severe pain that this woman complains of. Numbness is more typical of neurological pathology, and the fact that the hip has a good range of movement rules out major hip arthritis. This is more likely to be referred pain from the spine and plain X-ray may show degenerative change. Doing a hip replacement in this woman could be disastrous as it is a big operation and would not treat the pain.

5. D. Total knee replacement. This man has had a physical job for many years which has resulted in severe osteoarthritis of the knee. He cannot cope with his symptoms and further conservative treatment is not going to help. He should benefit from a total knee replacement.

Question 9

1. G. Epidural anaesthesia. The effect of this can last several hours (numb legs) and peripheral vasodilation causes pooling of fluid in the legs, which results in hypotension. Other causes of course must be sought before it is assumed that the cause of hypotension is the epidural, but all other parameters are normal in this case.

2. B. Sepsis. This man is in septic shock and requires an emergency hip washout to treat his septic hip. He has risk factors for infection, including type 2 diabetes mellitus and steroid treatment (immunosuppression).

3. D. Neurogenic shock. This man appears to have an isolated spinal injury based on his initial examination. This has resulted in loss of sympathetic tone to his legs and therefore hypotension. There is no evidence that he has any other injuries and therefore hypovolaemia secondary to blood loss is unlikely. In patients with spinal cord injury this blood pressure is acceptable and intravenous fluids should be given cautiously to avoid fluid overload.

4. E. Cardiogenic shock. This poor woman is having a myocardial infarction, confirmed on the ECG. This has caused left ventricular failure and therefore pulmonary oedema and hypotension. Thrombolysis is contraindicated here as she is only 4 days post surgery.

5. A. Hypovolaemia. Intraoperative haemorrhage has resulted in hypovolaemic shock and this man's blood pressure has not responded to fluids. He requires an urgent blood transfusion in order to prevent further deterioration. Hypotension within the first 48 hours of surgery is usually secondary to hypovolaemia.

Question 10

1. A. Anterior dislocation. In all, 95% of shoulder dislocations are anterior. This classically occurs when the arm is forced into abduction and external rotation (ball-throwing position). Her shoulder will require reduction under sedation in casualty. She should be warned that there is up to an 80% chance of recurrent dislocations in her age group.

2. B. Posterior dislocation, which accounts for 2% of shoulder dislocations and is associated with epileptic seizures and electrocutions. It should be suspected when the arm is held in fixed internal rotation.

3. D. Hill–Sachs lesion. Sometimes following anterior dislocation of the shoulder the humeral head impacts on the glenoid, causing a defect in the posterior part of the head. The articular surface is no longer congruent and so this defect catches on the glenoid in certain positions. This man requires bone grafting to restore the articular surface.

4. B. Fracture of proximal humerus. Common fracture, particularly in postmenopausal women. Treatment depends on the degree of displacement, ranging from conservative to operative fixation or even replacement.

5. E. Rotator cuff tear. History of settling injury but persistent weakness suggests rotator cuff tear. Examination findings indicate weakness of supraspinatus. Confirm with ultrasound or MRI.

Question 11

1. E. *Haemophilus influenzae*. This used to be the commonest cause of septic arthritis in infants but is now rare because of a successful vaccination programme. This unfortunate child is not up to date, however.

2. G. *Escherichia coli*. This woman has developed a septic arthritis of her hip. This has resulted from haematogenous spread of bacteria to the hip from her urinary tract infection (UTI) and *E. coli* is a common cause of UTIs. Always look for a source when diagnosing septic arthritis.

3. C. *Mycobacterium tuberculosis*. Travel to India may have exposed this woman to tuberculosis, which has remained dormant for many years. This has now become activated, however, and caused collapse of one of her thoracic vertebral bodies, resulting in a gibbus (sharp angulated kyphosis). She will need an MRI scan and then biposy of the lesion to confirm the diagnosis.

4. A. *Staphylococcus aureus*. This is the commonest cause of septic arthritis and osteomyelitis. This girl seems to have developed spontaneous osteomyelitis which will require antibiotics for 6 weeks and surgical debridement of the bone if indicated.

5. B. Anaerobic bacteria. This man has an open fracture which is potentially contaminated by cattle manure, amongst other things. Anaerobic bacterial and *Clostridium perfringens* (gas gangrene) infection is important to consider here based on the history. The fracture site should be irrigated and debrided urgently in theatre. Heavily soiled wounds should be covered with high-dose antibiotics,

including an intravenous cephalosporin, penicillin and metronidazole. Tetanus prophylaxis should be given if vaccinations are not up to date.

Question 12

1. A. Salter–Harris fracture. This is a fracture around the growth plate (physis) and these are common injuries in children.

2. C. Pathological fracture. This is a fracture through abnormal bone. The history alone is suspicious of this. This poor man has got lung cancer from smoking and now has metastasis to his right femur, which has been painful. This bone is therefore weak and low-energy activities such as walking result in fracture. Other primary malignancies that metastasize to bone are thyroid, kidney, breast and prostate.

3. F. Compartment syndrome. This is unlikely to be a fracture because he could initially walk on his leg. Compartment syndrome can occur with or without fractures and this man needs urgent fasciotomies to the compartments (within 6 hours of onset). Absent foot pulses is a very late sign and usually indicates that the limb needs to be amputated.

4. G. Non-accidental injury. The history is not consistent with a healing fracture. Be very suspicious of any fracture in children under 2 years. Take no chances, admit the child and inform the paediatricians.

5. D. Open fracture. Any wound, no matter how small, on the same limb as a fracture should be assumed to be open until proven otherwise. This woman has a puncture wound from when the bone burst through the skin when it was severely angulated. This woman needs urgent debridement of the wound, stabilization of the fracture and antibiotics to help prevent chronic osteomyelitis.

Question 13

1. E. Nerve conduction study. The distribution of the pain is in keeping with a median nerve lesion. The diagnosis is carpal tunnel syndrome. This is associated with other conditions such as diabetes mellitus and pregnancy. Usually this is confirmed with nerve conduction studies but if the diagnosis is very obvious the surgeon may proceed to do a carpal tunnel decompression without this.

2. B. MRI. This woman has sciatica, most likely from a disc prolapse in her lumbar spine at the level of L5/S1. X-ray may show an obvious cause of the pain, such as osteoarthritis, but is often unhelpful. MRI will provide detailed images of the soft tissues and vertebral discs. This is also a very useful investigation if sinister spinal disease such as malignancy is

suspected. CT is very good at showing detailed images of bones, e.g. for assessment of a complex vertebral body fracture.

3. G. Venous Doppler scan. The leg may just be swollen from surgery, but a total knee replacement puts the patient at high risk of deep vein thrombosis.

4. F. Ultrasound scan. This is likely to be a wrist ganglion. These are usually diagnosed clinically and excised if they cause problems, but if the clinician is unsure, an ultrasound scan is a simple, quick non-invasive test to provide more information. Ganglions are fluid-filled and therefore can change size depending on this. In the old days people were encouraged to bash them with a big book to rupture them!

5. C. Plain X-ray. This man may have metastasis to his ulna or radial shaft and a plain X-ray would normally show the diagnosis. Other malignancies that commonly metastasize to bone include thyroid, breast, lung and prostate.

Question 14

1. B. Cervical rib. Occurs in 1 in 200 people and may be bilateral. An extra rib from C7 (may just be a fibrous band) articulates with the first rib or may be free distally. This may cause vascular (subclavian artery) disturbance such as Raynaud phenomenon or neurological symptoms, normally in the distribution of C8/T1 dermatomes. The T1 myotome supplies the small muscles of the hand.

2. C. Pancoast tumour. An apical lung tumour has resulted in compression of the sympathetic nerves that arise from T1 and run up to supply the eye and forehead. This results in Horner syndrome (ipsilateral meiosis, ptosis and facial anhydrosis) on the affected side. The tumour is also compressing the T1 myotome.

3. F. Radial nerve palsy. The radial nerve runs in the spiral groove on the posterior aspect of the midshaft of the humerus. It is in direct contact with the bone at this point, which makes it prone to injury.

4. G. C6/C7 cervical disc prolapse. A disc at this level would compress the C7 nerve root, causing numbness and/or pain in the middle finger. C7 supplies the triceps and flexor carpi radialis and there is resultant weakness of elbow extension and flexion of the wrist.

5. E. Axillary nerve palsy. This man has sustained an anterior dislocation of his shoulder. The axillary nerve leaves the brachial plexus and winds around the surgical neck of the humerus to supply sensation to the army badge area over the upper lateral aspect of the upper arm, and motor function to the deltoid. This injury is normally a neuropraxia.

Question 15

1. B. Trendelenburg. This man has weakness of his left hip abductors so, when asked to stand on his left leg, his pelvis tilts down. This results in a Trendelenburg gait. Bilateral weakness of the abductors results in a waddling gait when the pelvis drops down with each step.

2. E. Foot drop. The policeman has purposefully hit the man over his common peroneal nerve to disable him. This nerve is very superficial as it winds around the fibula neck and supplies sensation to the dorsum of the foot and motor supply to the dorsiflexors of the toes and ankle. In order to prevent his toes dragging on the ground he compensates by lifting his foot high. Bilateral foot drop results in a high-stepping gait.

3. A. Ataxic. This boy has cerebral palsy secondary to meningitis as an infant. There is a loss of balance which is overcome by a broad-based gait.

4. D. Antalgic. Any painful condition results in an antalgic gait. This is characterized by a reduced-stance phase (less time is spent weight bearing on the affected side) during walking.

5. H. Spastic. This child has cerebral palsy. Children may display varying degrees of spasticity. Hip adductors contract, resulting in 'scissoring' of the legs. The equinus deformity of his feet will also worsen function. He may benefit from complex surgery to correct the deformities.

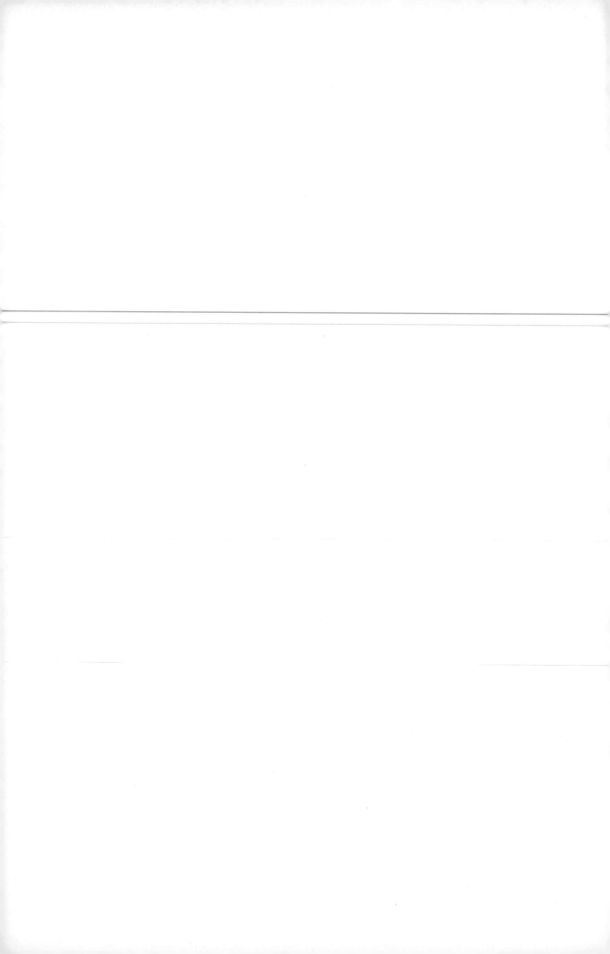

Glossary

Allodynia A painful response to stimulus that does not usually cause pain.

Arthrodesis Joint fusion surgery.

Arthroplasty Joint replacement surgery.

Baker cyst Synovial cyst in popliteal fossa, usually associated with knee arthritis (osteoarthritis or rheumatoid arthritis).

Bouchard node Bony swelling of proximal interphalangeal joint caused by osteoarthritis.

Boutonnière deformity Deformity of finger seen in rheumatoid arthritis, characterized by flexion of proximal interphalangeal joint and hyperextension of distal interphalangeal joint.

Bursitis Inflammation of a bursa.

Cauda equina syndrome Compression of central nerve roots in spinal canal causing bladder and bowel disturbance and saddle anaesthesia.

Chondrocalcinosis Presence of calcium pyrophosphate crystals in cartilage.

Chondrosarcoma Slow-growing malignant tumour of cartilaginous origin.

Codman triangle X-ray appearance when a bone tumour elevates the periosteum.

Compartment syndrome Pressure within myofascial compartment exceeds capillary pressure, resulting in compromised circulation to muscles and nerves within the compartment.

Crystal arthropathy Range of diseases of the joint resulting from crystal deposition, including gout and chondrocalcinosis.

Cytokine Intercellular messenger protein.

Dactylitis Swelling of whole digit in hand or foot, commonly found in spondyloarthropathies and sometimes referred to as 'sausage digit'.

Developmental dysplasia of the hip (DDH) Failure of acetabulum to develop normally, resulting in subluxation or dislocation of femoral head.

Diaphysis Shaft of long bone.

Dupuytren contracture Contracture of palmar fascia resulting in fixed flexion of digits (most commonly ring finger).

Enthesopathy Degeneration/inflammation of tendon or ligament where it inserts into bone.

Epiphysis Part of bone between physis and joint.

Ewing sarcoma Malignant tumour of connective tissue origin in children and young adults, typically affecting proximal long bones and pelvis.

Flail chest When two or more consecutive ribs are fractured in two or more places, resulting in a mobile segment which moves paradoxically with respiration and causes impaired ventilation.

Fracture Break in continuity in cortex of normal bone.

Ganglion Cystic lesion associated with joint or tendon.

Glasgow Coma Scale Objective measure of consciousness based on best eye opening, verbal and motor responses.

Haemarthrosis Blood in joint.

Haemothorax Blood in pleural cavity.

Hallux valgus Correct term for bunion deformity.

Heberden node Bony swelling of distal interphalangeal joint caused by osteoarthritis.

J sign Seen with lateral maltracking of patella.

Keratoderma blenorrhagica Pustular skin rash usually confined to palms and soles, associated with reactive arthritis.

Kyphosis Excessive forward curvature of the spine.

Lachmann test Test for anterior cruciate ligament rupture.

Lipoma Benign adipose tissue.

Livedo reticularis Reticular, purplish discoloration usually seen on extensor surfaces of legs.

Lymphoma Primary malignant tumour of lymphoid tissue.

Morton neuroma Painful nerve lesion in foot.

Open fracture Fracture associated with breach in overlying epithelium and dermis, allowing potential contamination of fracture site with bacteria.

Osgood–Schlatter disease Traction apophysitis of tibial tuberosity.

Osteochondritis dissecans Separation of subchondral bone and overlying cartilage (usually affects knee).

Osteochondroma (exostosis) Common benign bone tumour with thick cartilaginous cap.

Osteoid osteoma Painful benign bone tumour which is self-limiting.

Osteomyelitis Infection within bone.

Osteosarcoma Aggressive malignant primary bone tumour.

Pannus Inflamed synovial tissue that erodes articular cartilage in rheumatoid arthritis.

Pathological fracture Break in continuity of cortex of abnormal bone.

Perthes disease Segmental avascular necrosis of femoral head.

Pes planus Flat foot.

Phalen test Holding wrist in palmar flexion reproduces symptoms of carpal tunnel syndrome.

Physis Growth plate of bone.

Pneumothorax Air within pleural cavity.

Raynaud phenomenon Pallor, coolness, numbness and discomfort of extremity (commonly a digit) due to vasospasm.

Red flag signs Features of back pain suggesting sinister pathology.

Rheumatoid factor Antibody to Fc fragment of immunoglobulin G (IgG), commonly found in rheumatoid arthritis.

Rheumatoid nodules Subcutaneous swellings occurring in rheumatoid arthritis patients who test positive for rheumatoid factor.

Sarcoma Malignant neoplasm of connective tissue origin.

Schirmer test Test used to measure tear production in patients with dry eyes.

Schöber test Measurement of flexion at lumbar spine.

Sciatica Pain radiating down posterior aspect of leg below level of the knee.

Sclerodactyly Fibrotic thickening of skin over fingers seen in systemic sclerosis.

Scoliosis Lateral deviation of spine.

Shock Inadequate tissue perfusion and oxygenation due to acute circulatory failure.

Spinal claudication Spinal stenosis compressing spinal cord results in pain and numbness in back and legs, relieved by sitting forward.

Spinal shock Spinal injury causing temporary total loss of function distal to level of injury (different from neurogenic shock).

Spondylolisthesis Forward displacement of one vertebra on another.

Spondylolysis Defect in pars interarticularis. May result in spondylolisthesis.

Swan neck deformity Deformity of finger in rheumatoid arthritis characterized by flexion of metacarpophalangeal joint, hyperextension of proximal interphalangeal joint and flexion of distal interphalangeal joint.

Synovitis Inflammation of synovium.

Tarsal tunnel syndrome Painful foot condition in which posterior tibial nerve is compressed in tarsal tunnel.

Tenosynovitis Inflammation of synovial lining of tendon sheath.

Tension pneumothorax One-way valve develops in lung surface and allows air into pleural cavity during inspiration but closes during expiration, resulting in compression of mediastinal structures and requiring immediate decompression.

Tinel test Tapping over median nerve in wrist reproduces symptoms of carpal tunnel syndrome.

Thomas test Test for fixed flexion deformity of hip.

Tophus Hard deposit composed of monosodium urate crystals in or near joints in chronic gout.

Trendelenburg test Test for weak hip abductors.

Valgus Angulation away from midline.

Varus Angulation towards the midline.

Vasculitis Inflammation of blood vessels.

Yellow flag signs Psychosocial aspects of back pain associated with poor outcome.

Index

Notes: Page numbers followed by *f* indicate figures.

To save space in the index, the following abbreviations have been used:

ATLS - Advanced Trauma Life Support
DM - dermatomyositis
PM - polymyositis
SLE - systemic lupus erythematosus

A

Abduction, hip examination, 9*f*
Abductor pollicis longus, 193
Acetabulum, 120*f*
Aches, 3
ACL *see* Anterior cruciate ligament (ACL)
Acromioclavicular joint, 13*f*
Acromion, 13*f*
Acute anterior uveitis, 87
Acute gout, 113
  management, 115
Acute haematogenous osteomyelitis, 145–146
Acute hot swollen joints, 41–44
  associated symptoms, 41–42
  concurrent illness, 41
  differential diagnosis, 41
  drug history, 42
  examination, 43
  history, 41–42
  investigations, 43–44, 43*f*
  location, 41, 42*f*
  past medical history, 42
  social history, 42
Acute mechanical low back pain, 55
Acute myocardial infarction, 196, 211–212
Adalimumab, 83, 83*f*
Adduction, hip examination, 9*f*
Adjunctive treatment, SLE, 96
Advanced Trauma Life Support (ATLS), 139–140, 140*f*
  airway, 139, 140*f*
  breathing, 139, 140*f*
  cervical spine control, 139
  circulation, 139–140

disability/neurological state, 140, 140*f*
exposure/secondary survey, 140
pelvic fractures, 142
questions and answers, 193, 209
Age
  acute hot swollen joints, 41
  limps, 45
  tumours, 161–162
Airway
  ATLS, 139, 140*f*
  questions and answers, 193, 209
Alkaline phosphatase, paraneoplastic rheumatic syndrome, 36
Allopurinol, acute gout management, 115
Amyloidosis, ankylosing spondylitis, 87
Anaemia
  full blood count, 17
  rheumatoid arthritis, 80
Anaerobic bacteria infection, questions and answers, 203–204, 216
Anaesthesia, epidural, questions and answers, 203, 215
Analgesia
  mechanical low back pain, 57
  osteomyelitis management, 147
  septic arthritis, 149
Anal tone, lower limb examination, 4
Anaphylactic shock, 158–159
ANAs *see* Antinuclear antibodies (ANAs)
ANCAs *see* Antineutrophil cytoplasmic antibodies (ANCAs)
Angulation, fractures, 132*f*
Ankle
  examination *see* Ankle and foot examination
  fractures, 137
  pain *see* Ankle and foot pain
  reflexes, 4
  sprains, 179–180, 179*f*
Ankle and foot examination, 8–10
  feel, 10
  look, 8–10
  movement, 10
Ankle and foot pain, 27–29
  associated symptoms, 29
  characteristics, 29
  differential diagnosis, 29, 29*f*
  examination, 29

history, 29
investigations, 29
Ankylosing spondylitis, 85–88
  clinical features, 85
  drug treatment, 88
  extraskeletal features, 87
  HLA, 86*f*
  investigations, 87–88
  management, 88
  musculoskeletal features, 85–87, 86*f*
  physiotherapy, 88
  posture, 86*f*
  prevalence, 85
  questions and answers, 188, 197, 200–201, 207, 212, 213–214
  radiology, 87–88
  sacroiliac joints, 86
  Schober test, 86, 86*f*
Antalgic (painful) gait, 4, 4*f*
  questions and answers, 205, 217
Anterior cruciate ligament (ACL), 174*f*
  examination, 7–8
  injuries, 174–175, 175*f*
  questions and answers, 193, 199–200, 209, 213
  tear, 193, 209
Anterior drawer test, anterior cruciate ligament, 7–8
Anterior shoulder dislocation, 178, 178*f*
Anterior uveitis
  acute, 87
  questions and answers, 189, 208
Anteroposterior view, X-rays, 20
Antibiotic-resistant pathogens, osteomyelitis management, 147
Antibiotics
  discitis/vertebral osteomyelitis, 61
  osteomyelitis management, 147
Anticardiolipin antibodies
  antiphospholipid syndrome, 97
  questions and answers, 195, 196–197, 211, 212
  SLE, 95*f*
Anticentromere antibodies
  questions and answers, 196–197, 212
  systemic sclerosis, 103
Anticitrullinated peptide antibodies (ACPAs)
  rheumatoid arthritis, 81
  tests for, 18

Index

Index

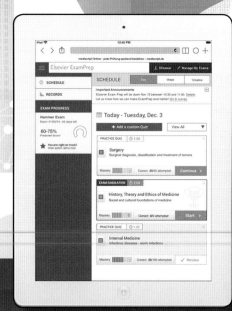